STRANGELYSTRANGE
but oddly normal

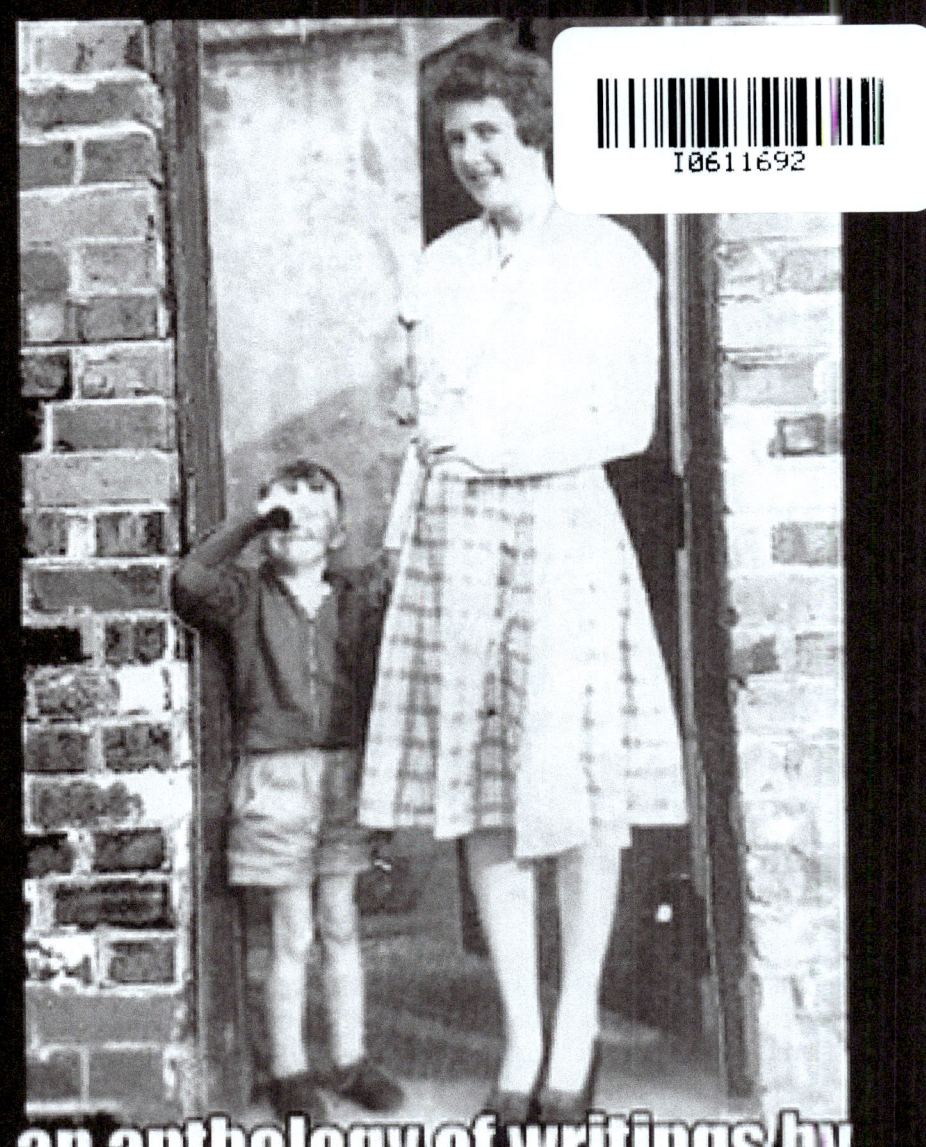

an anthology of writings by
ANDY ROBERTS

Typeset by Jonathan Downes,
Edited by Corinna Downes
Cover and Layout by SPiderKaT for CFZ Communications
Using Microsoft Word 2000, Microsoft , Publisher 2000, Adobe Photoshop CS.

Photographs © 2010 CFZ except where noted

First published in Great Britain by CFZ Press

**CFZ Press
Myrtle Cottage
Woolsery
Bideford
North Devon
EX39 5QR**

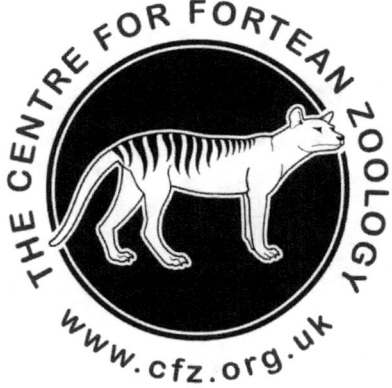

© CFZ MMX

ISBN: 978-1-905723-44-7

Dedication

To my mother, for being the cover girl. But most of all to my friend, partner. lover and cosmic companion, Gaynor.

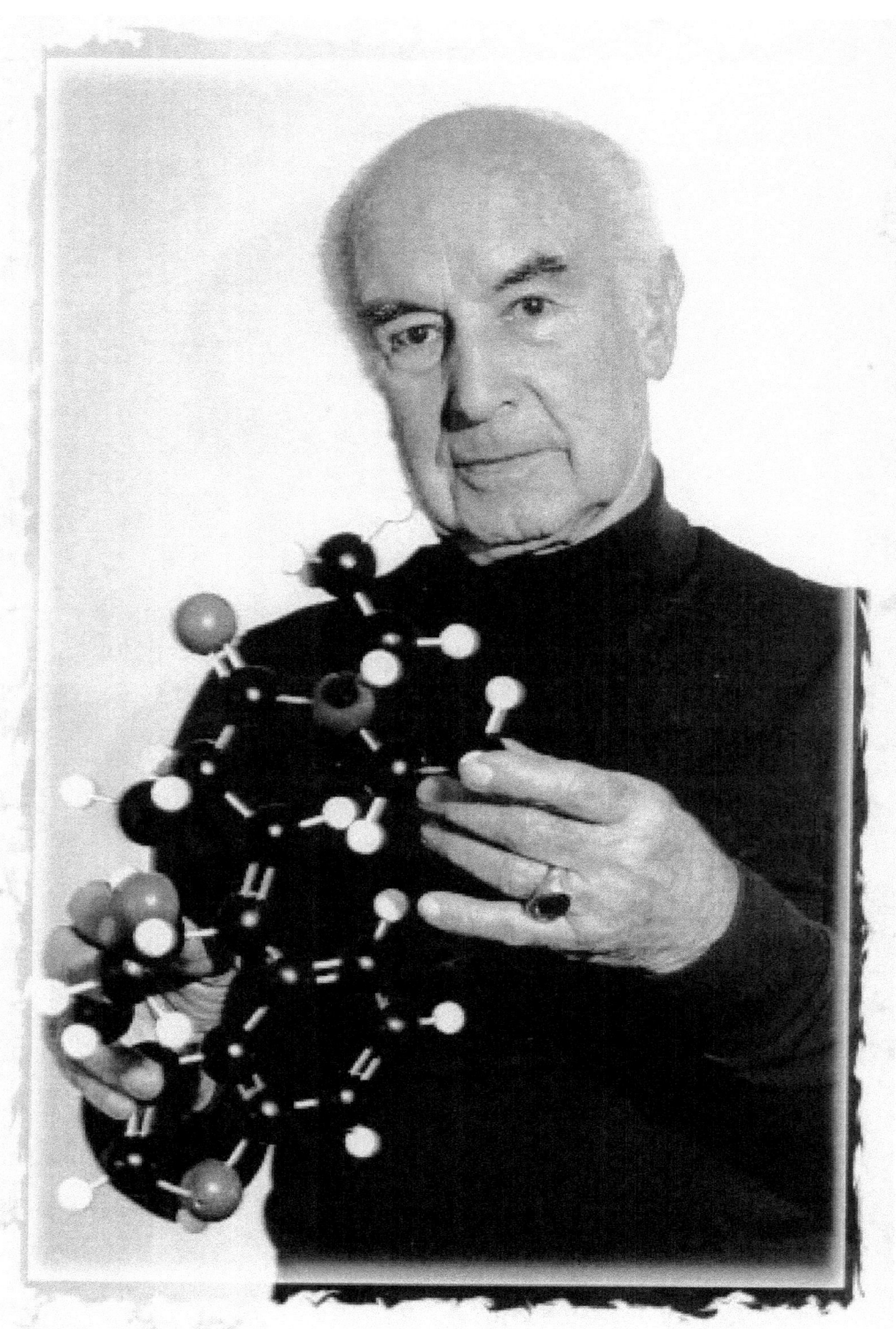

Albert Hofmann discoverer of LSD, and transformer of 20th Century culture

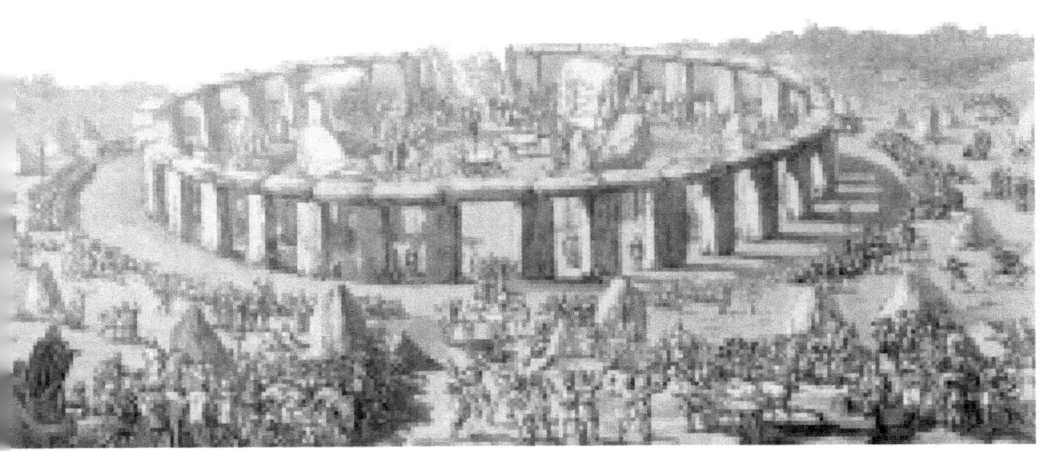

CONTENTS

7.   MY LIFE IN THE GUSH OF BOASTS - The Making of a Fortean
17.   TWO DAYS LATER
19.   THURSBITCH – VALLEY OF THE DEMON? Fiction, folklore and fact in Alan Garner's novel *Thursbitch*
29.   A SAUCERFUL OF SECRETS
37.   ALIENS STOLE MY BADGER'S RECTUM
39.   THE BIG GREY MAN OF BEN MACDHUI & Other Mountain Panics
65.   WWII DOCUMENT RESEARCH
69.   BETWEEN A ROCK AND A HARD PLACE The Cracoe UFO photograph
81.   THE ACID TEST FOR LSD
      A little known ESP experiment involving the *Grateful Dead* and LSD
87.   AN ENCOUNTER WITH FREYA
89.   DEATH RAY MATTHEWS
99.   ROCKING THE ALIEN
105. FOO FIGHTERS: THE STORY SO FAR
111. THE HANGMAN'S BEAUTIFUL DAUGHTER
117. FROM WORLDS AFAR: The Mollie Thompson Story
123. *ROLLING STONES* 27 AUGUST 2006, DON VALLEY STADIUM, SHEFFIELD
127. SYMPATHY FOR THE DEVIL
135. THE BERWYN MOUNTAIN UFO CRASH - A BRITISH ROSWELL?
147. TAKING LA PIS
149. THE JOHN KEEL INTERVIEW
161. THE LORD OF WEIR—A FAIRY STORY?
163. THE OLD STRAIGHT TRACK TO THE NEW AGE
175. An Interview with Andy Roberts
183. BY THE SAME AUTHOR

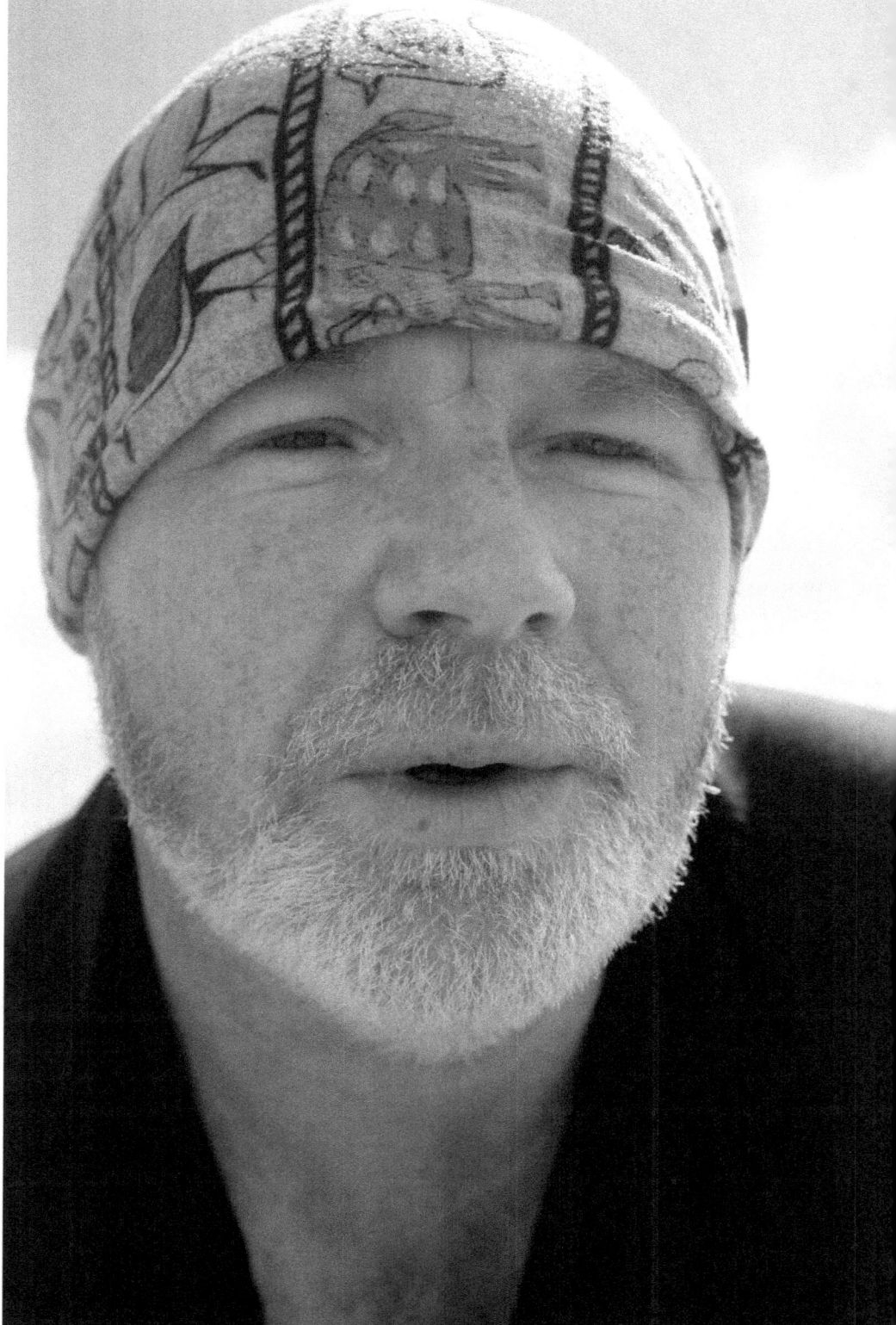

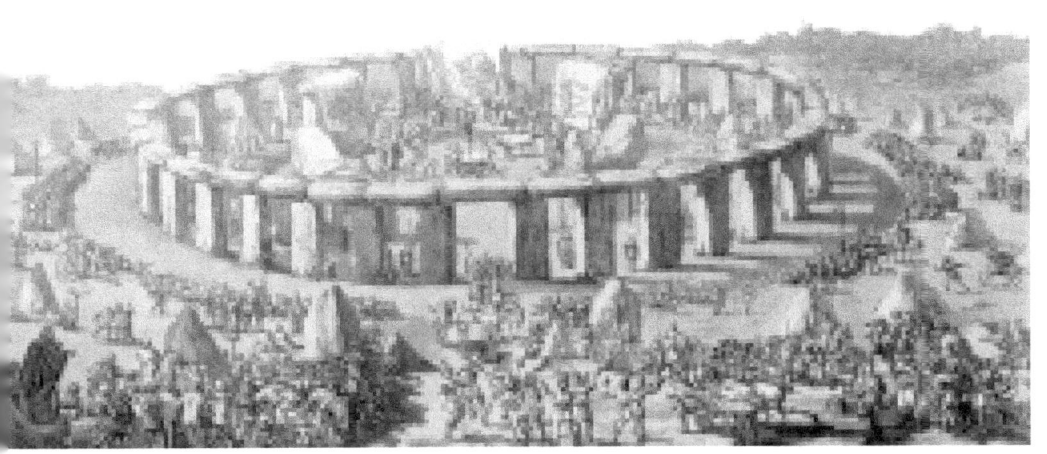

MY LIFE IN THE GUSH OF BOASTS
The Making of a Fortean

When, at the 2008 *Fortean Times* UnConvention, Jon Downes said he had a proposition for me, I quickly fumbled for my trusty phone to call the police, an exorcist and a specialised medical unit. Then I realised that he actually wanted me to collate into anthology form various articles I had written over the years. What a relief!

So, what, exactly, have you bought? Well, this book is a selection of articles, reviews, interviews and other writings dating back to 1974, although most are from the late 1980s to the present day. The subject matter of these pieces is largely Fortean in nature; the results of my investigations over the years into a wide variety of subjects.

The word 'Fortean', itself derived from the works of Charles Fort, carries many different meanings. For me it means holding an active interest in phenomena that is strange, out of place or which suggests the universe isn't quite as straightforward as we have been led to believe by the political, religious, scientific and social establishments who would have us believe their version of 'reality' is the only one.

By way of an introduction to this material I feel it is necessary to explain exactly how I became a Fortean and what has informed my view of Fortean phenomena. And to do that we must go back into the mists of childhood.

Overture & Beginners

Many people's world views are shaped or informed by their early religious experience. However I was fortunately spared the hideousness of a religious upbringing. Nominally Church of England, I did go to Sunday School for a while, but it had no effect on me whatsoever other than to induce a strong dislike of organised religion. In fact, my only memory is of us kids annoying the vicar so much that he threw his Bible on the floor in front of the altar. Very little control, these religious types! The way I saw the world was as a green playground, populated with amazing plants, animals and landscapes. What 'god' could possibly have created this perfection? Why was there any need for a 'higher being' or a creator? I just didn't get it at all. No, my Fortean world view has largely been informed and stimulated primarily by books, music, the natural world, and the psychedelic experience. It all begins a long, long time ago...

I was born in 1956, and during childhood and adolescence lived in various places on the rural fringes of Cleckheaton, a former mill town in West Yorkshire, famous for absolutely nothing at all. Childhood for me was a happy time; a blissful riot of reading, den building in the woods and railway embankments, playing `Japs and Commandos` and generally having fun in the outdoors.

Through the haze of childhood freedoms it seemed to me then, as it does now, that the physical world held no terrors, but the world of humans was full of them. From an early age I always believed we were living in the heart of a dream, a paradise which we could, if as a species we made a collective decision, make how we want it to be. Whatever there was, was here and now – why waste it? But unfortunately, humans tend to invent unnecessary difficulties and impose them on others, dressing them up in the moral, ethical, political or religious fashion of the day. I've never really fathomed why the vast majority of people either want to control others or are happy to be controlled. Robin Williamson of the *Incredible String Band* summed it up perfectly with:

> For rulers like to lay down laws
> And rebels like to break them
> The poor priests like to walk in chains
> And God likes to forsake them

When I was very young, I liked books such as Enid Blyton's `Secret Seven` and `Famous Five` series. These weren't Fortean stories as such but mysteries, populated with strange landscapes and enigmatic untrustworthy people. Here were hidden secrets that could be untangled by application of observation, logic and luck. I also devoured the historical, natural history and landscape fictions of Henry Treece and Rosemary Sutcliffe, Arthur Ransome, Henry Williamson and others like them.

Fast forward to when I was about ten or eleven years old. I'm in the northern Yorkshire coastal resort of Scarborough with my parents. As we passed a news-stand I noticed a magazine called *Flying Saucers*. I bought it immediately and my already fertile imagination entered another world; one of UFOs, aliens, and government cover ups. This was amazing stuff, and for at least a few hours I seriously entertained the possibility that craft from other worlds were visiting Earth.

Then I realised the utterly preposterous nature of that thought. To my young mind it seemed that even if civilisations from the stars had the technology to reach Earth why would they? Why would scientifically advanced extraterrestrials waste their time visiting a planet when even one cursory fly-past would show that its inhabitants were devoted to destroying not only each other, but the small blue dot they lived on? No, interesting as UFOs were, the extraterrestrial hypothesis was simplistic and didn't fit the available facts. Little did I know then that UFOs would later dominate my life for many years.

A year or two later, on holiday at Downderry in Cornwall, when I was bored of sitting on the beach dodging the sun with a towel on my head, my mother suggested I read some Dennis Wheatley. *The Devil Rides Out* and his other black magic novels were all I read for several months.

This was fantastic stuff and seemed much more believable than flying saucers. Wheatley gave us flawed human beings with base desires and the will to dominate others by black magic. Phew! Heady stuff and truly supernatural in nature.

Again, an interest Wheatley's subject matter sent me off down trails that would heavily influence me in later years.

Sometime in my early teens, I discovered the UFO and occult section in Cleckheaton library and came across John Keel's *Jadoo* and Jacques Vallee's *Passport to Magonia*. In *Jadoo* Keel spun stories of his adventures whilst travelling in Africa and Asia. I was fascinated by these tales of other cultures, which portrayed them as mysterious, and full of individuals with access to what Charles Fort had called 'wild talents'. I was equally fascinated by Keel's take on these phenomena. You never really knew what he really thought, and what was objectively real and what was subjective. There was no requirement for the reader to believe Keel, he wasn't selling a belief; just making observations on the strange world we all shared and having fun with the possibilities afforded by belief.

If someone had told me then, that I would in a few decades time, be involved in flying him to the UK for a conference at which I would interview him, I would have laughed and shaken my young head in utter disbelief.

I liked Keel's ambiguity very much. It allowed me to believe and not believe at the same time; a mental version of those optical illusions where you can see either a couple kissing or a goblet, but sometimes, when you know the trick, both at the same time. Keel blew me away and taught me that the real could be fantastic, and the fantastic real. The trick, it seemed, lay in how one perceived the world and I was slowly becoming aware that there were many ways of altering one's perception.

Passport to Magonia had a similar effect. Here were UFOs and aliens, but re-imagined as fairies and gnomes. It clicked in my teenage mind that whatever these phenomena were, they had always been with us here on Earth - only the names and appearance changed to suit the culture in which they appeared. Thus the 'flying shields' which were seen in the Middle Ages became the 'phantom airships' of the early 20th Century, which in turn made a brief appearance as 'mystery airplanes' in the 1920s and 30s, before becoming WWII 'foo fighters' and post-war 'ghost rockets'.

Fashion in supernatural experience changed and physical proof was nonexistent. But belief was constant, people confusing experience and perception with physical reality and holding an almost religious belief that these things were objectively real. Yet it seemed fairly obvious to me that none of these phenomena - and this included ghosts, elementals, devils, demons, fairies, the Loch Ness Monster, Yeti, angels and so on - had any literal, physical existence. At this point I should probably have thrown all these books away and started to think seriously about a career with Boredom Plc. Instead, I booked an appointment to see Dr Dim and Dr Strange.

Dismissing strange phenomena out of hand would have been wrong; throwing the baby out with the bathwater. To the witnesses - and to those who believed in the phenomena experienced by the witnesses - these things were real to them if to no-one else. And that belief created a separate reality; one which did indeed manifest itself in consensus reality in the form of cults, religion, folklore and so on.

I was also now fascinated by techniques which claimed they could change how one perceived reality; techniques such as Buddhism, magic, Wicca, hypnotism and mind control. I also had an interest in cults and outsiders and read widely about the Hells Angels and other biker gangs.

Hippie cultists such as Charles Manson also exerted a (quite probably) unhealthy hold on my developing consciousness. It was rapidly becoming clear to me that the world wasn't as clear cut as the 'straight' media or the blandishments and dogmas of politicians, scientists, and religious leaders would have it.

As I teetered on the edge of the 'grown up' world it seemed to me that the world was a fabulous, and unfathomable, mystery and I resolved I would carry that sense of mystery with me throughout my life. Boredom Plc had just lost a potential CEO, but Dr Strange had picked up a new and enthusiastic research assistant.

Adventures in a Yorkshire Landscape

All these things, and more, were fermenting in my mind as I arrived in the early 1970s, at the peak of what has become known as the counter culture. The hippie movement fascinated me, as did drugs, and long before I had any real understanding of what their impact on my life would be, I resolved to become part of it and taste its forbidden fruits.

The drug experience offered a radically different way of looking at and understanding the mystery of existence, and a more rapid way of accomplishing this than any of the available spiritual, religious or magical technologies. Let's face it, if you're 15 years old would you want to spend years training in, say Wicca, Buddhism or Cabalistic magic when you could take a herb or chemical and go direct, without the intermediaries of priesthood or scripture? It was a no-brainer, and my mental stage was set. I was going to get high and see what all the fuss was about.

I remember sometime in 1971 coming home after a school trip, and smoking some marijuana in my bedroom. I had high hopes! Unfortunately it had no discernable effect other than to put me to sleep, and nothing was delivered. I had yet to learn the secrets of set and setting, and that the effect of a drug is largely socially constructed. A lot of nonsense is talked about why people take drugs. I wasn't from a bad or poor family background, was never abused, nor did I suffer in any way when I was a child. I took drugs because I wanted to, because I liked their effects, and because I wanted be a part of the culture that used them. And that - dear reader - is why 99% of people take drugs. Anyone who tries to tell you any differently is lying. For millennia cultures across the globe have used plants and chemicals as a means to alter perception. What on earth gave the political establishment of the 20th Century the sovereign right to deny people access to these alchemical substances? This - to me - seemed like social control, and denial of individual freedoms on the worst possible scale.

'Freaks' (or 'heads', as we liked to call ourselves in those days) were - back then - sadly, few and far between in Cleckheaton, and so naturally gravitated together. Thus I eventually became good friends with a guy called Andy Holroyd. I'd been told he was into strange phenomena and drugs, and I should meet him. My first view of Holroyd was walking into his living room where he was rolling a joint. On the back of his denim jacket was written "Man's conception of reality is largely the construct of his own mind" which is - I think - a line from a Poul Anderson book, and was just what my 16-year-old brain needed. I was on the runway, engines idling, just waiting for takeoff.

Dope was one thing, but LSD – acid – was what I *really* wanted. The media painted LSD as a guaranteed first class ticket to heaven or hell, a complete rearrangement of the senses with the possibility of coming back from a trip changed, and with access to information denied to those who hadn't indulged. The fact that the price of admission to this Disneyland of the Gods was your mind didn't bother me too much. It was now only a matter of time, and so in the autumn of 1972, at a party at Holroyd's, I hooked up with destiny and an experience which completely and irrevocably changed my life overnight.

There were lots of people at the party, most of whom I didn't know, and it got progressively wilder and noisier as the night wore on. At some point G turned up and asked me if I wanted some acid. I did.

He sold me a green microdot, which I immediately ate. After half an hour or so nothing had happened, so I took another microdot. Any veteran acidheads reading this will be smiling and sagely shaking their head in anticipation of what was to come. This acid stuff isn't as good as it's cracked up to be, I thought, sitting on the back of a settee, talking to people. Then a guy called Tim Page said something to me and either hit me or pushed me. As I fell backwards my world changed forever.

In piecing together what happened over the next twelve hours I have settled on this version of events. My first recollection is of me being in the kitchen trying to put my head into the gas oven – presumably to harm myself, although that intention is missing from the memory. People were dragging me away and asking if was ok. I was too far gone to respond and was lost in the swirl of lights and noise. There was no fear, but there was no pleasure either, just jumbled sensory experience; the 'I', my consciousness and the entity known as Andy Roberts had left the building and the known universe.

Then I was out in the back garden. I could see rooftops and a clear, dark, starlit sky. High up over the rooftops mounted soldiers, taller than the sky, rode toward me. These were Ice Warriors, characters from the Michael Moorcock multiverse novels I was devouring at the time. Clad in steel blue ice-armour and carrying immense ice spears and shields, they came on in waves. This was fantastic beyond belief and I was enjoying it immensely but it was interrupted by people trying to move me again. I didn't want to go, and it apparently took several people to get me back inside (although I have no memory of this).

Suddenly I'm in the living room again. The party was over and just a few people remained asleep or sitting quietly in the glow of the street lamp outside. My mind spun off again and I became paranoid, convinced that someone had called the police, and that they and my parents had arrived to take me home.

This was very real and I was very frightened. But only the fear was real and this too passed and I came back to the room again. Now it was bathed in a red light – real or imaginary, and it was dead quiet. My consciousness was still very, very high, but I had some awareness of what was happening now and I didn't like it.

Dark thoughts began to arise and I was convinced I was in the presence of the ultimate, absolute, force of evil. This force was something waaaaaay beyond any trivial Satan the Christian church could conjure and more in line with the cosmic horror that author HP Lovecraft describes. The feeling of cosmic horror pervaded everything, every atom of every material object, every nuance of thought and every cell of my physical body. Evil was and there was no escape, evil was here now and in some way I was part of it.

Above me there was a ceiling lamp with a dish type glass shade. I looked up at it and could sense things dropping out of it onto me. They were maggot-like creatures and the lampshade was overflowing with them. As they dropped on me, I tried to get them off, and ripped frantically at my clothes, in a desperate attempt to remove them. I have a dim recollection of people preventing me from doing this and calming me down somewhat. I went back into myself again and continued the 'knowing' about the presence of evil and the how I was going to have to stay in that room until the maggots subsumed me back into the force of evil. I knew I must get away but knew equally well that if I did that I would still, at some time in my life, have to return to that room to face the maggots and the force of evil, so why not just stay there now and get it over with? This dialogue raged in my head for maybe a microsecond, maybe an hour. To me it was several lifetimes, several infinities. All time - everything - was both now, eternal and non-existent.

A decision formed deep within me and I decided I'd go for the live now pay later option and cross the bridge of having to deal with the ultimate evil only when it was absolutely necessary. It's a strategy I've stuck to ever since; if you don't like something, change it and if something bad is going to catch up with you, give it a good run for its money!

I often wonder what would have happened if I had not made that decision. Would I have gone mad? Or would I have developed some bizarre religious beliefs as I later saw other acid casualties do. Would I have died, either physically, mentally or spiritually, separately or in combination? I might not have lived my life as an acid casualty, but it's certainly been lived by the consequences of acid causality, and I wouldn't have had it any other way.

Reality, such as it is, slowly fell back into place and I set off home in the jingle-jangle morning. As I neared my house I realised the drug was still coursing strongly through my mind. I could see the house I lived in with my parents, but something wasn't quite right. Was it really my house or just part of the cosmic illusion I had been shown a few hours earlier? I stood in the field at the rear of the house for quite some time before going in to be met by my mother and father: Their son, unbeknownst to them, now a stranger in a strange land.

At this point, dear reader, if you're thinking that Andy Roberts is far too up himself, you'd probably be right. But the psychedelic experience was so fundamental, so overwhelming and so influential in my life that it requires some discussion to put my interest in Fortean phenomena into its correct context. It was the combination of my early reading and interests, coupled with my experiences of psychedelic drugs which led to this book having a physical reality.

I continued my exploration of psychedelics for some years. I had good trips and bad trips as well as some that were an amalgam of the two. These physical and mental excursions cannot easily be rendered into words. "Time has no meaning for days such as these" as Bill Nelson so correctly put it in *Adventures in a Yorkshire Landscape*. Some trips were alone, most with one or two other trusted psychonauts, every single one of them a life changing experience that I wouldn't have foregone. Acid was my generation's combat experience in the sense that the experience can really only be shared and understood by those who also went through it. LSD demonstrated to me, once and for all, that things are not always what they appear, and that realisation required further investigation.

But the psychedelic path is littered with problems and pitfalls and as with all spiritual technologies one requires a structure or a guru to provide guidance. That's how it was done in those days. And in late 1973 I was lucky enough to be introduced by G to L, a veteran acid head. L taught me how to respect and use the drug, and to use it for best effect. L also introduced me to the music of the *Incredible String Band* and *Dr Strangely Strange*; both of whose lyrics have also exerted a strong influence over my writing. Other hippies I hung out with at the time introduced me to the *Grateful Dead*, whose music and lyrics and attitude toward life has also heavily influenced my writing style and approach to the world.

The first time I took any acid with L was a mild trip but one which contained a very Fortean event. We decided to go out for a walk, and prior to doing so listened to *Pink Floyd*'s *Meddle*. Then we set out across some fields on a path I used regularly, and indeed had used earlier that same night.

There was a small wood on the path, enclosed by a stone wall and accessed by a stile. As we approached the stile we could see a glowing object which - as we neared - resolved itself into a piece of board on which was written in pink fluorescent paint PINK FLOYD. My tiny mind was blown. What were the chances of taking acid, listening to 'The Floyd' and then finding such a sign in the middle of nowhere? This meant everything and absolutely nothing. If it was a coincidence then it was proof that the universe is really a multiverse and far weirder than we can imagine. If it was evidence that L had planted the sign several hours earlier and navigated our trip to listening to PF and then coming out to find the sign, then that shows some genuine human psychedelic creativity. You will all have your own views on this but suffice to say it was tangible, evidence to me that the universe was just wilfully weird and that acid could turn up that weirdness well beyond number eleven!

A few hours later I walked home through that same wood. Of course, there was no sign and no evidence that there ever had been one! Sometimes you get shown the light, in the strangest of places, if you look at it right.

It was this strange experience that stimulated the first piece of my writing which has actually survived the passage of time. It's a brief account of the trip and forms the first piece in this anthology. It has not been edited in any way, and is exactly how I wrote it. Of course the language in it and the general tone and content of the piece is now extremely embarrassing. But hey, I was 17, young and naïve.

What matters is that is how it was then, for me.

I had many more psychedelic adventures with L and he taught me more than he will ever know about life, the multiverse and everything. He would laugh at the idea of being a guru, but would secretly like it. He was, and probably still is, a deeply flawed human being but as the cowboys used to say, I rode with him and I have no complaints.

Acid, music and Fortean phenomena were now the main focus of my life. At the Windsor Free Festival, in August 1974, I witnessed another acid-related Fortean event. This one showed me just how groups of people can create a reality visible to - and shared by - them, which is occulted from the rest of us.

Large quantities of high quality LSD were available at Windsor, and most people were flying high much of the time. One night, when I wasn't high, I was woken in the early hours by noises from a nearby tent. I looked out of my tent to see two males and a female sat on the grass staring at the sky, clearly under the influence of LSD, and chattering excitedly about what they could see. The sky was dark and cloudless with nothing but stars in view. Yet these hippies were watching and describing the landing of a UFO, from which a tall blond 'Venusian' appeared.

During the course of the hour or so I observed them, it was clear to me that for these three hippies the UFO and its occupant was 'real' to them. Although nothing was visible they were all having the same experience, subtly and unknowingly creating it between them, much in the same way that psychology describes the phenomenon known as a *folie a deux*.

The following day, when they had come down from their trip I questioned them about the event. They were adamant it actually took place, was utterly real to them, and couldn't understand why no-one else could see it. Analogues of this event can be found throughout Forteana. For instance in the numerous cases where groups of people have experienced the Blessed Virgin Mary yet, in the case of the BVM at Knock, for instance, observers merely saw them staring at a wall.

Wake up, down there!

Adolescence solidified into adulthood. The hideousness of work and having to make a living, together with marriage and buying a house, took me away from writing and strange phenomena for a few years. It was to be a death and a birth that re-vivified my interest in both.

My first wife, Helen, had our son Kai on 16 November 1982. Technically, he was our second child as Helen had undergone a full term neonatal death the previous year. I had given up my job as a gardener just after the stillbirth because Calderdale Council wouldn't allow me any time off to be with Helen. During that first year of Kai's existence I came across Jenny Randles' excellent book: *UFOs. A British Viewpoint* and I decided I wanted to engage with this mystery.

My introduction to WYUFORG was something of a disappointment. I had no idea whatsoever what to expect and found myself in an untidy flat in Idle, on the outskirts of Bradford. This was the home of Anne and Darren Chanter, who hosted WYUFORG meetings. It soon became painfully apparent that UFOs weren't really being discussed at all; it was all group admin, underpinned by the various beliefs of those involved. But they were the only people I knew who were into this stuff and so I hung around.

Paul Bennett edited the WYUFORG journal, *UFO Brigantia* - a photocopied, poorly edited monthly UFO journal distributed to maybe 30 people. After a couple of years Paul wanted to give the editorship up and so I took over. This was great stuff. Not only could I write scathing editorials, but I could write whatever else I wanted, and also accept or refuse the work of others. Publishers would send me stacks of free books to review. What thrills! What power! All at very little expense and to very little effect. But it was fun and slowly, as I became aware of the UK UFO subculture, I decided *UFO Brigantia* was going to be the only UFO magazine worth reading.

In the mid Eighties, long before the internet, there was a plethora of UFO magazines in the UK. Most were absolute rubbish, each claiming they knew the truth behind the UFO phenomenon. To counteract this nonsense, I modelled *UFO Brigantia* on hippie underground publications such as *International Times, Ink, Frendz* and *OZ*, as well as the gonzo journalism of Hunter S Thompson and music journos such as Charles Shaar Murray and Nick Kent.

I wanted *UFO Brigantia* to be rock'n'roll ufology; an outsider publication for those who were fascinated by ufology but not sucked into the vortices of the belief from which it was constructed. Of course we were as much a part of it as everyone else but so what? By the early 1990s I had managed to build *UFO Brigantia's* circulation up to around 1,000 every two months.

Alongside my ufological interests I was pursuing other areas of Fortean interest. The mystery Big Cat phenomena was slowly gaining in media coverage in the UK and as far as I could see there were very few people collecting info on this aspect of Forteana. So I decided to investigate a few sightings and thus did my first field investigations which resulted in a booklet called *Catflaps!*

As CFZ Press has very kindly re-published *Catflaps!* there are no examples from it in the present book. But it was my first sustained effort at Fortean writing and a genuine attempt to put information into the public domain which could be followed up by others, and to ensure that these mysteries were not lost forever in the newspaper archives.

What are words worth?

In the mid 1980s my interests in ufology led me to meet up with a young lad called David Clarke. He is of course now the internationally known UFO historian Dr David Clarke! Dave and I got on extremely well and have shared literally hundreds of Fortean investigations into ufology and folklore. We travelled tens of thousands of miles in search of UFO witnesses, the sites of unusual legends and folklore, and any other oddness that we fancied.

Dave's intensely practical, journalistic, approach meshed well with my psychedelically sceptical world-view, and we formed a writing and research partnership which continues to this day. I like to think I've changed Dave's mind about many things and he mine. We argue, and we bicker, but when it comes to researching a subject we never stinted to throw time, money and thought at it until we had drained it of every last nuance of information.

Dave and I managed to cut a swath through UK ufology, reinvestigating and solving a number of classic cases as we went. We also started to look seriously at the UFO files held by the UK Government since the 1950s, which bore fruit in *Out of the Shadows* and numerous articles. Dave's work with the UFO files held at the National Archives has brought him well deserved international acclaim and both he and I are widely hated in many corners of the UFO community because we burst the bubble of a government cover up. My friendship with Dave led to us conjuring up the idea for our first book, *Phantoms of the Sky*, after which we went on to write several books on various subjects either in tandem or individually. We also, again both together and separately, have done a great deal of TV and radio work, appearing as talking heads on many UFO documentaries and once also acting as consultants on BBC1's *Timewatch* documentary on UFOs.

The period from the mid 1980s to the present day have been a whirlwind of writing, researching and investigating a wide variety of Fortean phenomena, much of which you will find reflected in this book articles. Although ufology and its fringes are at the core of much of my work, you will also find articles on many other subjects including death rays, folklore, cryptozoology, cults, counter culture, ESP and much.

If you fondly imagine the life of a writer/researcher to be in any way glamorous, let me disabuse you of that belief. Maybe it is if you make enough money from your writing not to have to be a wageslave. But scepticism doesn't sell. I've had enormous fun, yes, oodles of it. I've been to some strange places, met some stranger people and been part of some weird scenes and have exerted an influence on ufology in the UK.

But any kind of writing, especially book writing, takes an immense toll. During the book gestation and writing period the book assumes a life of its own, an entity that lives in the brain making demands on thought, almost to the exclusion of everything else.

The physical act of writing and researching sucks time away from the rest of your life, often making me distant, withdrawn and irritable. Unless you have a particularly understanding partner (all mine have been fabulous and long-suffering) relationships can be put under strain and friendships cruelly tested in the crucible of research, writing and deadline. Ultimately, any writing is a selfish act, and all writing is really more about the writer than the subject matter.

Have I made any money? The amount of money I have spent on writing and researching outweighs, by a factor of at least ten, the money I have received in royalties. Keeping up with every known source on a particular subject might build an impressive library but it drains the bank balance. Travelling hundreds of miles to interview a witness from which only a few hundred words might make it to the finished product is not cost effective, yet it's necessary if the job is to be done right.

So, there y'go. I could tell you much more about my influences and how I got from there to here. But there's no time and I trust this brief, but candid, autobiographical sketch will - as we used to say - hip you to where I'm at. I hope you enjoy this eclectic selection of my writings. There is probably at least as much still hidden in obscure small circulation journals, some of which I've completely forgotten about. The writings anthologised here, especially the early articles and those written for little or no money, tend to be a tad shambolic, while those written for journals like *Fortean Times* are well polished. If you enjoy them, then perhaps you should take a chance and buy a few of my books? I'm always open to comments, criticism and correspondence and can be contacted at: andy@cfz.org.uk

Have fun
Happy Trails

Andy Roberts
July 2009

PUBLISHER'S NOTE: We would like to thank Andy, who is taking no payment for this, or indeed for *Catflaps!* and is donating the royalties from both books to the ongoing expenses of the Centre for Fortean Zoology (CFZ). Thanks mate. JD

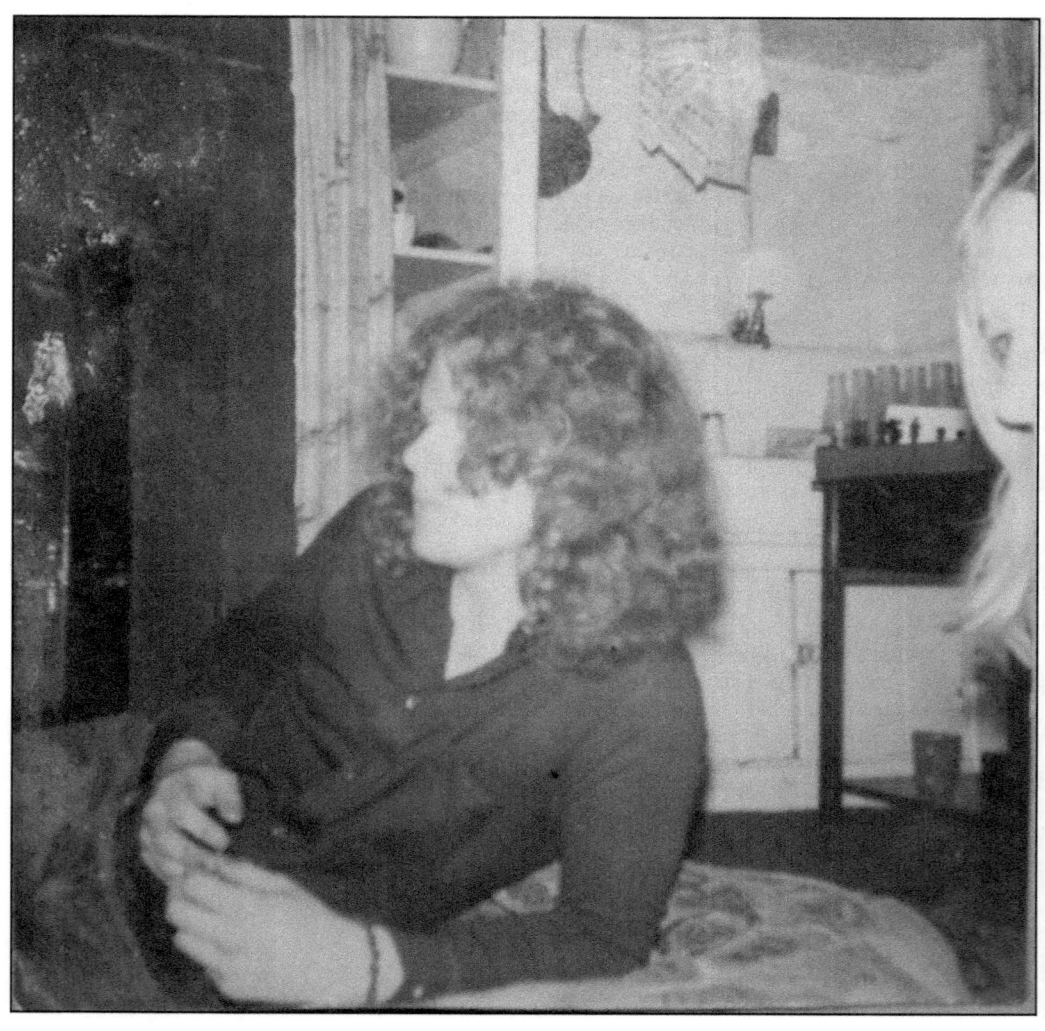

The young Andy Roberts, 1974 in the cottage of one of his hippie gurus

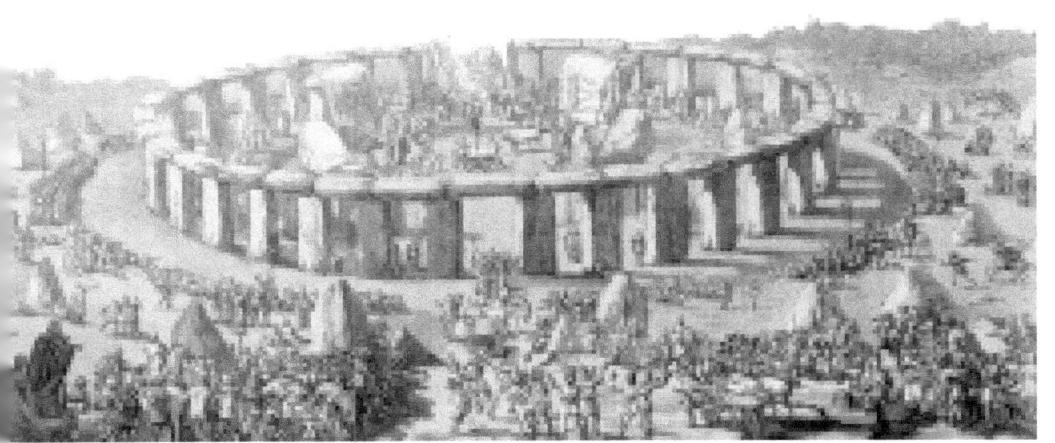

TWO DAYS LATER

The earliest extant piece of my writing. Written shortly after an influential LSD experience with my 'acid guru' and a good friend.

May 1974

I remember the music with no impression that I remembered and liked, A badger leading us through the fields to hug trees who love us with their breathing, watching the lites in the valley and realising how stupid it was that the lites lit the pollution up for us to see and realise its stupidity. The sign with *Pink Floyd* written on it dropped by the Intergalactic Drug Squad to freak and puzzle us.

Houses with lites on – who could be up at that time of night but people tripping? Raw toast and broken biscuits of which life is one long broken biscuit and I couldn't find the one I liked until the morning. An overcast dawn that I had waited to see that didn't matter when it arrived. My pineal gland being opened to the white lite by an earth creature with earth force who could crush my head with his power that no wizard could equal 'til now and only if he tries and he will because it's a path of many goals and he might find his source through it. And walking home through GREEN fields – Om-ing at the grave yard with little response from the dead who were tripped out on another plane above even the OM The grass running across the field and each noise separate until he looked into the mirror and realised his eyeballs were oh so huge and wondering what mother would say and she wouldn't understand it was good.

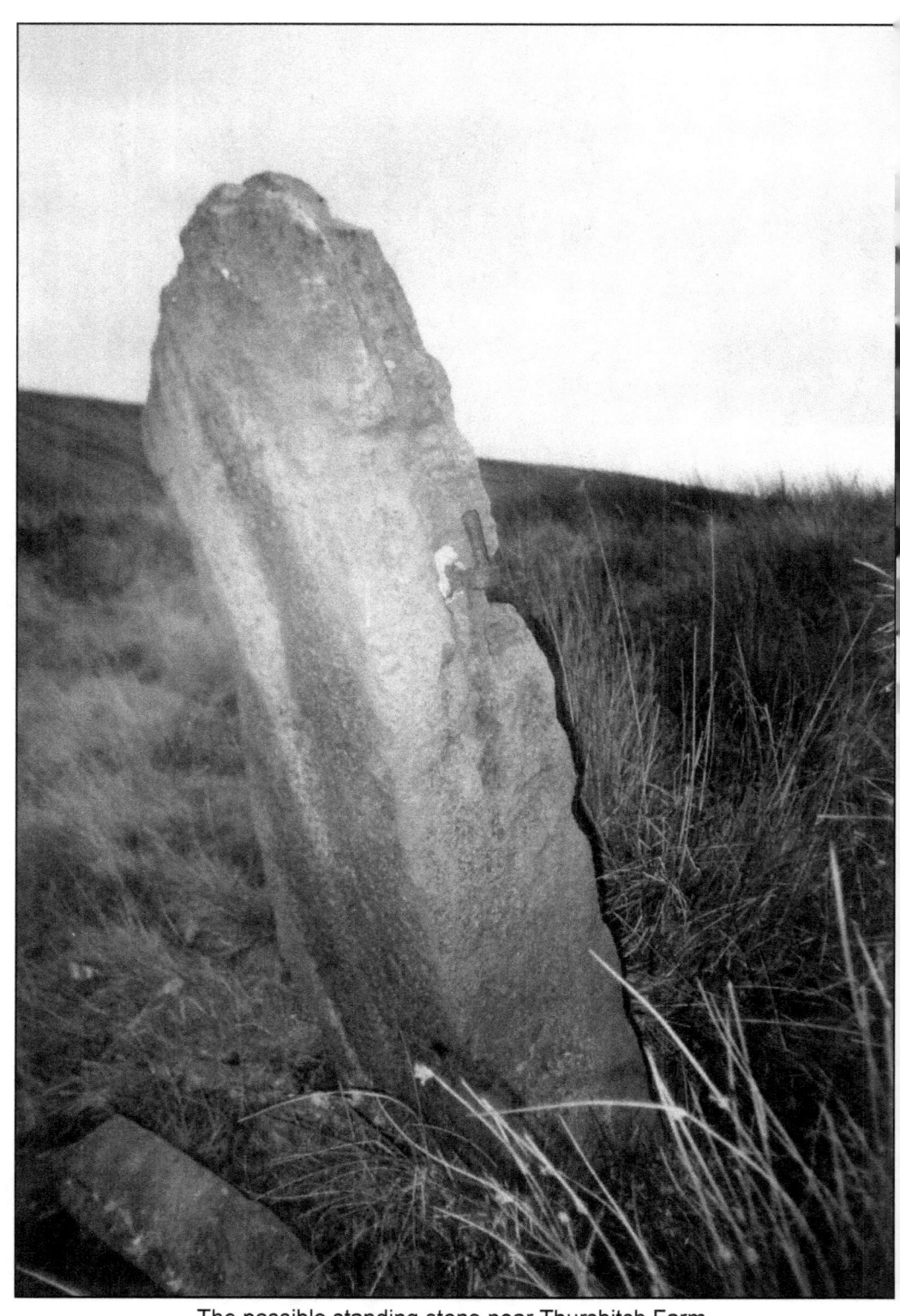

The possible standing stone near Thursbitch Farm.
Referred to in Garner's novel *Thursbitch* as Bully Thrumble

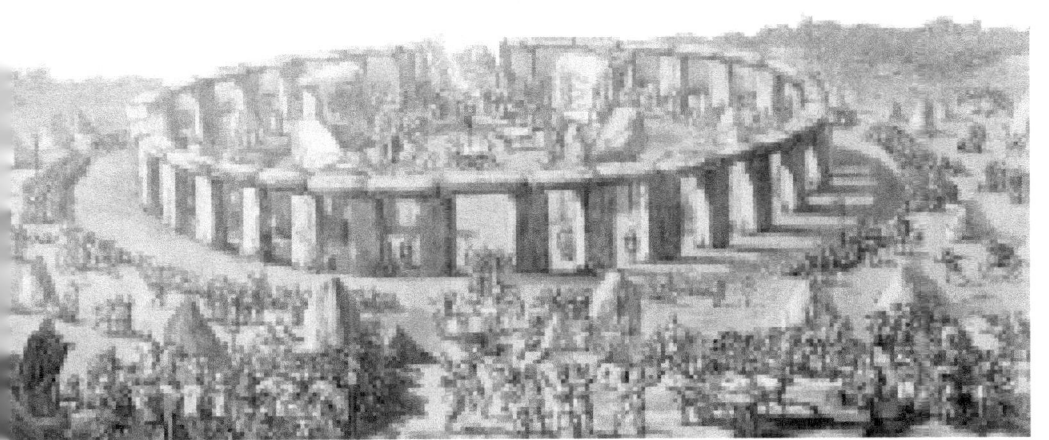

THURSBITCH – VALLEY OF THE DEMON?

Fiction, folklore and fact in Alan Garner's
novel *Thursbitch*

'What I was finding through research was more interlinked and unsafe than anything
I could structure as a novelist.'
Alan Garner Edinburgh, 22/8/04

This text is the basis of the Northern Earth Mysteries Group visit to *Thursbitch*,
on 11th September 2004, to look at the locations mentioned by Alan
Garner in his remarkable novel, *Thursbitch*. From being a physical tour it's
now a textual tour round the valley.

The source material is, of course, *Thursbitch* the novel, as well as numerous
interviews and articles with and by Alan Garner, his non-fiction writings
and his lectures, mixed in with local history and snippets of folklore
and archaeology which seem relevant.

This text is entirely unofficial, in that it is not in any way at all sanctioned by Garner, yet draws heavily on his material. Indeed, without his material it wouldn't exist. Every Garner scholar is aware that he isn't too keen on people rooting around in the backgrounds to his fiction, yet equally any Garner scholar loves the material so much that they really can't help but at least wonder...

At a recent lecture in Edinburgh Garner suggested the research and reality behind *Thursbitch*, and by implication all his novels, is a depth that the 'reader cannot, and should not know'. Personally I disagree with this. I would be more in agreement if Garner didn't freely discuss a lot of information about the background to his novels in his interviews and lectures, all of which beg many questions. I consider it an arrogance to wish to keep secret, yet give glimpses of any kind of knowledge, sacred or profane, in this way. Of course Garner believes himself to be involved in a family tradition belonging to a small area of land and he has stated that such knowledge and information '...is not a public matter. It has to be lived, in order to be won. There is no mystery; but there is a rightness'. Again this would be an acceptable, if questionable, attitude if it weren't for the fact that Garner is clearly happy to discuss his 'knowledge' with academics, yet restricts it in snippets to those less well placed in the academic pantheon.

Considering Garner's working class roots, I find this to be a curious dichotomy. If something really *is* worth keeping secret then secret it should be kept. There can be no half-measures. Garner clearly has a love and a reverence for the area and lore in which he has steeped himself. But he has a proprietorial attitude to those who share an interest in his source material, especially those who would choose, as he does, to write - albeit non-fictionally - about it. Writing in response to a request for information from an author in 1993 Garner wrote:

> 'You seem, indeed, to be coming into 'my' territory, but for a purpose I must not abet. It is 'my' territory in as much as I own it as it owns me, which lays the responsibility of mediator and stewardship on my function, as opposed to the journalist's, which is more the quarrying of the place as the sum of its usable reserves.'

This unequivocal statement is echoed and mirrored throughout all Garner's interviews and non-fiction essays, and the implication - to me at least - is that if it suits Garner to let slip gobbets of information for publicity or for the appraisal of academics, or to the public via the transient medium of the lecture then it's all well and good. For anyone else genuinely interested in the mysteries of our race, and the island we inhabit, to which we all - surely - are entitled to equal access, Garner uses his position to prevent access; a powerful guardian on the threshold, to prevent people looking further.

Thursbitch is complex and full of allusion and reference, to which I'm only going to touch upon here. There is much more, concerning pagan practices, archaeology, geology, astronomy, time anomalies, use of sacred plants, cattle fertility, and mythology and so on hinted at throughout *Thursbitch*. It's all there for the interested reader to find, and - if you've a mind to do so - to follow up. Nor will I mention what could be said about his use of boundaries, both of land, time, and states of consciousness and so on. Or his use of language and dialect. There are still things in there I sense but can't yet unravel properly and for that reason the nature of the Bull/Star/Snake/Bee/Hare/Stone relationship is barely hinted at here.

The interested reader can find an excellent range of articles/reviews about *Thursbitch* on the unofficial Alan Garner site at: http://alangarner.atspace.org/http://members.ozemail.com.au/~xenophon/, which will further illuminate them. Possibly not all that I've 'quarried' from *Thursbitch* and Thursbitch is entirely correct, but it's what I saw in the novel, and how I've come to see the valley, after Garner alerted me to it. I believe the mysteries shouldn't be kept secret, because the best way to keep a secret is to reveal it, on the grounds that there's none as blind as those that can't see! And those that can see deserve to be shown.

Although the novel deals with two very distinct centuries, I will be referring specifically in the main to the John/Jack Turner strand, which is the major story in the book, although inextricably linked to the contemporary Ian and Sal thread.

Garner mentions Thursbitch in a non-fiction context for the first time in his collection of essays *The Voice That Thunders*, where he says:

> 'As we went along the valley of the demon, my wife pointed out that the gateposts were too big, and shaped quite differently from the normal Pennine style, and many were of a different stone. Then, high in the valley, and away from the single ruin of human habitation, first there was a well, built of stone, going down into the ground, with a collapsed roof; then we

came to stones that had not been moved, and were pecked (worked by stone not metal) and the present evidence, which we are still collecting, is that it is a megalithic complex connected to a stellar cult, possibly of Orion.'

He makes the point in lectures and interviews that he believes many of the gateposts in Thursbitch are ancient standing stones. These, he believes, were re-used as gateposts, dating from The Enclosure Acts in the 18th and 19th Centuries. It's an intriguing, beguiling theory, and not a new one. Archaeologists and earth mysterians have argued about this problem for many years. Here, in Thursbitch, however I think Garner may have a point to one degree or another. As we will see, many of the gateposts to which he refers, and which he employs fictionally in the novel, appear to be substantially different to 'normal' gateposts. They are often ill paired, in that it seems that one of them was in existence as a separate stone and had another added to it to form a gate. Some of them are big, bigger than the one they are paired with and far too big to be a gatepost. Some are roughly worked, at variance to the newer ones which are neatly worked and much smaller. Some exist just as singular stones in walls and have never been employed as gateposts, and it seems obvious that they were there originally and the wall was simply built onto them. We will see at least one good example of this during the walk. Another reason Garner gives for some of the gatepost stones being older stones re-used is the fact that the majority of them have Ordnance Survey benchmarks on them. There seems to be a far greater distribution in Thursbitch than in neighbouring valleys and Garner makes the point that the O.S. only used stones etc which appeared to be permanent features of landscape.

If this is the case, and I have no idea if it is or not, then it is perhaps yet another indicator of the length of time that a stone has been used for this purpose. In my travels round and about Thursbitch, I have looked at other gateposts in neighbouring valleys, and once out of the valley, they tend to be well manicured, small, relatively modern stones. This discourse on the nature of gateposts may seem a little trivial, but it is central to any mystery or meaning there may be in *Thursbitch*.

THE HISTORY AND ORIGINS OF THURSBITCH

The name 'Thursbitch' dates from 1384, at a time when place names were, as Welsh, Gaelic and Irish place names are today, descriptive. The Old English word *thyrs*, means giant or demon. It occurs as such in the epic poem *Beowulf*. Batch or bitch means valley. Alan Garner believes that 'Thursbitch' means valley of the demon. Prior to 1742, the Thursbitch area was open land, after which it was walled during the time of the enclosures. This is relevant when considering stones Garner mentions, both fictionally and - as we will see - those which exist in reality. At some point in his ongoing investigations of the valley, Garner had an Alfred Watkins-like experience in which, 'the enclosures were stripped from (my) eyes, and I saw the valley as John Turner knew it', meaning he could see the standing stones in their original positions and relation, clear of the walls which now obscure them.

Thyrs doesn't always mean demon. It can also mean 'something big', a meaning which, considering the implications of what Garner has found in and was told about the valley of Thursbitch, works on many levels. Like Garner's books, the valley of Thursbitch and both its fictional and factual inhabitants are transtemporal, offering meaning from whatever age and standpoint they are viewed.

Thursbitch is, Garner believes, a 'sentient landscape'. This term is rarely used but its meaning is often implied in stories of the paranormal as they relate to landscape. I am a firm believer in the concept of sentient landscape, although it is an area from which researchers have shied because of its implications, all of which centre on the *genius loci*, or spirit of place, and how that is experienced. All landscapes have this quality, this possibility: some - for reasons as yet unknown - more than others. It's this latter group which seem to attract the strange experiences; the sacred sites and the sense that the landscape is in some way 'alive'. Though the idea of sentient landscape runs strongly through both strands of the book, it is first implied after one of Ian and Sal's visits. 'This place has had enough of us'.

As author Lawrence Durrell said, '...all landscapes ask the same question in the same whisper, 'I am watching you – are you watching yourself in me?''. I have done considerable research in this area, which is slowly gathering momentum towards a book, but which so far has been written up as a study of 'mountain panics'; wilderness experiences which have been codified as paranormal panics, and linked - at different locations - to local gods and goddesses, giants or spectral phenomena.

JENKIN CHAPEL

The simple date stone indicates the day and year of its consecration as 24th June 1733. But the story behind the chapel in both fiction and fact is far from simple.

The site, which was originally a meeting of tracks, is first recorded in 1364. A cross or pillar, possibly with prehistoric origins, called 'Jankin Cross' once stood here, on the opposite side of the road to the chapel. As is often the case with these sites, an annual fair was held here, in this case on the 24th of June. This date is old Midsummer's Day, and the Feast of St John the Baptist; a date central to many of the events in Thursbitch.

In or around 1732 the cross or standing stone was smashed by locals, led by Richard Turner. These same locals built what became the church, and Garner - both in the novel and in his lectures - links the two events, although there is no hard historical reference for this.

At first the church was a simple affair, lacking bell tower and chancel. According to Garner, the Bishops of Chester refused to consecrate the chapel for 61 years. When they finally did, it was - apparently - on condition that the dedication was changed to St John the Evangelist. Garner's take on this is that John the Baptist often has folkloric and pagan connotations, being linked with the Wodwo, Wodwose, or wildman and - in southern Europe - aspects of Dionysus. He has said 'is this why Chester refused to consecrate, or was it something other?' There is obviously a great deal of research to do, as I'm sure that - Garner's research notwithstanding - there must be some records in church archives which explain the situation more clearly.

Local historian Walter Smith, writing in 1932 said, 'We do not know...what use the chapel was put to... we do not know whether any services were held there or not.'. Locals apparently refer to Jenkin Chapel as 'the place where they marry the odd'. As Garner said, 'who, or what did they worship?' In *Thursbitch* this is the site of the standing stone called Jenkin, on which the stone head called Crom, taken from the well named 'Pearly Meg's', is placed in order to bear witness to the locals' pagan *Amanita muscaria* rites. Following Jack's madness when Nan dies, and after he smashes Jenkin, he leaves the valley for a year. When he returns, befuddled by evangelical preaching, his family build the chapel to contain the ever growing band of converts to Christianity. It's also the site where Jack eventually begins to come to his senses, slowly returning to the path he originally followed.

In *Thursbitch* it is alluded, but - like so many things never clarified - that the group rite celebrated at Jenkin, is connected to the major lunar standstill, which happens more or less every eighteen years, when the moon appears to be stationary for a period of a few days. And one such standstill takes place in the time period in the 17th Century in which the novel is set. This phenomenon was also noticed by many prehistoric peoples, and marked out by ceremony and ritual observance involving standing stones etc. When the rite takes place in Thursbitch the moon is the central feature, which reinforces this theory. This was one of the questions I specifically asked of Garner via his Press Officer, and which he declined to answer.

In 1999 Garner contacted the Anglican vicar then responsible for Jenkin Chapel, who had plenty to say about the building and the area. The vicar had - surprisingly - never been there, but he had been, among other things, told at his induction that 'it would not be safe for a man of the cloth to enter that valley'. Garner's notes from this conversation indicated that the churchwarden who inducted the vicar had been warned by inhabitants of the area that it was 'not right'. The vicar had also been told by locals that in 1985 Thursbitch was filled with 'a lot of electrical magic'.

Oddly, despite Garner's tale about the chapel only being consecrated after the dedication was changed, there doesn't seem to be any evidence of this. The chapel appears to be still called after John the Baptist, yet other sources also give the re-dedication account. For instance at www.wishful-thinking.org.uk/ genuki/ CHS/Saltersford/StJohn.html, a genealogy page, the author mentions the re-dedication and refers to the chapel as St. John the Evangelist.

MEMORIAL STONE

This is the stone which Garner says was the origin of the idea for *Thursbitch*. In lectures and interviews he says that he found the stone whilst out running, as a boy, on 19th July 1952. It was hidden in grass, set into the bank, with only one face visible.

> HERE JOHN TURNER WAS CAST AWAY IN A HEAVY SNOW STORM IN
> THE NIGHT IN OR ABOUT THE YEAR 1755.

Garner trapped his hand behind the stone and became aware the reverse also had lettering engraved on it.

Slowly he worked his fingers over the carved letters until he was able to make out the words:

> THE PRINT OF A WOMANS SHOE WAS FOUND BY HIS SIDE IN THE
> SNOW WERE HE LAY DEAD H

Alan Garner believes he was the first person to see the reverse side of the stone since it was first placed.

The current stone isn't the original; two others have been damaged and replaced since Garner relocated it, hence why it looks new and is at right angles to the bank. Note the letter H, seemingly out of place and pointless. This was missed out from the word W(H)ERE, and as masons were paid by the letter it was added at the bottom!

The image conjured by the stone and its eerie text 'the print of a woman's shoe' gave Garner the chills and he ran home somewhat scared. But the imagery stayed with him and is responsible for us standing here today!

But there's much more to the stone and the story which lays behind it, in all senses. Garner queries why, if a stone had been so carefully carved and erected the inscription was so vague, 'in or around' 1755'.

The field here on a tithe map dating from 1840 is called Osbaldestanecroft – which according to Garner meaning 'stone of the bright God'. The stone apparently exists somewhere and has not been removed or built into the wall.

One of Garner's informants, a farmer to whom he refers as 'Mr X', was a member of the Turner family. He told Garner the memorial stone was erected in the 19th Century by another member of the Turner lineage but the date was 1735 not 1755 and John Turner, referred to as Jack throughout *Thursbitch*, had died sometime on Christmas Eve.

Garner's informant gave some background to Jack's life. He was born in 1706 and became a packman or jagger, a name familiar throughout the Pennines and one which is still a common surname in the area. The area of Yorkshire from which I come, still has its fair share of Jagger surnames and many vestiges of the packhorse trade. Jack Turner transported salt from Chester and Northwich in Cheshire, to Derby, from where he returned with other goods. Besides this, in the novel, he is the link between the valley and the outside world, and he brings news, information and artefacts from the outside world to isolated hill farms of the Cheshire Pennines. He lived at Saltersford in both fiction and fact, and in both his father was the tenant farmer Richard Turner.

Jack died when he was 29, on Christmas Eve. Garner makes the point that he shouldn't have died then as he was a fit young packman with masses of outdoor experience. Not only that but he must have recently just passed through the farmyard of Buxter Stoops Farm and could have sought help if he had needed it.

He was found, as both folklore and fiction relate, on Christmas Day itself, a day not without folkloric significance, in deep snow with the print of one woman's shoe at his side. Of course he could have died of a heart attack or many other causes but of course that would spoil a good tale and in any case doesn't detract from what Garner has discovered in and around the valley of Thursbitch.

Garner states that the local people believe that Jack Turner was a real antecedent who lived and died, as is recorded in the oral tradition handed down through the generations. Yet when Garner tried to find a papertrail to validate Turner's existence, he ran up against a dead end. There is no mention of a Jack (or John) Turner in any of the birth, marriage, or death registers. Nor is a Jack Turner recorded at the Public Record Office, where the records of all packhorse men are kept; the 18th Century version of the Inland Revenue being very keen to register the packhorse trade. Other than the memorial stone, there are no physical records of Jack Turner's life whatsoever.

THE STONE AT HOWLERSKNOWL FARM

This is the stone in Thursbitch that Garner refers to as the Belderstone. It is the stone to which the Bull - which is both real and imaginary in the book, worshipped and torn apart - is attached in the communal *Amanita muscaria* rite. It doesn't appear to be a standing stone, although it is a little odd that it has been left in the middle of a field. Perhaps it once held some arcane significance, and that's the reason it wasn't uprooted. Or perhaps it was merely left as a cattle rubbingstone. Whatever the case here, in his lectures Garner tells an interesting story about the stone, which - if true, and we have no reason to doubt it - is proof of the supernatural.

Garner tells of how in his researches for *Thursbitch,* he and his wife came upon the stone. The Garners first spotted it in 1999: 'At first I thought it was a sheep. I went across to look at it, and saw that it had a shiny steel or iron ring hammered into it. I was intrigued by the fact that the ring wasn't rusty'. He then photographed the rock with the ring set in it, and shows the slide in his lecture.

However, the next time he and his wife visited the stone, there was no ring in it, nor any trace of there *ever* having been a ring there. It seems logical that if a ring had once existed, and had been removed, there would at least have been some trace, yet there was none. Nowadays there is neither ring in the rock, nor any sign of there ever being one. So, was Garner lying? Blending fact into fiction to create a good 'back story' for his book? If so, did he go to the trouble of faking a picture of the stone with the ring in it? Or was the ring really there, as Garner's lecture slide shows? And had it really vanished on his second visit, leaving no trace? Those are the only two options available to us. One implies dishonesty; the other implies a genuine supernatural occurrence and all that entails. The choice is yours.

THURSBITCH

The ruined farm of Thursbitch is the centre of the valley. Up on the eastern hillside you can see a large stone. This is the stone Garner calls 'Thoon' in the novel.

In his lectures Garner tells quite a few stories he has gathered about Thursbitch via his anonymous (to us) informants. The previously mentioned Mr X, on another visit, asked Garner somewhat enigmatically as he was leaving the room, 'what's wrong with the valley Alan, what's wrong?'. Very Lovecraftian! On a later visit Mr X made the passing comment, 'they never should have buried that baby in Thursbitch'.

Another informant, who once spoke to Garner after a lecture, told him that he had once been a General Practitioner in the area of Thursbitch. He had always 'dreaded' a night visit to Saltersford.'

Mr Y, a former tenant of Saltersford Hall told Garner he wanted him down off Andrew's Edge before dusk, and he wanted Garner to tell him he was down off the edge. 'You see, there isn't a farmer in all these hills around as'll open his doors after dark, not even to cross the yard, without he's got his gun. Not that it would be any use.' This always raises a laugh in the lectures but, having spoken to a few dour hill farmers who had tales to tell I can assure you it's a sobering moment when a sane, practical outdoorsman tells you he is frightened of a particular area or landscape or a landscape feature. Such is the power of the *genius loci.*

On the ground at Thursbitch there are several things to look at. Firstly there is a huge gate-post, which may or may not have been a standing stone at one time or another. It's odd because it's large and doesn't appear to have a purpose or a matching stone. Then there is the well. This is basically a stone run off trough to capture water. The significance of this will be more relevant later.

BULLY THRUMBLE

This stone is another central feature of the fiction - and fact - of Thursbitch.

- It is where Nan tells Jack she is pregnant,
- where Jack ritually catches the hare ('old goibert' in local dialect),
- where Ian and Sal spend the night watching the celestial parade, and expounding Garner's theory among other events.

A close examination will reveal - Ian and Sal noted in the book - that it has been lightly carved to give it a phallic appearance. Garner believes the markings on the stone indicate it was 'pecked', worked by stone not metal tools, which would put its carving - I was going to say erection but thought better of it - in the Neolithic or early Bronze Age. Garner claims that this has been verified by a stonemason from photographs.

Whilst I don't doubt this, once again it's something which needs investigating further, preferably by an archaeologist experienced in dating stone carving techniques.

If it were once a standing stone then its position at the confluence of two streams would have had some importance. We know from other folk, and from pagan traditions, that the confluence of streams was of significance. Many standing stones and artefacts from prehistory have been placed at the confluence of streams or rivers. In the Derbyshire Pennines in the valley of Longdendale, only a few miles from here, a pagan tradition which existed until the late 20th Century held a special veneration for the confluence of streams.

This is also the site from which Ian and Sal make their celestial observations, and Garner believes may be one of the locations pre-historic man used as an observatory.

Across the field to the east, almost hidden in the wall that is the boundary between valley and open moor land is another stone.

This is named Biggening Brom in *Thursbitch*, and is the effect to Bully Thrumble's cause. I am 100% certain that this, irrespective of what we may think of the other stones, is a genuine prehistoric standing stone. It has no remnants of gatepost fastenings or holes, it is roughly carved (and could well be said to resemble a pregnant woman) and is built into a wall as though it were there when the enclosures took place and was allowed to remain *in situ*.

It also marks the route from Thursbitch to Thoon.

THE WELL

The well in Thursbitch is central to the tale. In both fact and fiction it is a Holy Well, sacred to people in the area. Garner fictionalises it as Pearly Meg's, and it's where Jack goes for a variety of reasons. It's where the stone head Crom is kept, and it's where John takes the Blue John cup of water back up to Thoon to give to Nan. In the fictional valley legends the water is said to be poisonous once a year and it is on the night John collects it for Nan. The water kills her and the valley takes its sacrifice.

The Garners discovered the actual well, and it's sturdily constructed. Steps are visible, and someone, at some time went to great deal of trouble to build it here. As the only habitation for at least a mile in each direction is Thursbitch Farm, the question must be asked who, and why?

Thursbitch itself, as we've seen, has an open tank for a well, and easy access to the stream. That well is marked on the OS map. This one isn't. Once again, who and why?

Apparently this well once belonged to the Turner's farm at Saltersford. They refused to allow the tenants of Thursbitch to use it, hence the comparitively poor run-off tank at Thursbitch Farm. One of Garner's informants recalled being sent to put butter on a shelf in the well as a child. At the time he believed this was for refrigeration purposes.

Yet the farm was over a mile away. This is clearly a vestige of the tradition of leaving an offering at wells and other locations. This is still practiced in out of the way places throughout the British Isles, to this day. Folklorists Janet and Colin Bord, in their book *Sacred Waters* mention two Butter Wells, and milk and dairy products are a common motif in Holy Well lore.

The Bords also note the tradition of Holy Wells being potent only on certain nights of the year and - as with the events of *Thursbitch* the novel - St. John's Eve is one of those nights.

THE WALL TO THE WATERSHED

This wall, part of the 1742 enclosures has - quite unusually - three benchmarked stones within half a mile, at fairly regular intervals. These stones may also once have been standing stones. Garner states that the stone row is 11° 30 min east of north. In the late Neolithic/early Bronze Age, would have pointed to the Pole Star.

At that time the Pole Star was Alpha Draconis, or The Snake: yet *more* celestial and serpentine imagery which exists both in novel and landscape, and which Garner has expertly and seamlessly conjoined.

THOON

This landscape feature is one of the centrepieces of *Thursbitch*, and a physical punctuation mark on the edge of the valley. It's clearly and strikingly visible from many places within Thursbitch, yet from the Shining Tor ridge is barely noticeable. In the novel it is - among other things - the site of Jack and Nan's pagan handfasting, the placement of the stone head Crom for the three days of the major lunar standstill, and immediately before the rite at Jenkin, and finally of Sal's exit from the world.

On the top is an ambiguous mark which may be said to resemble a woman's footprint, and the inference for the novel is obvious. Footprints in stone are a common folkloric motif in the UK, as they are in other countries, and veteran folklorist Janet Bord has recently written a book on this subject. The stone is cave-like, but entirely natural, and a logical place from which to view the valley. The shape of the little cave lends itself to interpretation of a beehive and Garner uses this to great effect in the novel, which is replete with references to bees in one form or other, physical, metaphorical, celestial and mythological.

The farm of Thursbitch, the well, and most of the standing stones and farms are visible from here. Garner states that the location of a cave above a confluence of waters is the natural habitat of a Thyrs or demon.

Garner also suggests that this stone was a sighting stone, which was used for astronomical observations from standing stones in the valley. A look at the *Red Shift* astronomy programme reveals that Taurus, Orion, the Moon, and several other astronomical bodies, rise from (and fall behind) this ridge at various times of year. Garner employs this fact to spin the cosmology of the valley, as revealed by Jack Turner in the novel.

As Jack prepares to meet his snowy fate at the pillar of Osbalderstone he talks his dog through what is happening as he 'puts the stars and moon to rights', his seasonal, ritual observance which he hopes will end the troubles he and the valley have been under, which has culminated with the advent of the 'land man' and the coming of the enclosures. This rite, as with others in which Jack participates, is fuelled by 'corbel bread', the fictional name for the fungus *Amanita muscaria*, which propels Jack into an altered state of consciousness. It goes without saying that the use of *Amanita muscaria* and other hallucinogenic fungi is widespread across the Northern Hemisphere, and is the tradition from which Garner drew in his descriptions of its preparation and use. This is extremely well done, even down to the container Jack uses for keeping the *Amanita* in, carved with the entoptic imagery that is often experienced during mushroom visions. Garner's description of the effects of the drug on a group of people is also very well drawn from reality; with the mushroom sending them into a trance-like state, before the full hallucinogenic effects hit.

And of the course one of the first scenes in the book, later repeated, where Jack gives his urine, 'piddle juice' to someone to drink is entirely factual; Siberian shamans in particular practised this method of passing the effects of the drug on within their tribe. The only query about this aspect of the book is why Garner employed *Amanita muscaria*, which is not particularly prevalent in the area, rather than the much more common and equally powerful *Psilocybe semilanceata*. Another question I posed, but which - sadly - Garner was too busy to answer!

The story Garner tells through Jack is just one variation on the many celestial myths told by indigenous peoples throughout the world. Whether any real people living in Thursbitch made these observations, or indeed whether any of the stones - natural or man-hewn, and placed - were ever used as archaeo-astronomical markers, we will probably never know. But in *Thursbitch*, at the end of the book, as Jack nears his fate, he reveals all. And weaving in and about this, Sal too states her identification with the valley, 'If you must know, I would stay here. Here is my place of understanding'.

The meaning and impact of Thursbitch to all who can sense it is amplified by Sal when Garner has her quote from the English mystic Thomas Traherne's *Dumbness*, 'And every stone and every star a tongue. 'And every gale of wind a curious song'.

Jack then looks from the stone towards Old Gate Nick on the eastern horizon, and then watches the mythological sky drama unfold, recounting the story as it belongs to him and his. Firstly the star cluster of the Pleiades makes its appearance in the Nick, the 'bees on Bull's shoulder'.

Then the red eye of Taurus, Aldebaran appears in the sky. This particular star system is also central to the archaeoastronomical plot of Peter Ackroyd's novel *First Light*, which I highly recommend. Taurus, the Bull rises, and is followed by the 'Big Chap', Orion, with his club. As Orion 'strides' toward Shining Tor 'old goibert' emerges. This is the tiny constellation of Lepus, the hare. Then rises Canis Minor, 'The Big Chap's gotten a dog', which goes after the hare. Taurus, pursued by Orion then starts to set and Jack weaves his tale around them.

Jack's valediction on the final page is beautiful; a summing up of a man knowing his place in his chosen landscape. And there, for now, the story of Thursbitch ends. But the mystery continues.

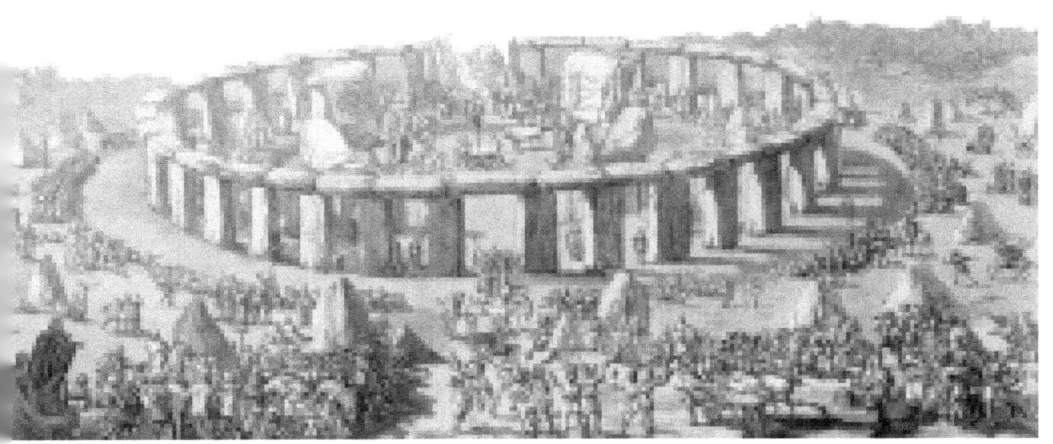

A SAUCERFUL OF SECRETS

"... UFOs were not just in the air, they'd become a religion and the word a common sacrament to everyone who'd tripped." -

Neil Oram

The word hippie conjures up intense visions of brightly clad youth rebelling against society while advocating peace, free love and the right to alter their consciousnesses in whatever way they chose. But behind the fashions and fads, the hippie underground movement in the UK was solely responsible for the greatest expansion of interest and belief in Fortean phenomena in history. Social historians invariably associate the hippie movement with Eastern religions such as Buddhism and Hinduism, sources of both inspiration and imagery, and the hippies' interest in these belief systems has been well documented.

But there was another alternative to the blinkered Western worldview of the 1960s already deeply embedded in the British cultural psyche, and already present in the lives of those who would form the movement known as the Underground – the flying saucer culture. In the mid-1960s, although flying saucers were being discussed among the influential group of post beatniks and modern mystics who would form the core of the Underground, the nascent movement lacked a voice. A figurehead was needed; someone who could breathe life into the background hum of belief in flying saucers, and articulate it for the burgeoning subculture.

Cover art from Oz No. 9, an issue which became known as *Flying Saucer Oz*, but horrified founder and editor Richard Neville.

That voice came in the form of the late John Michell [**], whose influence on the Underground and

[**] As this book was being prepared, John Frederick Carden Michell died on 24 April 2009 at the age of 76. He was a good friend of CFZ Press and we shall miss him greatly.

Forteana in general, cannot be overestimated. Like many of his generation, Michell was disillusioned by the acquisitive post-war society:

> "When I was at Cambridge, the whole atmosphere was extremely rationalistic, materialistic. Everyone believed the current academic orthodoxies of the time and there seemed no way of questioning them."

UFOs first caught Michell's imagination in the 1950s when he noticed that

> "it was quite obvious that people were having experiences that weren't allowed for within the context of our education. There was a split between the view of the world we'd been taught and accepted unquestioningly and the world of actual experience."

To Michell, flying saucers were more than just 'nuts-and-bolts' craft; they were one of a whole number of phenomena which became attached to the 'Matter of Britain'. This corpus of belief largely concerned itself with the canon of legends of King Arthur and the Holy Grail and was focused on the Somerset town of Glastonbury.

The View Over Glastonbury

Glastonbury is firmly embedded in the public consciousness as a centre of all things strange. Since the early 20th Century, it has been the pulse of alternative Britain and has seen wave after wave of settlers arrive there, each seeking their personal Holy Grail. This vortex of the weird was well known to John Michell, who decided to experience the 'Glastonbury Effect' for himself:

> "It was, I think, in 1966 that I first went to Glastonbury, in the company of Harry Fainlight We had no very definite reason for going there, but it had something to do with strange lights in the sky, new music, and our conviction that the world was about to flip over on its axis so that heresy would become orthodoxy and an entirely new world order would shortly be revealed.

> "At that time I was writing the first of my published books, *The Flying Saucer Vision*. It followed up the idea, first put forward by CG Jung in his 1959 book on flying saucers, that the strange lights and other phenomena of the post-war period were portents of a radical change in human consciousness coinciding with the dawn of the Aquarian Age. A theme in my book was the connection between 'unidentified flying objects' and ancient sites, as evidenced both in folklore and in contemporary experience."

In this statement, Michell encapsulated an entirely new way of looking at the subject of flying saucers and their meaning. Michell may have been the catalyst and helmsman for the hippies' interests in flying saucers but the motive power was provided by the drug LSD, which had hit London during 1964–5. LSD, or acid as it was popularly known, was quickly taken up by the countercultural mystic vanguard and suddenly everything was not only possible, it was likely!

Art gallery owner and Underground luminary Barry Miles (usually known only by his surname) summed up the effect of the drug on the hippies:

"From the mid-Sixties onwards you have what would have to be called a sort of LSD consciousness permeating the whole of the counterculture side of British society. And you get it in the songs of Pink Floyd all these bands incorporate LSD-inspired imagery, and that of course was not the normal imagery of love songs and picking up girls, it was much more to do with a sort of specifically British form of psychedelia which involved dancing gnomes and flying saucers".

The combination of a new generation of seekers with powerful psychedelic drugs revivified Glastonbury as a spiritual centre. Now, in addition to the mythos of King Arthur, the terrestrial zodiacs and other landscape legends, flying saucers were also woven into the tapestry of belief. The debut edition of the Underground magazine *Albion*, edited by Michell, provides the visual clues; dragons and UFOs appear in the skies over Glastonbury Tor, while swords, serpents and geomantic imagery are visible in the Earth below. A new meaning for flying saucers was being forged, and to the Underground this rich blend of saucers, sacred sites and mythology was a damn sight more interesting than the nuts-and-bolts, sci-fi derived vision of the UFO orthodoxy.

Barry Miles was also aware of the attraction Glastonbury held for those in the counterculture:

"The King's Road led straight to Glastonbury in those days. The people we knew led double lives, experimenting with acid, spending entire evenings discussing flying saucers, ley lines and the court of King Arthur. Other people waited patiently at Arthur's Tor for flying saucers to land."

And as word got around that Glastonbury was the new 'window area' for UFO sightings, more and more hippies made it a place of pilgrimage. According to Michell,

"UFOs were constantly being sighted over St Michael's Tower on Glastonbury Tor. Mark Palmer, Maldwyn Thomas and their group were then travelling with horses and carts on pilgrimages across England. They often camped near the Tor, and while I was with them we used to watch the nightly manoeuvrings of lights in the sky. Jung's prophecy of aerial portents being followed by a change in consciousness was evidently being fulfilled."

Craig Sams, who set up England's first macrobiotic restaurant, was also a Glastonbury enthusiast:

"I didn't see a flying saucer till October 1967 when I went to Glastonbury. One day I got a 'phone call from Mark Palmer saying that it would be a good idea to come down, that there was a lot of UFO activity, that John Michell, who had just written *The Flying Saucer Vision*, was camping down there, and Michael Rainey. So here we are in the field and up come the UFOs. We weren't tripping, I'd given up acid. I was completely normal, maybe I'd had a cup of tea about half an hour before Mark Palmer saw them – they were definitely there. They were in the classic cigar-shaped mother-ship form. Little lights emanating from them. Then at one point you saw these other lights coming up towards them and the smaller lights just shot into the cigar-shaped mother-ship, which then just disappeared at high speed. The other lights had been RAF jets. It was obvious that the RAF had scrambled some jets."

It would be easy to dismiss the Underground's fascination with saucers if it weren't for the fact that 1967 was a huge 'flap' year for UFO sightings across the UK. This wasn't just a 'hippie thing' – it was even happening to policemen, who chased them for hours in their patrol cars. The MOD was so inundated by UFO reports it radically changed its UFO policy and set up a team of investigators to interview civilian UFO witnesses, the first time this had been done.

Saucer Rock

As flying saucers became further embedded in popular culture, rock musicians were becoming interested in them as a means of expressing the psychedelic experience. Music promoter Joe Boyd consolidated the link between drugs, music and flying saucers when he named one of the first hippie clubs, on London's Tottenham Court Road, 'UFO'. Although 'Unidentified Flying Object' was only one of its meanings, advertisements in *International Times* (*it*) showed a flying saucer hovering over the head of a dancing hippie. Most musical histories of the psychedelic era tend to cite Eastern influences – sitars and raga-like instrumentals – as the primary indicator of how groovy, fab and 'far out' the music was. But there was another aspect of psychedelia steeped in saucers and space.

Pink Floyd's first album *The Piper at the Gates of Dawn* included the atmospheric pæan to deep space *Astronomy Domine*, possibly the first song to use outer space as a metaphor for inner space. By their second album, *Pink Floyd* had further absorbed saucer culture, entitling it *A Saucerful of Secrets*, and were mixing ideas of UFOs and the secrets of the mind (with, perhaps, a nod toward a particularly potent batch of LSD called 'flying saucers').

The sleeve artwork left fans in no doubt that space – inner or outer – was the place: swirling universes and spinning discs mixed with signs of the zodiac (adapted from the Marvel Comics encounter between Dr Strange and the Living Tribunal). The album's keynote song, *Set The Controls For The Heart Of The Sun*, became the backdrop for many psychedelic journeys toward dawn.

Even the *Rolling Stones* – possibly the least spiritual band of the Sixties generation – took an interest in saucers. John Michell accompanied them on a saucer-spotting mission to Stonehenge, while singer Marianne Faithfull recalls the Stones' ill-starred rhythm guitarist Brian Jones taking a great interest in Michell's ideas on the subject;

> "Like a lot of people at the time, myself included, he was convinced there was a mystic link between druidic monuments and flying saucers. Extraterrestrials were going to read these signs from their spaceship windows and get the message. It was the local credo: Glastonbury, ley lines and intelligent life in outer space..."

Similarly, the Stones' Keith Richards was more than curious about saucers: "I've seen a few, but nothing any of the ministries would believe," he told a *Melody Maker* journalist.

> "I believe they exist – plenty of people have seen them. They are tied up with a lot of things, like the dawn of man, for example. It's not just a matter of people spotting a flying saucer. I'm not an expert. I'm still trying to understand what's going on."

Throughout his career, David Bowie flirted with the idea of 'the alien', often mentioning extraterrestrials in songs such as *Starman*, and creating the 'Ziggy Stardust' persona. In the late 1960s, before he was catapulted to fame with the single *Space Oddity*, he claimed to have been closely involved with flying saucer research. In 1975, he revealed to *Creem* magazine:

> "I used to work for two guys who put out a UFO magazine in England about six years

ago. And I made sightings six, seven times a night for about a year, when I was in the observatory. We had regular cruises that came over. We knew the 6.15 was coming in and would meet up with another one. And they would be stationary for about half an hour, and then after verifying what they'd been doing that day, they'd shoot off."

The fact that the '6.15' was so regular over south London should have given Bowie a hint that it might have been an aircraft rather than a UFO! Bowie's active interest in UFO research dwindled as his fame as a performer grew, but it can't have been helped by this event, recounted in a recent issue of *The Word*:

"An early attempt, while living in Beckenham, to attract extraterrestrials involved standing on his roof at dusk pointing a coat hanger into the skies. He gave up, dejectedly, when a passer-by enquired, 'Do you get BBC2?'"

Notes From the Underground

If music was one way of spreading the flying saucer message through the Underground, then poster art was another powerful method. Artists such as Martin Sharp and the English/Weymouth collaboration as *Hapshash and the Coloured Coat* created lavish posters for even the smallest-scale event, incorporating the myths, signs and symbols of the era with visual images of the music and musicians. Barry Miles recalled:

"The symbol of the flying saucer on the posters of Michael English and Nigel Weymouth and the references in all of the songs wasn't just used as a graphic symbol or a convenient lyrical device. People did feel that flying saucers were shorthand for a wider, deeper under-standing, a sort of god figure I suppose or a sense of an external spiritual deity of some sort. There was one clothes shop called *Hung On You* that Michael Rainey had, and he very much believed in flying saucers, and there was a lot of flying saucer imagery all over the shop."

As saucers permeated the hippie subculture, they began to appear more frequently in the underground press. *International Times* featured many articles and book reviews concerning saucers, engaging John Michell as its 'UFO correspondent'. In the 16 June 1967 issue, it reviewed *Anatomy of a Phenomenon*, the first UFO book by French scientist and influential ufologist Jacques Vallee. Reviewer Greg Sams used the argot of the period to express what a significant book it was:

"Do you believe in flying saucers? Most people with even a slightly open mind accept their existence, if only because so many reliable people have seen them. The book itself doesn't turn you on. You must read the book and turn yourself on. If you are just beginning to be interested in saucers then read his book. If you are already convinced and want a beautiful rave with your mind, read other further out authors."

Quite!

Oz was less keen on UFOs. Editor Richard Neville was more interested in provoking the establishment through explorations of radical politics or sex than through modern myths. But when Neville took his eye off the ball for issue nine, leaving the work to poster artist Martin Sharp and designer John Goodchild, he was shocked at the result: "To my embarrassment, it was devoted to flying saucers." Enraged, he asked Sharp, "How can you indulge your intergalactic delusions, when Asia is a bloodbath?" Sharp's reply typified the zeitgeist: "There are far more things in heaven and earth, Richard, than are dreamt of in your philosophy".

The cover of *Flying Saucer Oz*, as it became known, featured a large flying disc, taken from a collage by the Dadaist/Surrealist Max Ernst, with six coloured pages featuring a variety of quotes about the saucer phenomenon from 'hip' people ranging from Charles Fort to Mick Jagger.

John Michell's influence on the hippie movement, coupled with his erudition, was such that the 'establishment' couldn't just ignore him. Following the screening of *UFOs and the People Who See Them* on BBC1 on 9 May 1968, *The Listener* devoted most of that week's issue to a discussion of flying saucers. Michell was asked to contribute an essay, simply entitled Flying Saucers, which clearly laid out the hippie philosophy in relation to aerial phenomena – a blend of sightings of inexplicable lights in the sky, snippets of folklore, Glastonbury, ley and dragon lines and other ephemera from the Underground's dream world.

Listener editor Karl Miller contributed a critical piece, *Midsummer Nights' Dreams*, analysing the 'UFO cult' and more importantly Michell's place within it. "He is less a hippie, perhaps," opined Miller, "than a hippie's counsellor, one of their junior Merlins.' Recognising Michell's influence, but critical of his stance, Miller wrote that:

> "Michell behaves like a visionary, though his language doesn't always avoid the current jargon of the pads and barricades. He likes to talk about how the light from the midsummer sunrise shot across the land, travelling a line from holy place to holy place, starting the crops, bathing the feasts and fairs that saluted its passage. I would say that his book is relatively weak, busying itself with sundry mysteries like that of the Mary Celeste and converting them to extraterrestrial proofs."

'Straight' society was intrigued by the hippie take on flying saucers but then - as now - could see no real evidence it could take seriously.

Just as straight society quickly dissociated itself from the hippies, mainstream UFO enthusiasts kept their distance too, the nuts-and-bolts saucer buffs considering the newcomers to be just a bunch of drug takers with strange views (the irony that mainstream society viewed the nuts-and-bolts crowd as being equally strange was completely lost on them!)

Saucer Camp

Nevertheless, some influential individuals from the orthodoxy saw that the hippies were receptive to new ideas, and that mercurial aristocrat of flying saucer culture, Desmond Leslie, decided to organise the UK's first flying saucer convention for them (see FT225:40–47). The conference, which was held during the summer of 1968 on Lusty Beg Island on Lower Lough Erne in County Fermanagh, Northern Ireland, was jointly organised by Desmond Leslie and Camilla, Countess of Erne - a wealthy socialite with an interest in flying saucers who frequented the edges of the Underground.

The Lusty Beg event was small, with attendance estimated at about 80 people, but many of those who attended were influential movers and shakers from the Underground, including Nicholas Saunders, editor of *Alternative London* and founder of the Neal's Yard shopping complex in Covent Garden. Saunders recalled:

> "I was fascinated by what John Michell was saying about UFOs and leylines and so on, but felt pretty guarded about it too. I did go to a Flying Saucer conference on an island

in the middle of a lake in the northwest of Ireland. There were all these people plodding about in the rain and the mud and there were very serious talks by people who either said that flying saucers had visited, that they'd been on flights themselves or that they'd seen them."

Another key member of the Underground, Neil Oram (See FT217:44–49), was also there. Oram had morphed from beatnik wanderer to hippie philosopher, later writing his semi-fictional memoirs as *The Warp* trilogy. In *Lemmings On the Edge*, he describes the scene as he arrived at the shores of Lough Erne:

"At the water's edge, we were met by Michael Roner, who took us across the choppy lake in a battered rowing boat which was equipped with a noisy, erratic outboard motor. Apart from the big white house on the lawn, the rest of the island was overgrown, without a trace of permanent habitation. Although now there were camp fires and tents scattered all over the wooded hills, which rose quite steeply from the beach."

Desmond Leslie was responsible for organising the conference lectures, which were held each evening in a large marquee. Scant information now exists as to exactly who spoke, but Neil Oram remarks that they consisted of "rather dull pronouncements of what lay in store for the human race". According to Oram, "It wasn't until the fourth night that we were given some real information, by an ex-Australian Air Force radar expert." This impressed Oram:

"It made my hair stand on end when we learnt that he'd picked up unidentified craft, whose estimated diameter was in the region of three hundred miles! MILES! Travelling in excess of one hundred THOUSAND miles an hour!"

Johan Quanjar, another attendee, recalled:

"[D]ozens of people had descended on the island for fun, jollity and invocation of higher energies. By the end of the week, the entire hippie UFO community had gone native. They had formed separate tribes with some not speaking to others."

This event was as close as the hippies ever got to organising the subculture's fascination with flying saucers, but they were rapidly losing interest. Too many other gloriously fantastic possibilities vied for their attention, and when you'd explored inner space, the wastes of outer space could seem positively tedious. Essentially, those among the Underground who took an avid interest in flying saucers did so not out of certain belief, but from a desire to explore the possibilities. When the flying saucer experience didn't deliver the goods or, as the hippies saw on Lusty Beg, it descended into conflict and argument, they didn't want to know. Poet and author Barry Gifford, whose novel *Wild at Heart* was used by David Lynch as the basis for his film, sojourned as a hippie in late 1960s London. In *The Duke of Earls Court*, Gifford writes of his interest in UFOs and refers to an incident in which a friend called Ace invited the editor of *Flying Saucer Review* to dinner. The clash of cultures was inevitable:

"It was obvious upon his entrance that the editor, an ordinary-looking, balding, middle-aged man in a dark grey three-piece suit, was visibly shaken by the den of freaks to which he had unwittingly lent his presence. He had no idea, he said, attempting to smile, that the dinner was to be such an event.

After answering a few desultory questions about saucers, it was clear that the editor wanted to be anywhere else but with those people. The food was macrobiotic and when he enquired what was in the meal was told, 'Brown rice, kasha, bulgur, soy, miso. The food of the people. It makes you high'. Mention of the word 'high' caused the editor to drop his fork, obviously afraid that the meal had been spiked with drugs of some form. He left soon afterwards, pleading a prior engagement."

Selling Saucers by the Pound

Flying saucers continued to be courted by the Underground in the dying embers of the 60s, but by 1970 the hippie movement had become subsumed into the broader spectrum of youth culture: now, you could buy kaftans in Marks & Spencer, and like all youth movements, it had been diluted and repackaged by commercial interests; it was being sold rather than invented. Those who had been heavily involved in saucerdom moved swiftly on. For everyone else, the subject of UFOs was now just another hip belief to be 'into'; the publishing floodgates opened and books on Earth Mysteries, witchcraft, folklore, astrology, occultism and mysticism offered other ways of thinking and being.

But were it not for the hippies' interest in flying saucers, nurtured by John Michell, it's doubtful that the continuing interest in such subjects would be part of our cultural landscape in the 21st Century. This brief burst of drug-fuelled exploration cross-pollinated many Fortean subjects, the results of which we see today.

Where mainstream ufology was mired in the yes/no argument about the physical reality of UFOs, the hippies treated the subject as just one in a long line of possibly useful ideas. This difference of attitude between the hippie and straight views of saucers was aptly summed up in an exchange between Barry Gifford and his friend, after the FSR editor had fled their dinner party. Referring to the editor's 'stuffy' attitude Ace pointed out to Gifford:

"But it's OK man, it really is; he's a dedicated cat. I mean he's never seen one, but he really believes in them flying saucers."

"So do you," Gifford said.

Ace nodded. "Sure, man, sure I do. The difference between him and me is that I'm not so bloody serious about it."

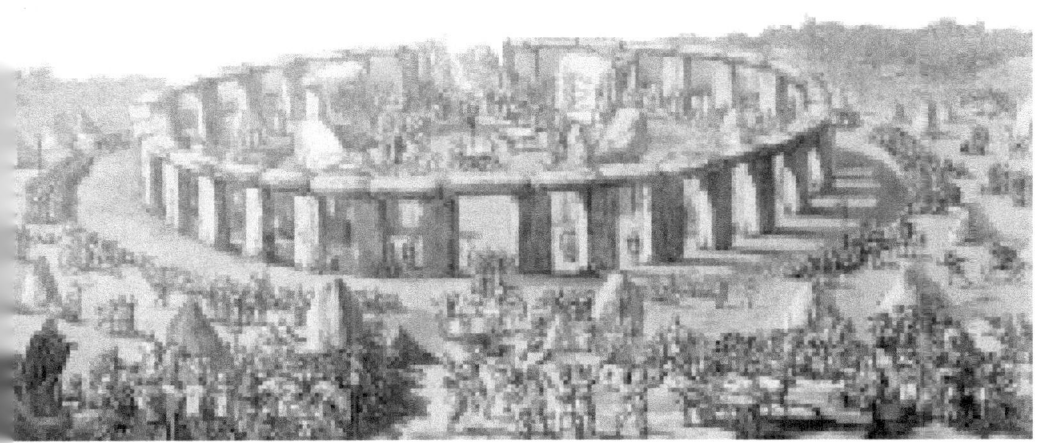

ALIENS STOLE MY BADGER'S RECTUM

First published in *Fortean Times* 101, summer 1997

Men in Black, those besuited and dissonant spectres of ufolore who put the frighteners on witnesses, are very much in the news again. The comedy sci-fi film *Men in Black* is out on 1 August and Jenny Randles' book, entitled simply *MIB,* came out on 14 June and is a thorough overview of the legend, updating it and unveiling much new information. Whereas once considered to be from the outer reaches of the belief system, MIB are slowly - but surely - being rehabilitated into mainstream ufology.

This is not entirely without at least some justification it seems. Besides Randles' revelations, a new piece of evidence has recently been unearthed at the Public Records Office by researcher Nick Redfern. The case in question concerns PC Colin Perks of Wilmslow in Cheshire, whose 7 January 1966 sighting of a classic domed saucer-type UFO was duly reported to the MOD through police channels. The MOD deemed the sighting to be of sufficient calibre to be passed on from the usual UFO desk, S4F to a 'specialist unit' known as DI61. Less than a month after Perks' sighting, on 1 February a gentleman of that persuasion was dispatched to quiz Perks about his experience. Was he asked, as per the myth, to keep schtum about their visit? Very possibly, because in numerous subsequent newspaper interviews and in his report filed with the British UFO Research Association he strangely chose not to mention 'the Men from the Ministry'.

Perhaps he simply forgot about them.

This information is something of a breakthrough as until now it was accepted wisdom among serious ufologists that the government did not make any special attempts to question UFO witnesses. Nick Pope, ex MOD UFO desk jockey and author of *Open Skies, Closed Minds,* has always fervently claimed that there were no departments, beyond his, who took an interest in UFO phenomena, and that any witnesses who did claim to have been visited by officialdom had merely been hoaxed by convenient 'Walter Mitty'-type civilian characters out for a jape. Oh dear, Nick has obviously not been telling all because when Jenny Randles proved to him that DSTI *did* exist he went quite pale and refused to discuss the matter further! A more detailed examination of this case and other fruits of Nick Redfern's meticulous research will appear in his book, *A Covert Agenda,* published by Simon & Schuster later this summer. According to some ufologists, we might be close to a solution to the Alien Big Cat mystery. For years now the Scarborough area of the east coast of Yorkshire has been plagued by sightings of these creatures and in just one instance during February 1997, nine dead sheep were found on Pauline Sandiman's farm at Snainton, all with their stomachs ripped open. Close encounters of the furred kind? Not according to the ufologists. Genuine terrestrial alien big cats (ABCs) not being strange enough for them, certain UFO investigators have drawn their own mazy conclusions. David Kenneally of Global Investigation Systems believes the slayings to be the work of a 'Morph', which is an alien able to shape shift at will. According to Kenneally, this naturally explains why there is no evidence left at the scene. Are we seeing here, in embryonic form, a new twist to ufology in Great Britain? One in which the still unsolved ABC sightings - and the killings attributed to them - subtly become `cattle mutilations' caused by aliens and therefore part of the UFO mythos? We're watching.

But something weird does seem to be going on in this area; a view amplified at a lecture given by ex-police sergeant and veteran ufologist Tony Dodd in March. ** Dodd spun an everyday story of a region gripped by fear and panic, with mutilated creatures being discovered on an almost daily basis. Cows, sheep, horses, deer and other animals had all been found dead he claimed, all victims of the same sinister *modus operandi*. Whoever - or whatever - is leaving its prey with a single hole in their head and without their rectums. Unfortunately Tony's slides weren't available and the best evidence he could offer, besides the alarming narratives, was of the "and then my mate said come and look at this" variety. A disbelieving colleague in the audience whispered "it'll be voles next" and in an eerily telepathic instant, Tony cited a case where a mouse had been found with ventilated cranium and missing rectum. The sceptics among you might rightly question why anyone, alien or human, would want to do this to defenceless woodland creatures and what use the missing parts could be put to in any case.

But who are we to question alien behaviour? After all if it is *truly* alien, both motive and method should be totally incomprehensible to us. Then again, perhaps crunchy deer ring piece is something of a delicacy on Zeta Reticuli. Levity was not on Tony's agenda however as he hinted at dark motives and darker agencies against which we mere mortals appear to be powerless. Just when the audience couldn't get any more agog, Tony cranked the credulometer right up to number eleven. He had allegedly been told by several witnesses that some of the animals had actually been seen falling from the sky in their mutilated state. One man had narrowly escaped being hit by a descending badger; another had been obliged to drag sundry livestock out of the road to get his car past.

This animal roadblock had been dropped not a minute previously from 'something' with immensely bright lights which had swished overhead. Tony's conclusion? Aliens, flying in giant football-pitch sized craft, who collect the animals Noah's Ark-style, perform their grisly business while aboard and callously discard them haphazardly on the highways and byways of North Yorkshire. Just why this Earth-shattering information was not on the front page of *The Times* or the lead story on *Newsnight* wasn't quite clear. But whether due to cover-up or couldn't-care-less on behalf of the authorities, Dodd claims that these barbarous acts *are* taking place on a regular basis in this area. So if you're thinking of somewhere to take a break and spend some time sky watching, or want to try your arm at investigating an active mystery which, if any part of it is true, has enormous implications, then the Scarborough area is the place to go.

** Tony Dodd (1935-2009) became interested in UFOs in the 1950s and fell hook line and sinker for the myth of physical extraterrestrials. In his police career Dodd lived in the Yorkshire Dales where he claimed to have seen over 200 UFOs, becoming convinced they had bases under the moors. Dodd was highly active within the Yorkshire UFO Society, which spawned *UFO Magazine* - the UK's first newsstand saucer publication - and was obsessed with the alleged government cover up of UFO information. For many years he exerted a subtle and pervasive influence on UK ufology which continues to this day.

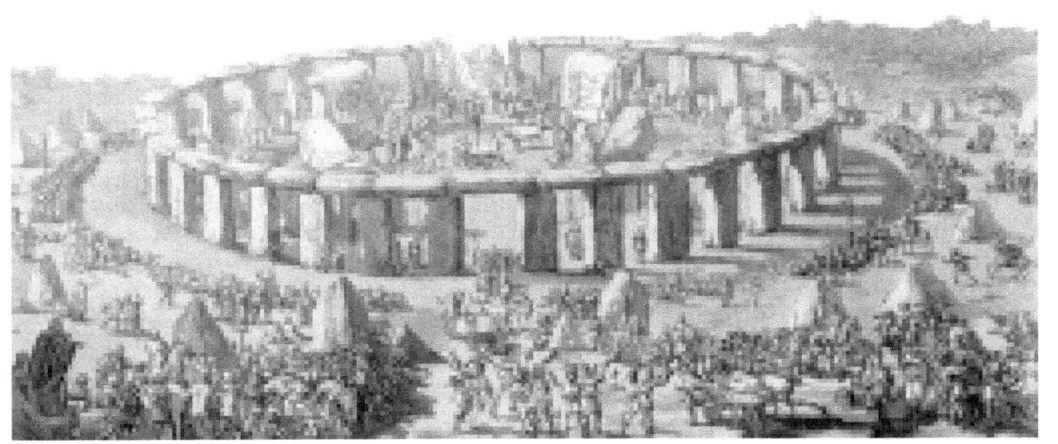

THE BIG GREY MAN OF BEN MACDHUI

& *Other Mountain Panics*

*'Though your nerves be of steel, and your mind says it cannot be,
you will be acquainted with that fear without a name, that
intense dread of the unknown that has pursued mankind from
the very dawn of time.'*

Richard Frere [1]

The past eighty years has seen The Big Grey Man of Ben Macdhui become a staple for authors and journalists writing about Scottish legends. With the exceptions of the Loch Ness Monster and the Bonnybridge UFO hotspot it is arguably Scotland's best known example of strange phenomena. So much has been written about the Big Grey Man that one could be forgiven for believing it is a well-attested experience with tens if not hundreds of witnesses. If only it were really that simple!

When put under the microscope, away from the conventions of storytelling or the obligations of having to make a profit, the Big Grey Man of Ben Macdhui (BGM), like most other Fortean phenomena, takes on a completely different appearance. It's not my intention here to go over every last word which has been written about the BGM, nor to list each and every possible sighting and theory, rather to give an overview of the phenomenon, and an analysis of the main sightings and proffered explanations. Nor is it my intention to 'explain away' or to 'debunk' the phenomenon completely. Rather, I wish to broaden the discussion with some completely new case material and ideas which may shift encounters with the BGM into a class of experience to that which it occupies at the moment.

Witnesses to the phenomenon which is known as the Big Grey Man describe how they have variously encountered footsteps, a sensation of 'presence', sightings of a large hominid and an overpowering sense of panic whilst on the mountain called Ben Macdhui. The experience is terrifying enough to compel witnesses to flee in blind panic, sometimes for several miles. Given that this all takes place on rocky and dangerous ground, and often in weather conditions of mist and snow, we should not underestimate the power of the experience. The phenomenon is usually, but not always, experienced by solitary witnesses. Accounts, incidents and theories of this phenomenon have been detailed in numerous books, magazines and newspapers from 1925 to as recently as 1998. Anyone wishing to gain a more general insight into the phenomenon and surrounding issues is advised to follow up the references given in this article and to certainly obtain Affleck Gray's excellent, if unstructured, book on the subject, which is written in the spirit of true Fortean enquiry. [2]

Ben Macdhui, at 1309 metres (4296 ft), is the second highest mountain in the U.K. and lies in the heart of the high mountain range known as the Cairngorms. The mountain comprises of a high plateau with a subarctic climate and is often covered in snow for months at a time. Weather conditions can be extreme and unpredictable. Sadly the Cairngorms have been defaced by ski-lifts and restaurants but until recently have remained remote, requiring considerable physical effort and mountaincraft to navigate successfully. The wild nature and relative inaccessibility of the area has undoubtedly contributed to their popularity and the Cairngorms have been a playground for climbers, walkers, skiers, naturalists and those who love the high and lonely places for hundreds of years. Ben Macdhui has several spellings and its English translation is Gaelic for hill of the son of duff. [3]

Like any other area of land be it mountain, plain, or urban town-scape Ben Macdhui and its environs have a large body of oral and written folklore which encompass phenomena which broadly fall into the Fortean and paranormal fields [4]. The majority of folklore from the Cairngorm area refers to disparate phenomena which need not concern us here, save to recognise that the BGM does not exist as a discrete phenomenon.

Although the first recorded Big Grey Man experience as described earlier did not take place until 1891, and was not made public until 1925, there are antecedents to the matter which set the phenomenon into some geographic, folkloric and historical context. In 1791 the poet James Hogg, sometimes known as the 'Ettrick Shepherd', described seeing a huge figure on Ben Macdhui whilst tending his sheep. As he watched the halo which had formed around him due to the combination of sunshine and mist he suddenly noticed a huge, looming figure. It was vaguely human in shape and he imagined it to be the devil. Hogg fled in terror, not stopping until he reached fellow shepherds.

The next day he saw the same figure under similar climatic conditions.

> 'It was a giant blackamoor, at least thirty feet high, and equally proportioned, and very near me. I was actually struck powerless with astonishment and terror. My first resolution was, if I could keep the power of my limbs, to run home and hide myself below the blankets with the Bible beneath my head.'

But instead of fleeing he stood his ground, determined to trace the source of the figure. Fear gave way to astonishment when he removed his hat and found the 'devil' mimicking this and his subsequent actions. Hogg believed that the phenomenon, which initiated the terror a day earlier, was in fact an uncommon natural phenomena known as the 'Brocken Spectre'. [5]

The Brocken Spectre, so named because the summit of the Brocken in Germany's Harz Mountains was one of the places it was first recorded from, is a dramatic natural effect with many variations. Essentially it is formed when the observer's shadow is cast onto mist by sunlight. The experience is dependent on the relationship between factors such as the brightness and angle of the sun, the thickness of the mist, presence and intensity of rain or wind and the position of the observers. The resulting effect can range from the simple 'shadow' effect of the viewer to grossly distorted, moving images of what appears to be one or more giants. In all cases, however dramatic or terrifying to the witness, the Brocken Spectre is just one of nature's free light shows. It has been invoked by many writers to 'explain' the BGM and may have some relevance in a number of the experiences. But the Brocken Spectre is only a small part of the whole story. [6]

Several writers on the BGM have referred to an article which originally appeared in the 1831 edition of the Edinburgh New Philosophical Journal. The witnesses, Sir Thomas Lauder and some friends were descending Macdhui in mist when initially they each saw their own Brocken Spectre, but not that of their two companions.

This effect is due to the fact that a body of mist is not an opaque surface, but a constantly shifting matrix of water particles. Thus the witnesses' position will determine how many Brockens they will see. At fifty yards apart, Lauder and his companions could only see their own Brocken. When they moved closer together they could all see each other's. [7]

In *The Cairngorm Mountains* John Hill evocatively manages to describe the Cairngorm Experience, skilfully mixing perceptions of natural phenomena with the creative imagination of the mountain goer, finally querying how the traveller would feel

> '...if he shall discover that he has been accompanied in every step and motion by a shadowy figure of huge proportions and savage mien, flourishing in his hand a great pine tree....Such are the spirits of the air haunting this howling wilderness...' [8]

Both Hill and Hogg refer to the legend of the 'fahm' as being prevalent in the Ben Macdhui area. A line in one of Hogg's Cairngorm poems tells of a man who, 'Beheld the fahm glide o'er the fell'. [9 Hill notes of the fahm that 'sometimes the phantom's head is large and his body small'. The legend of the fahm seems to have been first recorded in the Statistical Account of Scotland, in the section dealing with the area around Kirkmichael, which also includes Loch Avon and the eastern environs of Ben Macdhui.

However, far from being a giant, this version of the fahm legend describes,

> '...small quadruped which they call famh. In summer mornings it issue from its lurking places emitting a kind of glutinous matter fatal to horses.....It is somewhat larger than a mole, of a brownish colour, with a large head disproportionate to the body. From this deformed appearance and its noxious quality the word seems to have been transformed to denote a monster, a cruel mischievous person who, in the Gaelic language is usually called famh-fhear.' [10]

Hastie, in his Scottish Mountaineering Club Journal article on the BGM notes that both Hill and Hogg's interpretation of the legend probably derive from this source. Hastie suggests the word 'fahm' (which doesn't exists in Gaelic) being a misreading of famh, which means mole, and that Grant may well have mistaken the Gaelic word for giant - fanhair - as fhear. [11] Hence we have a the initial recording of the legend of a giant mole-like creature whose etymology and representation has been grossly distorted in less than a century, from supernatural poisonous mole-creature into a giant stick-wielding figure which stalks the mountain plateau.

However there are also legends of giants in the Cairngorms which may have informed Hill and Hogg's poetic speculations. High above Loch Einich, on the slopes of Sgor Gaoith, to the west of Ben Macdhui, is a natural feature called Am Bodach, the Old Man. There is also another stone bearing the name A'Chailleach, the Old Woman. One of the legends attached to these stone giants is that they are locked in eternal combat, doomed to hurl stones at each other. [12] Stones bearing these names are very common in Scotland and the legends pertaining to them are similar. The notion of giants in and on the landscape, either personified by rock formations or as creatures from mythology is entrenched in the folklore of these Isles. With the Big Grey Man of Ben Macdhui we have one of the few which is part of a living tradition. Whether it is a breathing entity remains to be seen.

Hugh Welsh, camping with his brother by the summit cairn of Ben Macdhui in 1904 heard the type of footsteps which later became synonymous with the BGM. They heard the noise both at night and in daylight describing it as being like '....slurring footsteps as if someone was walking through water-saturated gravel.' Welsh also recalled they were 'Frequently conscious of 'something' near us, an eerie sensation of apprehension, but not of fear as others seem to have experienced'. They questioned the Head Stalker at Derry Lodge who told them, 'That would have been the Fear Liath Mor you heard.' [13]

Fear Liath Mor is Gaelic for 'Big Grey Man' and if this account is true it is the first known reference to the BGM by name. That it was proffered as an explanation by a local stalker may indicate a larger body of tradition regarding the Big Grey Man which has gone unrecorded.

Moving further into the twentieth century, George Hall - in his book *Leaves From A Rambler's Diary* - recounts the experience of an unnamed friend who worked in the Cairngorms. Hall gives few details, remember this was prior to any wide public knowledge of or interest in the Big Grey Man, but it seems his friend had an odd experience on Ben Macdhui involving a 'presence' which frightened him to such an extent that he left the mountain, after which the sensation faded. [14]

The *Cairngorm Club Journal* for 1921 noted a recent letter to the *Aberdeen Free Press* in which the writer, '....called attention to a myth prevalent in Upper Deeside to the effect that a big spectral figure has been seen at various times during the last five years walking about on the tops of the Cairngorms. When approached, so the story goes, the figure disappears. Moreover, it has got a name - 'Ferlie More', to wit.' [15] Obviously the name 'Ferlie More' is a derivative of the Gaelic Fear Liath Mor, or Big Grey Man, again perhaps suggesting the tradition of a local giant.

In 1924 Dr Ernest A Baker's book *The Highlands With Rope and Rucksack* appeared. Here Baker relates the experience of a friend whose job took him into the mountains - a deer stalker or perhaps a shepherd. Alone on Ben Macdhui one day he slowly became aware of a terrifying presence which - as Affleck Gray recounts - 'disturbed him in a manner which was beyond his experience'. Gray makes the point that this was no ordinary fear but something so powerful that Baker's friend fled Ben Macdhui, the terror only subsiding when he reached low ground. Baker also reports how one mountain climber had told him that he would under no circumstances spend any time on Ben Macdhui alone, even in daylight. [16]

That's the pre-history of the BGM. When you take all the evidence into consideration, it seems that prior to Collie's 1925 unveiling of his 1891 experience there *was* a tradition of a giant figure, and of 'presences' which cause fear in the Cairngorm regions. Whether any of the foregoing was a template onto which later BGM reports were hung on to or expanded from is debatable.

In discussing the BGM the researcher is immediately confronted with the problem of exactly what can be admitted as evidence for its existence. Affleck Gray's book lists numerous alleged BGM encounters and draws in a plethora of other ghosts and paranormal phenomenon encountered on Ben Macdhui. [17] This heady mix gives the impression there are far more BGM encounters than there actually are. There is also the problem relating to the geography of the mystery. Many encounters and experiences attributed to the BGM are not actually on Ben Macdhui but from surrounding mountains and valleys. So the first step in any discussion about the BGM is to define what constitutes a BGM experience.

My definition, based on all available sources, is as follows: The experience must contain any or all parts of the core phenomenon. This core phenomenon consists of the following elements:

• Footsteps being heard.
• A sensation of terror or panic, strong enough to cause flight.
• The experience must have taken place on the mountain of Ben Macdhui or in its immediate environs.
• A giant figure [18]

This immediately discounts much of the phenomena discussed in Gray's book such as the many odd sounds, singing, chanting, musical notes etc as well as the sightings of figures (especially the ones that are described as of human size) at a distance and unaccompanied by other phenomena. The sounds are almost certainly attributable to natural phenomenon such as the actions of wind, snow and water in an extreme environment. The 'figures' seen at a distance are just that and may well be other climbers. Gray discussed this problem at length and eventually accepts this is likely to be the case. [19]

This definition could be construed as being unnecessarily dismissive of what might be seen as supporting evidence. I will be the first to admit its inadequacies, but when dealing with a phenomenon as mutable (both by witnesses and its commentators) as the BGM it is essential to have some parameters within which to work.

> Anyone who has spent any time in wild, mountainous or open country will be well aware of the problems of visual and aural perception. Particularly when alone, especially in poor visibility or in bad weather. The mountaineering literature is scattered with many good examples of these perceptual tricks, of figures being seen, of presences being felt and so on. As an example it is worth quoting the experience of veteran Scottish mountaineer and author W.H.Murray which also took place in the Cairngorms. 'When we started on the last rise to Cairn Toul there came a wider clearance than usual. Suddenly Mortimer gripped my arm and pointed uphill through the misty chasm. "Look!" he exclaimed, "Two men crossing to Glen Einich." Upon looking up at the slope I was duly surprised to see two climbers a long way ahead of us.....I watched them traverse a full fifty feet from east to west across the snow-slope, one about ten yards in front of the other.....We advanced and saw them halt, apparently to wait for us. At a hundred yards range they turned out to be two black boulders. So great was our astonishment that we failed even to laugh at ourselves.' [20]

On a similar note J.A. Rennie writes that, 'Stefannson, the Arctic explorer, tells of an instance when drifting sea mist once so magnified a tiny lemming that he raised his rifle in the belief that he had come upon a musk-ox.'[21]

The sense of hearing is also widely affected by environmental factors. I recall a backpacking trip in the Lake District back during the summer of 1976 when I heard my first name being repeatedly called from behind a wall as I toiled up the Kirkstone Pass at 6 a.m.. Looking over the wall, fully expecting to find tangible evidence of some supernatural agency, I was highly amused to find a sheep bleating! For further evidence of the frequent unreliability of the senses, in mountain environments, and their concomitant interpretations, I wholeheartedly recommend Dr Helen Ross' book which deals with this and with other related matters. [22]

Returning to the definition of the BGM, and by using this definition, an analysis of the BGM literature using primary and secondary sources but discounting rumour and anecdote, reveals the following factors:

- There are only six 'good' first or well attested accounts which fit the criteria.
- Of these only three took place on the summit or summit plateau of Ben Macdhui.
- Only two of the six include a 'Big Grey Man', or similar figure.
- Of those, one was later relegated by the witness to either being imagined or as a confabulation of panic and mist.

This interpretation is obviously my own and open to argument but I would suggest that however the sources are looked at none of the factors above would differ by more than one, either way. So bearing that in mind, let's look at the source material. Despite rumours that the BGM was experienced frequently by climbers in the late 19th Century, the only firm record from that century is that of Professor Norman Collie's 1891 encounter. This experience is the one most often quoted by writers on the subject and the one which brought the BGM to the general public's attention. Collie was Professor of Organic Chemistry at University College, London. A climbing contemporary of Aleister Crowley he was a keen all-weather mountaineer who was well used to the rigours of the Himalayas, Alps, Rockies and Scotland. Collie was a rigorous scientist who was closely involved with the discovery of the gas neon, and was responsible for taking the first X-ray for surgical purposes. [23]

Collie did not go public with his experience until 1925, although there is circumstantial evidence his was the tale recounted in Baker's book, as the two were climbing partners [24]. Speaking at the Annual Dinner of the Cairngorm Club on November 28th that year, he recounted his frightening experience on Ben Macdhui. His story was published within days by an Aberdeen newspaper and shortly afterwards in the *Cairngorm Club Journal*. The account in the *Press and Journal* read:

> 'I was returning from the cairn on the summit in a mist when I began to think I heard something else than merely the noise of my own footsteps. For every few steps I took I heard a crunch, and then another crunch as if someone was walking after me but taking steps three or four times the length of my own. I said to myself 'This is all nonsense'. I listened and heard it again but could see nothing in the mist. As I walked on and the eerie crunch, crunch, sounded behind me I was seized with terror and took to my heels, staggering blindly among the boulders for four or five miles nearly down to Rothiemurchus Forest.

> Whatever you make of it I do not know, but there is something very queer about the top of Ben Macdhui and I will not go back there by myself I know.' [25]

The only other first person account of his experience seems to come from the obituary that was published following Collie's death in 1942.

> 'One day at Eastertime I was climbing Ben Macdhui. It was very misty and I was only able to see a few yards from me when not very far from the summit, I suddenly heard footsteps on the snow behind me. Confident that some man was following me, I waited for him to join me, but the moment I stopped the footsteps also stopped. When I started on my way again, once more I heard the footsteps clearly. More than ever convinced that some man was on my track I turned and ran back for some distance, but found no-one. Once again I started on my way to the summit and once again I heard footsteps which stopped whenever I stopped. When at last I reached the summit the footsteps did not stop but came nearer and nearer until they came right up to me. At that instant I was seized with an intolerable fright and I ran my hardest down the mountainside. No power on earth will ever take me up Ben Macdhui again. [26]

According to his biographer, Collie was true to his word and never climbed Ben Macdhui again. [27] Baly, Collie's obituarist had, at times, worked and climbed with him and his unreferenced account gives the impression it was obtained verbatim from Collie. But it differs slightly from the account in both the *Press and Journal* and the *Cairngorm Club Journal*, changing the story slightly. The *Press and Journal* article and Baly's obituary have been the two sources from which all subsequent retellings of Collie's experience have been taken.

Another element often used by writers dealing with the BGM is to suggest that although Collie didn't speak publicly about his experience in the U.K. until 1925, he had originally revealed his story in an obscure New Zealand newspaper at the turn of the century. Despite no one having seen or referenced the original source - usually given as an article entitled A Professor's Panic - it is nevertheless used to add weight to the story. It is first mentioned in an article about the BGM by Ronald W. Clark in *Scotland's Magazine*, November 1961. But there is no evidence, according to his biographer, that Collie visited New Zealand until the 1930s.[28]

Yet another variation which has crept into the Collie story is that he saw the 'something' which was causing the footsteps. This canard stems from Seton Gordon's retelling of the experience. Gordon used the phrase 'Collie encountered this spectre', seeming to infer a visual encounter. But this statement is not backed up by Collie's 1925 account, and it is very clear from Gordon's overall context that Collie saw nothing [29]. His experience was purely the hearing of footsteps, followed by blind panic.

It has been suggested that Collie invented the whole story having, according to Rennie McOwen, 'a mild reputation as a prankster'. [30] But again, accounts differ. Affleck Gray believed him to be 'sardonic and dry as dust, he did not suffer fools gladly'. [31] In her biography Mills notes that despite his scientific rigour Collie was a bit of a nature mystic who believed in the Loch Ness Monster. [32]

Whatever his character, and whatever the minor variations in the story it appears that Collie did indeed have a terrifying experience and one which had a dramatic effect on him. He was convinced that there was 'something very strange' about the summit of Ben Macdhui, something that he clearly believed was supernatural in origin. His biographer spoke to Collie's niece about the matter and she confirmed that she had heard the story from him many times and that 'Uncle Nor believed in it completely'. [33]

Collie, for all his science, was not a reductionist though, and well understood the atmospheres created by wild places. Years prior to revealing his Ben Macdhui experience he wrote '...there are places that one dreads, when one trembles and is afraid, one knows not why and fears stand in the way'. [34] In her discussion of the matter Collie's biographer concludes that, 'Collie remained emphatic - something beyond the wit of man haunted that mountain'. [35]

Shortly after the newspaper coverage of Collie's Cairngorm Club speech. the *Press & Journal* ran an article entitled *Opinions on the Elusive "Big Grey Man"*. Cairngorm Club members, with hundreds of Ben Macdhui ascents between them, opined on the legend. Robert Clarke claimed he had heard the story direct from Collie in 1915 and as a result made enquiries in the area among the older deer stalkers and crofters. He found that it was virtually unknown on Deeside to the south but that it was 'still current among the older residents on Speyside, where it had apparently had its rise'. [36].

William Gordon, then the president of the Cairngorm Club, regarded such stories as 'perfect nonsense', although having heard the story direct from Collie himself. Gordon is quoted as saying 'It was not even a tradition entertained, as such, among the members of the club, nor had he ever encountered residents on the Deeside or Speyside districts, abutting upon the Cairngorms who gave forth the story or hinted at anything of the kind.' [37] Arguments as to whether or not there was a pre-existent tradition of the BGM raged in newspapers, magazines and climbing journals for the next few years or so but no specific oral or written tradition pre-dating Collie's experience has ever surfaced.

The second account of the BGM originates from another mountaineer and medical colleague, Dr Henry Kellas. Unfortunately neither he nor his brother, with him at the time, ever recorded their experience and Henry Kellas died on the 1921 Mount Everest Reconnaissance Expedition. Their account, which is also widely featured in the BGM legend featured, first appeared in print as a letter in the pages of the *Press and Journal* in December 1925, following hot on the heels of Collie's speech to the Cairngorm Club. The account
read:

> 'The correspondence in your paper on the subject of the Ferla Mohr has encouraged me to state the story as given to me by the late Mr Henry Kellas, my lifelong friend, with whom I once climbed Ben Macdhui. He and his brother, Dr Kellas, had been chipping for crystals in the late afternoon well below the cairn, and were together on the slope of a fold of the hill. Suddenly they became aware of a giant figure coming down towards them from the cairn. They saw it pass out of sight in the dip on the side of the fold remote from themselves, and awaited its reappearance. But fear possessed them ere it did reach the top, and they fled. They were aware it was following them, and tore down by Corrie Etchachan to escape it. Mr Kellas said there was a mist on part of the hill, but refused to believe that the figure could be the shadow of either his brother or himself, causing an optical illusion. He asked why not two figures if that had been the case. But he never spoke of 'crunching' or of footsteps being heard by either himself or his brother.' [38]

This is not a primary source for the story, and must not be treated as such. But if we are to allow for it being a genuine account with a degree of accuracy, it is still the first recorded sighting of a giant figure. Kellas' certainty that it couldn't be a Brocken Spectre because there were two separate witnesses to one phenomenon is not borne out by the factors which govern the Brocken's appearance and would have depended on where he was standing relative to his brother. The conditions of mist and light mentioned in the account would have been optimum for a Brocken to be seen. But Brockens only actually move if the observer or observers do so, and going on the details given it is difficult to ascertain whether Kellas and his brother were standing or moving.

Given that they were chipping for crystals the likelihood is that they were stationary at the time. The date of the Kellas brothers' experience is unclear. Affleck Gray points to it being twelve years after Collie's encounter, placing it in 1903. There is also some confusion as to the exact circumstances. The *Press & Journal* account gives it as being on a late afternoon. Gray mentions that it was late on a clear June night. A clear June night in those latitudes, even after midnight, would have been very light. Gray does not reference his alternate version and I have been unable to contact him or locate his papers on the subject.

But the panic that was engendered by the experience, whatever its origin, seemed to be real enough, and like Collie the Kellas brothers fled. And not just a few yards, or even hundreds of yards, but several miles, risking life and limb over rough and dangerous terrain. Mountaineer Alexander Tewnion wrote an account of his 1943 BGM experience for *The Scots Magazine*:

> 'Of all the experiences that have come my way, one stands out above all others in its strangeness. This was when I shot the Fear Liath Mor, the Big Grey Man of Ben Macdhui. It happened like this. In October 1943 I spent a ten day leave climbing alone in the

Cairngorms. Rations were short then, and I carried a revolver and ammunition to shoot any hares or ptarmigan that came my way. One afternoon, just as I reached the summit cairn of Ben Macdhui, mist swirled across the Lairig Ghru and enveloped the mountain. The atmosphere became dark and oppressive, a fierce, bitter wind whisked among the boulders, and, fearing a storm was imminent, I took hurriedly to the Coire Etchachan path. Above Loch Etchachan the path angles easily downhill. I was swinging along at about five miles an hour when an odd sound echoed through the mist - a loud footstep, it seemed. Then another, and another. Spaced at long intervals!'

'I am not unduly imaginative, but my thoughts flashed instantly to the well-known story of Professor Norman Collie and the Fear Liath Mor. Then I felt the reassuring weight of the loaded revolver in my pocket. Grasping the butt I peered about in the mist, here rent and tattered by eddies of wind. A strange shape loomed up, receded, came charging at me! Without hesitation I whipped out the revolver and fired three times at the figure.

When it still came on I turned and hared down the path, reaching Glen Derry in a time I have never bettered since. You may ask, was it really the Fear Liath Mor? Frankly, I think it was. Many times since then I have traversed Macdhui in mist, bivouacked on it in the open, camped near its summit for days on end on different occasions - often alone, and always with an easy mind. For on that day I am convinced I shot the only Fear Liath Mor my imagination will ever see.' [39]

Tewnion's experience is widely quoted in the BGM literature. The fact that someone would be so scared as to pull a gun and fire on the phenomenon, gives considerable weight to the 'reality' of the experience.

It also contains all the criteria for a BGM experience. It cannot easily be explained in terms of a Brocken Spectre. Yet few writers quote Tewnion's letter to Affleck Gray in 1966 when he wrote:

'To this day I am convinced that I saw something but I am equally convinced that something was only a towering wisp of mist which I imagined to be a menacing ghost.' [40]

Peter Densham recounted his BGM experience verbally to many friends but did not write an account himself. Eventually it was recorded by his friend, mountaineer and author Richard Frere. The encounter took place in May 1945 when Densham was in charge of aeroplane rescue in the Cairngorms during WWII. Densham arrived at the summit around mid-day and settled down to eat his sandwiches and:

'.......was eating a piece of chocolate a little later when I had the sudden impression there was someone near me - an impression which is sometimes experienced by mountaineers. I did not pay much attention to the impression knowing it was fairly common. After a little I had the impression of something cold on the top of my neck. I had the hood of my anorak down. I thought this feeling of cold was due to the air having become more moist, but I still seemed to feel a pressure on my neck. I stood up and was conscious of a crunching noise from the direction of the cairn on my left. I went forward to investigate this noise.

When I got near to this cairn I began to think of the Grey Man and his footsteps. I thought this experience very interesting and until within a few feet of the apparent source of the sound I was not the least frightened. Suddenly, however, I was overcome by a feeling of apprehension and after a little my overpowering wish was to get off the mountain. I found myself running at an incredible pace, and then realised that I was running in the direction of Lurcher's Crag. I tried to stop myself and found this was extremely difficult to do. It was as if somebody was pushing me. I managed to deflect my course, but with a great deal of difficulty, and I managed to strike the direction between the left of the Lairig Ghru and Coire an Lochain. I ran down the ridge all the way to the Allt Mor Bridge, and all the way past Glenmore, and I was right on the other side of the loch before I stopped running.' [41]

Densham's account flags up several points. The most significant is that although his experience is firmly enshrined within BGM lore like Collie he did not see anything at all. Densham's experience consisted solely of feeling a presence and being gripped by a fear. As with other BGM experients the fear was so compelling that it caused him to run blindly for several miles, narrowly avoiding certain death if he had run over Lurcher's Crag. The phrase 'I found myself running at an incredible speed' suggests he was fully aware of what was happening, yet so overpowered by it he could not stop it. Also, according to Affleck Gray, Densham was aware of the BGM legend and 'scornful' of any power which could make a man flee in terror. [42]

He later had another unusual experience on Ben Macdhui involving phantom voices. He attributed both incidents to a 'psychic' origin, the 'effect on his consciousness of undefined properties of the mountain' and contended that Ben Macdhui was '...the most mysterious mountain I have ever been on.' [43]

These four accounts are the most important ones relating to the BGM which have come to light as being from Ben Macdhui and which incorporate elements of the core phenomenon. There are however a couple of tales from the vicinity of Ben Macdhui which may have some relevance to the mystery.

Joan Grant, spending the stalking season of 1928 in the Cairngorms with her husband, set off walking through the Rothiemurchus Forest towards the Cairngorms. The day was too hot for any serious climbing and so after a while they set off back down to Aviemore.

'Nothing could have been farther from my mind than spooks when suddenly I was seized with such terror that I turned and in panic fled back along the path. Leslie ran after me, imploring me to tell him what was wrong. I could only spare breath to tell him to run faster, faster. Something - utterly malign, four-legged and yet obscenely human, invisible and yet solid enough for me to hear the pounding of its hooves, was trying to reach me. If it did I should die, for I was far too frightened to know how to defend myself . I had about half a mile when I burst through an invisible barrier behind which I was safe. I knew I was safe now, though a second before I had been in mortal danger; knew it as certainly as though I were a torero who has jumped the barrier in front of a charging bull.' [44]

Grant's account frequently becomes entangled in BGM lore even though it took place several miles from the summit of Ben Macdhui, did not involve a sighting and was not witnessed by, or even conveyed to, her companion. Grant was a writer of historical fantasy who had a strong belief in reincarnation and similar ideas and it has been suggested that her encounter was more the product of a fertile mind than of any genuine experience.

Grant also notes that:

'A year later one of my Father's professors described an almost exactly similar experience he had when bug-hunting in the Cairngorms. He was a materialist, but he had been so profoundly startled that he wrote to *The Times* - and received a letter from a reader who had also been pursued by the 'Thing'.'[45]

Affleck Gray checked *The Times* for the relevant period and I have done so myself. No account similar to the one mentioned by Grant appears to exist. This does not of course mean it was never printed, but it is typical of the sort of unfindable information which accretes around accounts of a Fortean nature, where a key piece of information has been seen but then 'mysteriously' is untraceable. Allegations that Collie's experience appeared in a New Zealand newspaper are of a similar order. In the wider Fortean field a good example is the mystery surrounding the famous 'Thunderbird' photograph, the search for which has become an item of Fortean interest in itself! [46]

Speyside author Wendy Wood also had a bizarre experience below Ben Macdhui in the Lairig Ghru pass. This took place in 1940. Wood claims she heard '..an enormous echoing voice which seemed to use Gaelic words. It occurred to her that it might be the barking of a deer magnified by a freak echo. Latterly, the sound seemed to come from beneath her feet.' Although half convinced that the sound had a natural origin Wood circled the area in case it was from an injured climber. As she did so she '...had an uneasy feeling of someone following her and taking gigantic strides. She ran away and did not pause until close to Whitwell when the barking of a dog brought her to her senses'. [47]

I have included this account for a number of reasons. It shows how easily experiences become connected to the BGM legend even when they start with something such as an undefined noise. Wood claimed no knowledge of Collie or Kellas' experiences at the time and yet, if we believe her account, developed a similar experience leading her to panic and flee.

These accounts are the main body of experiences comprising the BGM experiences. Explanations for the BGM have been tossed to and fro in numerous editions of many Scottish newspapers as the interest in the BGM has risen and fallen. Books such as Gray's, detail theories which range from the BGM as space-visitor or faerie-like elemental to outright hoax. No real evidence is ever put forward to back these claims up and they rest entirely on belief and speculation. One of the main contentions has been that the experiences are evidence of a flesh and blood creature of the same type as the Yeti, Bigfoot or Alma [48]. I doubt this very much. Even being charitable with and broadening the content of acceptable cases to include anecdotal and third and fourth hand stories within a twenty mile radius of Ben Macdhui, it is almost certain that the BGM is not a corporeal creature. There are no photographs, no bones, no fur or skin samples, no evidence of a family group, no droppings, no evidence of any predatory action on the local mammal population. There is not even a reasonable number of good consistent accounts seen within a defined area.

Although the Cairngorm plateau is a wild, oft-inhospitable place, since the boom in outdoor activities of the last thirty years or so the area is frequently visited by relatively large numbers of people at all times of day, night and year. It seems logical that if the BGM was physical in nature some tangible evidence would have come to light by now. When dealing with the possibility of other large relict hominids such as the Yeti and Bigfoot etc. being flesh and blood creatures, the argument is considerably strengthened by the existence, however ambiguous, of photographs, videos, footprint casts, skin and hair samples etc. None of these exist in respect of the BGM and until they do it is reasonable to assume that we are not dealing with a physical creature.

However, when considering any physical evidence connected to the BGM it is worth noting that some accounts refer to photographs of unknown footprints taken in the Spey Valley. [49] Although the location of the photographs is some fifteen miles from the summit of Ben Macdhui it has been claimed or inferred by some writers that they may be of the BGM. Indeed Rennie cites a ghillie as having said (upon seeing the footprints) they were 'Bodach tracks' [50]. This comment, made by a local man, may indicate the survival of a tradition connecting unexplained phenomena to the legendary 'Bodach' or old man, familiar from wider Scottish legend. As these tracks have indeed been proffered as physical evidence for the BGM in the literature they and their possible origins need addressing.

The source of these photographs is the book *Romantic Speyside*, by J.A. Rennie. Rennie describes how on December 2nd 1952 about a mile outside the village of Cromdale, he came across mysterious tracks which:

> '...were running across a stretch of snow covered moorland, each print 19 inches long by about 14 inches wide and there must have been all of seven feet between each "stride". There was no differentiation between a left and a right foot, and they preceded in an approximately single line.' [51]

Rennie likens them to the mysterious 'Devil's Hoofprints' found in Devon during the winter of 1855, which have a been a Fortean staple for years. [52] Rennie followed the tracks for about half a mile, until they 'terminated at the foot of a pine tree, for all the world as though the strange creature making them had leapt up into the foliage of the tree.' Twenty yards further on he picked the tracks up again, and he followed them across a field and down to the river's edge where they terminated opposite the village churchyard. Rennie rushed home for his camera and showed the resulting photographs to baffled locals.

Writers often cite Rennie's photographs as evidence for the BGM case but fail to quote further from his account at this point, which is regrettable because he goes on to give highly useful information. Whilst working in Northern Canada in the 1920s Rennie came across similar tracks whilst crossing a frozen lake. These tracks reduced his French-Canadian companion to a state of gibbering terror as he believed them to belong to the Wendygo, [sic] a Bigfoot-like creature [**]. Rennie was baffled by the tracks until later that winter when he saw the mysterious tracks for the second time. But on this occasion he saw them being made.

> 'There on the flawless, smooth white of the snow, a whole succession of tracks in "lineastern" were appearing miraculously before my eyes. No sign of life anywhere, no movement even, other than the drifting clouds overhead and those tracks springing suddenly into being as they came inexorably towards me. I stood stock-still, filled with reasonless panic. The tracks were being made within 50 yards of me -20-10-then, smack! I swung round brushing the water from my eyes, and saw the tracks continuing across the

---

[**] The Wendigo is known by many names, Windigo, Weendigo and Witiko being just a few of the 37 variations. It haunts the legends of the Algonquin Indians of Eastern Canada. The beast itself is supposed to be a pallid, emaciated giant. Some say it has a skeleton and heart of ice. The Wendigo is generally hairless save for a wild mane of white hair about the head. Its eyes are owl-like or sunken with glimmering points of light like indigo stars. The gaping lipless mouth is fringed with teeth like a forest of icicles. The beast is a personification of hunger and winter. It thirsts endlessly for human flesh and with each person it devours, it gets larger, so that its ravening appetite is never sated. It is constantly hungry and constantly searching for prey. Some say the Wendigo can fly or 'walk on the winds' travelling miles in search of its human prey. But this dire spirit is doubly dangerous as it can also possess human beings. This can be done in three ways. An evil shaman can call down the Wendigo to possess himself or another. The creature can reach out with its own baleful influence into the minds of people, filling them with the urge to eat human flesh. Finally, and most horrifically, if a person is compelled to eat human meat, even for their own survival, they will 'go Wendigo' or be possessed by the terrible spirit. **Richard Freeman**

lake. In that moment I knew that the Wendygo, [sic] Abominable Snow-man, Bodach Mor, or what have you, was forever explained so far as I was concerned.' [53]

Rennie went on to give his explanation of the cause both of those tracks and the ones he had seen many years later in Speyside.

'Some freakish current of warm air, coming in contact with the low tempera-ture, had set up condensation which was projected earthwards in the form of water blobs. When these landed in the snow they left tracks like those of some fabulous animal.' [54]

Given that Rennie saw these tracks being made, and felt water falling from the air it is reasonable to assume that both the Canadian tracks and the tracks seen near the Cairngorms were the result of a rare meteorological condition. This 'explanation' may be applicable to the origin of other 'mystery' tracks such as the 'Devil's Hoofprints'. On the other hand a rare and invisible water throwing creature may be at large.

It has also been suggested that because witnesses to the BGM have heard what they interpreted as 'footsteps' as part of the experience these footsteps must have caused by something with a foot! In other words another contention for the physical existence of a Big Grey Man. Affleck Gray in his book on the BGM devotes a whole chapter to this matter [55]. BGM witnesses and other visitors to Ben Macdhui have experienced phenomena which has been interpreted as being footsteps. These have been heard in winter conditions with snow underfoot and also in high summer, when the terrain is of bare rock with little or no vegetation. A review of both the mountaineering and paranormal literature suggests that the sound of 'footsteps' being heard on mountains, but with no evidence for their origin, are a relatively common phenomenon. Dependent on the context they are often attributed to the unknown, usually in the form of 'ghosts', or to natural phenomena such as unusual echoes. However in all these cases, as well as those concerning the BGM they have also been heard when the witnesses have been stationary and when no-one else seems to have been in the area. Gray can find no fitting and comprehensive explanation for the footsteps. In the context of the BGM though nothing has ever been seen to make the sound of footsteps, no footprints have ever been discovered which could be connected with the sounds. Walter Reid, in the *Aberdeen Press & Journal* the week after Collie's account was first made public, is reported as having '....often experienced the "crunch crunch" noise in the snow which Professor Collie described. He had got it when he was on the mountaintop alone and when there was perfect silence, but he attributed it to a weird echo effect.' [56].

It is possible that some form of meteorological phenomenon similar to that which J.A. Rennie witnessed in Canada could be responsible. Echoes or other people in the same general area may also account for some of the footsteps heard, but it is impossible to isolate any consistent phenomena, be they natural or paranormal which causes them. As evidence for the physical existence of the BGM though the 'footsteps' do not stand up to scrutiny, even though they remain largely unexplained.

During the writing of this piece I asked Loren Coleman, an American cryptozoologist, for his opinion on the BGM. Coleman believes that whilst much of the evidence attributed to the BGM may be natural or psychological in origin a percentage is paranormal and physical in origin:

'I think that a cryptozoological specimen may be related to SOME of the reports...especially of the ones where tall hairy creatures are seen and large footprints are left in the snow.' Coleman goes on to say ' I tend to think that ancient European tales of Big Grey Men and Grendels are evidence of a memory of humans who coexisted with "True Giants" - real hominoids that may be Gigantopithecus. Some relict populations of these species may have survived in wilderness areas of Europe into the middle of this [20th] Century.' [57]

This may be the case elsewhere in Europe but almost certainly not with the BGM. There are no footprints at all, and the evidence for visual sightings is, as we have seen, slim to say the least. In dealing with accounts of the Big Grey Man of Ben Macdhui all we really have are the accounts given by the people who have had the experience. No physical evidence exists. The experiences appear to be random in location and time. They do not happen to everyone who visits Ben Macdhui, even those people who go to the exact spots where previous witnesses have had the experience. Nor do they appear to happen to the same people twice. The experiences appear to be non-physical in origin, spontaneous and transitory in nature. They seem to be as likely to happen to people who know nothing about the BGM legend as they do to hardened and knowledgeable mountaineers who scoff at the supernatural.

It would be easy to suggest, in the cold light of day, that the BGM legend appears to be little more than a few unusual experiences moulded by the media into a localised folktale. But a number of people have had unusual experiences on and in the vicinity of Ben Macdhui. They have been experiences which have caused rational and hard headed mountaineers to risk their lives in fleeing highly across dangerous ground. Something, physical or non-physical, must have caused those experiences. And that's where the whole subject begins to get very slippery indeed!

Going back to the BGM accounts, a close, analytical, reading reveals one underlying, constant motif. All the witnesses in the 'good' accounts report some form of extreme, uncontrollable panic reaction, leading them to flee in blind terror, often for miles. Fair enough, you might say, anyone would panic if they saw the BGM. But some of the 'panics' take place prior to any 'sighting', and in the majority of cases the whole experience is solely a panic, the trimmings of BGM legend being tacked on later by either writer or witness because of the geographical context of the experience.

So is there a genuine mystery after all? Well, if this core phenomenon were isolated to the Cairngorms and the BGM legend we could probably discount it as an artefact of the storytelling process. But the accounts of being gripped by an uncontrollable panic, and furthermore, one which results in fleeing to the point of exhaustion or narrowly avoiding death by falling over cliffs intrigued me. In digging into both the paranormal and mountaineering literature I discovered that this core experience is relatively widespread in wild or mountainous areas, but has been either ignored or subsumed into the broader, and more 'exciting', area of 'ghost' stories. This is a mistake because, whether paranormal or psychological in origin, there appears to be a very real phenomenon at work.

With the specific evidence for a BGM being so sparse, but the core phenomenon being so consistent and evidenced elsewhere, it would be a mistake to continue to see the BGM phenomenon in either isolation or terms of being caused by an encounter with a physical entity. The evidence I have gathered suggests that the BGM experience and others can be re-framed as mountain panics onto which local folklore is grafted. Bear with me while I take an excursion to the mountains of madness and speculate on what lives there. May 1954. Intending to make use of the excellent weather on his day off, water company surveyor Clive Elliot decided to walk the hills from Kilmuir to Staffin, on the Isle of Skye. Everything was fine until he reached a stream in Glen Sneosdale. He jumped across and:

'.....immediately, as if I'd stepped into another world, my mind just went to pieces. I cannot describe the feeling, one of total, absolute, blind terror. I didn't look round to see what was happening, I just went up the hill and I remember pulling myself against the grass and boosting myself as hard as I could. I've never felt anything like that in my life before and please god I never do again'.[58]

The feeling stopped after a few hundred yards and Elliot's day continued with no further problems.

Clive Elliot's account is self-explanatory, a one-off experience totally out of character which has puzzled him intensely over the years. The italics are mine, stressing the terror and wonder Elliot put into the words when I interviewed him twenty two years later. Had Elliot's experience taken place within the Ben Macdhui area his account would surely have been part of the overall legend. The fact that he did not reveal his experience to anyone until 1996 and did not attempt to connect with any legendary creature suggests that we have got the data as 'raw' as possible. Perhaps there is something about northern Skye because the following two accounts both originate from
within a few miles of Clive Elliot's experience.

On a visit to Skye in June 1971 veteran hill walker Brian Miller headed south from the Staffin-Uig road. After passing the top of Bioda Buidhe he began to feel distinctly uneasy, intimidated and depressed. It was as though something - some *thing* perhaps - were watching him. He continued, but was becoming increasingly convinced that 'something malignant was watching and waiting for a chance to spring'. After another half mile he descended into a small hollow and, '......really felt fear, for all the world as if something was hiding behind the last rise and would spring if I took my eyes off the route I had taken.' Miller turned and retreated to his car in panic. [59]

Miller returned to Skye the following year and on one outing walked over the tops toward Baca Ruadh. 'Before I'd gone more than three hundred yards I was assailed again by a feeling of unease.' Miller told me. He pressed on but once again, '...the old feeling of being watched by something malignant became overpowering'. The feeling of panic intensified and he again abandoned the walk. [60]

Intrigued by these out of character panic attacks Miller did some research and discovered Swire's book on the legends of Skye. In its pages he found the area round the Quaraing (about two miles from his first experience) described as having 'an atmosphere which can never be captured. Perhaps it can best be summed up by saying that it is as if 'the terror that walketh in darkness' here walks by day.' Swire also recounts being told by two men that the '...Baca Ruadh....which they visited at different times, gives just this same feeling of terror and potent, living evil. All other Skye hills are friendly, but not the Baca Ruach.'.[61]

Both Elliot's and Miller's experiences took place in northern Skye, within a few miles of each other. Both experiences were reported to me independently and the witnesses do not know each other. Another correspondent, Mr J. Craig, told me of an incident which took place on Bennachie near Aberdeen. He and his two friends were resting below the summit when, '....we all stopped talking and a most horrid feeling of unease and then absolute terror swept over us. As one person the three of us fled down through heather, boulders, with no thought except 'get away, get away'.' They didn't stop running until they reached the foot of the mountain. [62] There was no forewarning of this 'terror' happening and, oddly, Craig nor his companions mentioned the experience to each other for years afterwards. Bennachie has a legend connected to a giant who protects the mountain, known as Jock o' Bennachie. Craig is convinced he and his friends experienced the power of Jock o'Bennachie.Long distance walker Chris Townsend, in his book *Walking the Munroes and Tops,* recalls an experience which occurred by the Allt Innis a'Mhuill in Glen Strathfarrar when he '....suddenly had a strong feeling of a presence nearby, of something or someone waiting and watching...'. Townsend sensed what he described as a 'hint of hostility' in this presence and, 'for a second or two I felt frightened.' [63]

Was Townsend's experience just the results of isolation and a hard day on the hill? Or was it something primeval and brooding, indigenous to the landscape? I contacted Townsend, who commented:

> 'I never thought my brief experience would be noticed. I haven't really anything to add to the description but your email did set me thinking. I don't think isolation or a hard day were anything to do with it. I've walked thousands of miles alone in much remoter places than the Highlands and I often have long days. Much of that walking has been in Western North America where I would have put such a feeling down to there being a bear nearby - and felt much more frightened! Whether it was supernatural terror or not I don't know. Overall I tend towards the sceptical but I can't think of what could have made me feel like that.' [64]

Sensations of 'presence' and extreme panic are clearly not restricted to the confines of Ben Macdhui or even the broader area of the Cairngorms. They can occur in any mountainous or wild area. They do not fall into any easy category, which makes their reporting difficult. After all, who wants to announce that they have been terrified to the point of flight by something they cannot see, hear or feel? Therefore these experiences are often ignored or go unreported until they are noticed as passing remarks in the literature or when they are specifically hunted out by researchers. When these experiences are reported they often become subsumed into local folklore, attached to ghost stories, hauntings and so on. The form that the experience is given by witness or commentator, i.e. giant, ghost, faerie, elemental or whatever supersedes the core phenomenon and becomes the motif for the experience. This makes for an interesting story but, I think, lays a false trail.

Ghost hunter and author Thurston Hopkins received a letter which recounted an undated experience not dissimilar to many of the BGM and other panics discussed so far. The writer told of an experience which took place whilst visiting the hills above Rhossilly Bay in South Wales. As he climbed higher he became aware of feeling uneasy, a sensation which increased until he

> '....sat still and waited-then looked from side to side. I was being WATCHED. Slowly, painfully, in an agony of horror I turned my head to see I knew not what....' He continued his climb, all the time aware of the sensation of being observed. 'Then horror, violent sickening seized me. A huge menacing form enveloped rather than touched me. I prayed and shrieked aloud, and began to run - run madly down the steep to the sea.' The following day he made enquiries locally to be told 'Many a one has been frightened badly up there. It's got an evil name. Some say the old Stone Men used to live up there...' [65]

Another account dating from 1965 and also from south Wales recounts how a local man was walking on the slopes of Foel Feddau, when:

> 'Suddenly, as though a curtain had fallen, all about him changed completely and he felt the raw edge of fear. He felt that he was in the presence of the unknown........He became aware that evil, invisible eyes were upon him.' ....and he '...rushed away from that accursed spot' [66]

Whilst research was being undertaken for a book dealing with landscape mysteries one informant told of a mountain experience from the early 1960s which tops even the 'best' account from Ben Macdhui. The informant was a boy at the time, out on the 2000 foot Bleaklow plateau in the Derbyshire Peak District, with a friend to investigate one of the many WWII aircraft wrecks which litter the area. After visiting the crash site he heard his friend shout and....

> 'I looked and saw, all in one instant, grouse exploding out of the heather towards us, sheep and hares stampeding towards us and behind them, rolling at a rapid rate towards is from the direction of Hern Clough, a low bank of cloud or fog......but what was truly terrifying was that in the leading edge of the cloud bank - in it and striding purposefully towards us, was a huge shadow-figure, a man-like silhouette, but far bigger than a man - as high as the cloudbank, as high as a house. And the terror that hit me and was driving the birds and the animals and my friend was utterly overwhelming - like a physical blow - and I have never felt the like since!'

Needless to say both lads fled '....in mindless terror...and all the sheep and wildlife that could run or fly went careering down with us in utter panic.' [67]

A giant figure looming from mist? Uncontrollable panic? Why, it's the Big Grey Man of Ben Macdhui on holiday! The two boys had never heard of the Big Grey Man and his friend attributed this terrifying incident to 'Th'owd Lad', a Pennine appellation for the devil. Had this incident happened within a twenty mile radius of Ben Macdhui it would be the jewel in the legend's crown.

But what was it? It would be hard to explain this incident in purely psychological terms as it has two witnesses and, most significantly of all, reports of wildlife also responding panicked to the stimulus. Unfortunately the other witness has not been traced so I have been unable to follow that line of enquiry. Even if we ignore reports of strange clouds, fleeing wildlife and giant figures we are still left with an experience of extreme panic leading the witnesses to flee in terror.

The informant concluded the experience.

> 'We fled. We plunged over the crags above Gathering Hill - and every time I go back and look at those crags, I wonder why we didn't break our necks. We fled in mindless terror down that mountainside towards the Shelf Brook and Doctors Gate - and all the sheep and wildlife that could run or fly went careering down with us in utter panic. And then, about half way down, we seemed to run out into the sunlight - and it was all over! All the panic gone. The sheep stopped, put their heads down, and started to graze. Everything returned at once to normal. But back up there, on Higher Shelf Stones, wisps of mist were still coiling round.....' [68]

The informant had his own views about the cause of this particular mountain panic and of attempts to 'explain'

> 'Don't ask me to rationalise. Or rationalise it away - which is what it amounts to. I've come to the conclusion that sort of thing amounts to no more than a cop-out, a late twentieth century defensive mechanism - it's safe if it can be explained. As if 'explaining away' were like defusing a bomb. I do think that every now and then, some of us - maybe all of us - stumble into an encounter with elements deeper and older than we are, and they are not, by their nature,

benevolent, though they may be. This certainly wasn't. [69]

Experienced mountaineer Bill Steele wrote to me detailing an experience which took place on Mt. Giluwe on Papua New Guinea. Several kilometres above the tree line Steele and his German climbing partner, casting about for a suitable campsite, stopped at the mouth of a cave for lunch. Over to Steele:

> 'As we finished we discussed whether to make a base camp there and push on to the peak with a light pack. At this time I suddenly felt an intense feeling of my impending death, there was a sense of being watched by something evil that seemed to be drawing near and about to pounce. Although there was nothing to be seen apart from the pleasant shelter and it was a bright dry day I knew I must get away immediately from that place. When I called to Dieter to grab our stuff and run he thought I must have somehow lost all reason as he felt nothing unusual at all. I then panicked and said he could do what he liked but I was off! I threw the pack over my shoulder and ran as fast as I could down the track and only slowed down when I reached the treeline several kilometres away.'

Steele also commented that he felt safer the further away he got from the cave mouth, echoing other accounts where witnesses have felt the feeling increase or decrease as they moved across the landscape. [70] There are many, many more similar accounts from across the world. All include isolated areas and mountain panics. Some, like those on Ben Macdhui and Bennachie, seem to have become attached to and synonymous with entities said to cause the panic. Some appear to be in clusters, like those of Northern Skye, but remain as yet 'unnamed'. Others stand alone, as one-off, random experiences in space and time. All the witnesses were profoundly terrified by their encounters with this unknown terror. There is genuine mystery here. But once identified, even a possibly new genre of anomalous experience becomes just another 'interesting' story for the Fortean equivalent of stamp collectors unless some attempt is made to untangle possible cause or to put the phenomena in context.

As several of the experiences have taken place in the same general area it is tempting to suggest that the origin for the experiences are intimately connected to, and possibly caused by, the area itself. The Earth Mysterians, nature mystics and fringe scientists have long suggested there are 'energies' locked into the landscape.

Energies which can be tapped into intentionally or accidentally and which are responsible for a wide variety of strange phenomena from fairies to ghosts to UFOs. It is also claimed that these energies can cause illness, stress, unease and a whole range of psychological and physiological symptoms. This idea is echoed in the Chinese concept of *feng shui* where landscapes or dwellings would be physically altered to aid the flow of an earth-energy called *ch'i*, which in turn affects people's well-being. So could it be unspecified 'energies' of this nature which are causing mountain panics?

Archaeologist and dowser Tom Lethbridge thought so and referred to these incidents as 'ghouls'. As a teenager he and his mother had experienced 'a horrible feeling of gloom and depression' in some woods, which lead them to hurry away. Later a suicide was found almost at the spot. When married both Lethbridge and his wife experienced a similar ghoul independently at Ladram Bay in Devon. This seems to be one of the spots where the experience is replicable as they felt it again, together. His wife walked into it again at the top of a cliff and 'Moreover she had an odd feeling, as if someone - or something - was urging her to jump over.' Shades of the fleeing panics which have been detailed so far. Lethbridge attributed this phenomenon to a 'place-field' caused by underground water producing changes in the earth's magnetic field and thus affecting the brain of anyone who happened to be in the right place at the right time. [71]

'Repeater' spots like the Cairngorms, North Skye, Ladram Bay and so on may, if investigated further, yield positive evidence of 'energies' which lead to panics and possibly suicides. The Christian church has certainly held this view and accident black spots and regular suicide locations have been exorcised to rid them of the perceived demonic influence. Many of these locations are said to create effects which temporarily unbalance the human mind. As an example of how they include the type of 'panic' I am discussing here, an earth mysteries journal printed the following letter from Michael Cook in which he describes a car journey home along familiar, well travelled roads.

> 'As I was driving around a not particularly sharp bend, and not too quickly, I suddenly felt seized by panic; I felt I was being dragged off the road and would not negotiate the bend. It took a considerable effort of willpower to keep to the road. In a short while the panic disappeared and my confidence returned.' [72]

Cook had driven over that same stretch of road many times before and after his experience with nothing untoward happening. On the surface this seems to be exactly the same type of phenomena experienced by BGM witnesses and others who have encountered a random and meaningless 'panic'. In his classic study of the fear which gripped West Virginia during 1966 John Keel describes his encounter with a panic zone. Whilst out driving alone after midnight in the 'TNT area' Keel had, as he puts it.

> '....one curious experience. As I passed a certain point on one of the isolated roads I was suddenly engulfed in fear. I stepped on the gas and after I went a few yards my fear vanished as quickly as it came.'

He noted the exact spot and drove through it twice more, with exactly the same effect. Keel stopped his car and '..walked back to the 'zone of fear' slowly, alert for any rustle of bushes, measuring my own breathing and emotions. I was perfectly calm until I took one step too many and was back in the zone. I almost panicked and ran, but I forced myself to look around and proceed slowly.' Keel determined the 'zone' was about fifteen feet across, and walked back through it to reach his car. He concluded he was 'probably walking through a beam of ultrasonic waves.' Returning to the spot in the morning he found the 'zone' had gone, and there was nothing in the area to account for it. [74]

Researchers Albert Budden and Paul Devereux have both written extensively about 'energies' which can have the type of effect we are discussing here. Devereux suggests consciousness affecting energy can originate via natural radioactivity and electro-magnetic fields. His books list numerous examples of anomalous experiences he believes have occurred after an encounter with these energies [75]. Budden contends that modern electro-magnetic pollution as well as natural electro-magnetism can have a radical and often deleterious effect on people [76].

None of this is completely proven but Lethbridge, Devereux, Budden and other researchers are building a persuasive case for the earth's natural energies playing a part as being at least the stimulus for 'paranormal' experiences. Critics will have none of this. Even the kindest would say they are replacing old folk tales with a new age techno folklore, claiming that allegations of these 'energies' are rooted in unverifiable narrative and on science which is at best tenuous, at worst specious. But there is no doubt that the forces of natural radiation, electro-magnetism exist and reasonable to speculate they can have an effect on consciousness.

With or without the acceptance of 'fringe' energies there are other ways of looking at the causation and interpretation of 'panics'. Being among mountains and other wild places is frequently an awe inspiring experience where the difference between the natural and supernatural is often really only a matter of perception. Perhaps senses stretched by exertion, heightened by beauty and isolation create psychological phenomena which causes panic of the type outlined in this article. Or perhaps the psychologists are wrong and there is another reason. In his book *Gulfs of Blue Air* Jim Crumley lists ten 'More Reasons For Hills'. Number six is because, 'They accommodate the gods of the ancients'. A clue? [77]

In the contemporary western world it is our predilection as a society to interpret any unknown experience as psychological or paranormal in nature, as if that designation explains it all. Frequently we use one unknown to 'explain' another and explanations change with the times. The nature based cosmologies of our ancestors in these Isles would have no problem with the experiences I have recounted here. They believed every facet of the landscape had a presence, and was a personification of a god or spirit, the genius loci. Anomalous or visionary experiences here would have been interpreted as belonging to that particular rock, valley, cliff etc and symbolised in a form relevant to local mythology or folklore. Whether the experience was repeated or not, the very idea of the *genius loci* inhabiting that particular spot would become embedded in and handed down through the local tradition. My dictionary defines *genius loci* as the spirit dwelling in a particular spot, or the characteristic atmosphere of a place. Does that sound a little familiar? So in a way the BGM and giant of Bennachie and so could be described as *genius loci*, still being experienced, irrespective of any pre-existing traditions concerning them.

So perhaps these mountain panics are just the direct experience of a location's *genius loci*. But that's as unprovable a concept as the 'earth energies' theory, or as pointless as a reductionist psychological view-point. Visionary experiences, mountain panics, and earth 'energies' can also be seen as metaphors for spontaneous psychic or psychological experiences, which in turn are only metaphors themselves for any experience in which human consciousness comes up against the forces of nature. Not nature as described by the aesthetics of landscape appreciation via art or literature. Or nature as in the form of a scientific understanding via the various relevant "ology's". All those are just temporary ways of describing. I mean what Cairngorm poet Nan Shepherd refers to as the 'experience of nature in the raw, a primitive thing, and utterly, utterly baffling'. [77]

To even begin to understand that we must go back to the description of experiences given by witnesses to all these phenomena and the core of that description seems to be one of 'panic'.

The word 'panic' which the witnesses to these strange experiences often use derives, of course, from the Greek god Pan. According to one book on mythology, 'The feeling of solitude and lonesomeness which weighs upon travellers in wild mountain places....was ascribed to the presence of Pan.....And thus anxiety and alarm, arising from no visible or intelligible cause, came to be called 'panic fear', that is, such fear as is produced by the agitating presence of Pan.' [78]

A typical description, which pretty much describes all the BGM accounts and other mountain panics listed here. Another writer has it that, 'Pan is unlimited in movement or scope of action - in the original Greek he is literally 'everywhere'.....The apparent form, again, is symbolic, rather than representational of any physical entity. The elemental archetype is more often sensed than seen.' [79] All descriptions of encounters with Pan speak of the same criteria and phenomena; lonely, often mountainous or wilderness areas, the core phenomenon being randomly triggered and frequently experienced or later described in terms of a physical entity, which isn't really 'there'.

So have all the witnesses to 'panics' met Pan, and isn't that just another bonkers explanation anyway? The clue to it is to get away from notions of entities, nature spirits, energies and so on as being in any sense objectively real, and to look at 'panics' and the Pan experience as yet another metaphor for the interpretation of 'raw nature' when it overrides our normal waking consciousness.

Perhaps the clearest synthesis of the panic experience and one with the most relevance here is that given by Jungian analyst James Hillman who wrote:

> 'Panic, especially at night when the citadel darkens and the heroic ego sleeps, is a direct participation mystique in nature, a fundamental, even ontological experience of the world as alive and in dread. Objects become subjects; they move with life while one is oneself paralysed with fear. When existence is experienced through instinctual levels of fear, aggression, hunger or sexuality, images take on a compelling life of their own. The imaginal is never more vivid than when we are connected with it instinctually. The world alive is of course animism; that this living world is divine and imagined by different gods with attributes and characteristics is polytheistic pantheism. That fear, dread, horror are natural is wisdom. In Whitehead's term nature alive means Pan, and panic flings open a door into this reality.' [80]

An apt description of exactly what happens. In wild or mountainous country the solitude, exertion and oft overpowering awe of the surroundings together with realisation (consciously or otherwise) of being a fragile entity in an awesome and ultimately unknowable landscape could be said to overpower the 'heroic', or rational, ego. The 'objects', ie the environment and its contents, become the subjects - mist becomes BGM, areas of landscape become threatening, noises assume and infer preternatural origin, and then existence in all its forms is encountered directly. Human consciousness is not prepared for this and panic results, the witness fleeing until the spell is broken, often by contact with other human beings or a familiar sound or location.

What triggers this? Well as we've seen it could be any or all of the 'energy' theories put forward by Devereux et al. Or just the age-old call of the wild. Recall how Tewnion's shooting of the BGM was, according to him, just a panic response to mist, or how Wendy Wood believed her terror could have started with a deer bark? Or how the Bleaklow informant could only see wisps of mist when the panic had subsided, the 'giant' has long since receded into the imaginal realm. Whilst they must still remain a possibility for the trigger we need not even invoke mysterious energies as the cause of these panics as the following episode, from the Cairngorms near Ben Macdhui, illustrates:

> 'I was coming home round about 1.00am along the Revoan road when my nerve suddenly gave way. It was a fine winter's night, fairly clear, and I was belting along it when it suddenly hit me. Exactly what triggered it off I don't know - maybe the call of a vixen or a wild cat, the hoot of an owl or the bark of a roe-buck. Anyhow, I trembled. I ran whiles and walked fast, looking over my shoulder till I got home in the small hours.. soaked with perspira-tion......A doctor told me it could happen to any fit man and he could not account for it.' [81]

That experience occurred to a naturalist and forester with long experience in the more remote areas of the Cairngorms. Like many of the other witnesses he was a hardened hill man, knowledgeable about - yet sceptical of - local ghost lore and the like. In other areas of Fortean study, say ufology or ghost-hunting, these witnesses would have their experience as observers and scepticism used to support the objective reality of their experience. But that's the myth of the credible witness. We're all fallible and susceptible and like the doctor said, 'it could happen to any fit man.' And apparently does. Fans of the more occult explanations for mountain panics and their ilk may like to consider Marshall's remedy for this form of psychic experience. Upon returning home he, '..stripped to the buff, had a good rub down, swallowed a stiff dram and lashings of tea, and slept like a log till 7.am.' Who needs exorcists, psychologists or shamen!

Irrespective of whether these experiences are caused by the mind suddenly glimpsing the immensity of nature in the raw, or whether they are caused by as yet unknown forces in nature, they amount to then same thing - the direct experience of the overpowering force of nature and existence, to be fled from, to be personified as the BGM, a giant, the devil, *genius loci* or whatever.

As a final example of the random nature of these panics and of how these panics can seriously affect others consider author John Buchan's (writing as Lord Tweedsmuir) unscheduled meeting with Pan.

> 'We do not hear so much to-day of the goat-foot god.....But the experience which was the basis of the myth does not go unrecorded. In wild places or in wild weather, men are still awed by a sense of the immensity and pitilessness of Nature. There is a *Natura rnaligna* as well as the Wordsworthian *Natura benigna*....... Sometimes, too, there come moments when one feels a kind of personal malevolence, the sense of a hostile will which almost takes bodily form, and which sets the nerves fluttering in despite of the reason. In such moments one sees - or at any rate feels - what the ancients meant by Pan.' [82]

Buchan goes on to relate an experience from 1911 in the Bavarian Highlands. Returning down from the summit of the Alpspitze he noticed his guide had:

> '.....fallen silent and, glancing at him, was amazed to see that his face was dead white, that sweat stood in beads on his forehead, and that his eyes were staring ahead as if he were in an agony of fear - as if terror were all around him so that he dared not look one way rather than another. Suddenly he began to run, and I ran too, some power not myself constraining me. Terror had seized me also, but I did not know what I dreaded. It was like the epidemic of giggling which overcomes children who have no wish to laugh. We ran-we ran like demented bacchanals, tearing down the glades, leaping rocks, bursting through thickets, colliding with trees, sometimes colliding with each other, and all the time we never uttered a sound. At last we fetched up beside the much-frequented high-way, where we lay for a time utterly exhausted. For the rest of the road home we did not speak; we did not even dare look at each other. ' [83]

Buchan concluded, 'What was the cause? I suppose it was panic. Sebastian had seen the goat-foot god or something of the kind...and he had made me feel his terror.' [84] Buchan's guide had experienced 'Pan' and therefore panic, which had been transmitted to him as a form of contagion. This experience is very like Craig's experience on Bennachie, even down to the fact of the percipients not discussing the event afterwards.

Buchan in passing makes a very important point, that 'Pan' can be experienced as a terror or sometimes as it's opposite, a benign force. And again a trawl through the canon of mountaineering literature reveals a plethora of experiences where people have experienced Wordsworthian raptures as an exact opposite to the malevolence personified by the BGM and the other nameless terrors I have described.

We've come a long way. From the possibility that odd experiences on a Scottish mountain may have been caused by an indigenous relict hominid, to a plethora of core experiences which I have termed 'mountain panics'. I make no claims for absolute truth here and indeed I am mindful that categorising these experiences, suggesting that one unknowable may have the same cause as another, similar one, is fraught with problems.

All I can say for sure about this research is that the core experience appears very similar in all cases, and that there is no one single occurrence which triggers it. I am also wary about needlessly creating another Fortean pigeon-hole, that of mountain panic, for unexplained phenomena. But based on the evidence I have reviewed both new and old, I think this is a very real psychological or psychic phenomenon and one which may lie at the core of many so called 'paranormal' experiences. Its triggers may be many but they all stem from the human instrument's perception of and relationship with the reality we live in. As one commentator wrote to Affleck Gray '..the most mysterious thing to be found among mountains was the human brain'. [85]

In the end we can but speculate. It's entertaining and quite informative. But only the witnesses who have experienced these panics, witnessed the Fear Liath Mor and its brethren know for sure what it's like and what the experience means for them. There is a vast gulf between those who know and those of us who speculate. Huge Corrie's letter to Affleck Gray summed up both the experience and the difference well:

> 'Sometimes in dark days, in wild places, Skye in dense mist and rain, in desert, mountains and jungle, I have thought that I got a hint or two. From our fancied and narrow security, I know, having looked out upon the wilderness in turmoil where there could be no help and no witness of our undoing, where the gleams were fleeting, as though the daylight itself were riven and collapsing, that I saw the filmy shapes of those things which darken and affright the minds of primitives. While the sky is changeful and menacing, and there are storms at sea, when our fellows are absent, when shades take their hour of ease and voices whisper in wood and stone, and mischance and death are veiled, but here we shall have gods and ghosts. The sharp sighted collectors of old-train lumber, and similar curios may still keep busy, and tie up their dry bundles of mythology and superstitions; but I myself - and any Scottish hillman could make plenty more.' [86]

References

1. Quoted in Affleck Gray, *The Big Grey Man of Ben Macdhui*, Birlinn, Edinburgh, 1994 p.9.
2. Gray, op. cit.
3. Adam Watson, *The Cairngorms*, Scottish Mountaineering Trust, Edinburgh 1992
4. *Fortean Studies 3* dealing with Pendle Hill and its environs. Gives a overview of the warp and weft of anomalous experiences which can be found in one region. This principle could be applied to any area.
5. Hogg, quoted in Gray, op. cit. p. 39-40.
6. Dr Helen Ross, *Behaviour and Perception in Strange Environments*, George Allen & Unwin, London, 1974. p. 54-56.
7. Edinburgh New Philosophical Journal, Edinburgh 1831

8. Quoted in Gray, op. cit. p.21.
9. Quoted in Gray, op. cit. p 22.
10. Rev. John Grant, Statistical Account of Scotland, 1790, quoted in Gray, op. cit. p 21.
11. Jack Hastie, "Big Grey Man - The Evidence", *Scottish Mountaineering Club Journal*, 1998, p. 507-513
12. Jim Crumley, *The Heart of the Cairngorms*, Colin Baxter Photography, Grantown-on-Spey, 1997. p.22-27.
13. Quoted in Gray, op. cit. p???
14. George Hall, *Leaves From A Rambler's Diary*.
15. Cairngorm Club Journal, Vol. X. No. 56, January 1921, p.86
16. Dr Ernest A Baker's book *The Highlands With Rope and Rucksack*, Quoted in Gray, op. cit. p.89.
17. Gray, op. cit.
18. See also Hastie, op cit., for a similar definition
19. Gray, op. cit.
20. W.H. Murray, Mountaineering in Scotland, Dent, London, 1947, p.140 and 214.
21. J.A.Rennie, *Romantic Strathspey*, Robert Hale, London 1956, p.83.
22. Ross, op cit.
23. Christine Mill, *Norman Collie: A Life In Two Worlds*, Aberdeen University Press, Aberdeen, 1987
24. 'Mountain Climbers and the 'ghost' of Ben Macdhui', *Aberdeen Press & Journal*, 12 December 1925.
25. *Aberdeen Press and Journal*, 30 November 1925. 'The Ben Macdhui Spectre', *The Cairngorm Club Journal*, vol. 11, July 1926. p. 214-215.
26. E. C. C. Baly, Obituaries of the Fellows of the Royal Society, London, 1942, p. 347-348.
27. Mills, op. cit., p 97.
28. Mills, op. cit.
29. Seton Gordon, *Highways and Byways of the Central Highlands*, MacMillan, 1949, p 344.
30. Rennie McOwan, Magic Mountains, Mainstream, Edinburgh, 1996, p 20
31. Gray, op.cit.. p
32. Mills, op. cit. p 96
33. Mills, op. cit. p 97
34. J.N. Collie, "Dreams", *Cairngorm Club Journal*, vol. 15, p 214.
35. Mills, op. cit. p 97.
36. 'Mountain Climbers and the 'ghost' of Ben Macdhui', *Aberdeen Press & Journal*, 12 December 1925.
37. 'Mountain Climbers and the 'ghost' of Ben Macdhui', *Aberdeen Press & Journal*, 12 December 1925.
38. *Aberdeen Press & Journal*, 15 December 1925.
39. Alex Tewnion, 'A Shot in the Mist', *The Scots Magazine*, 1958, p 227.
40. Gray, op. cit. p. 107.
41. Edinburgh Psychic College, The Big Grey Man of Ben Macdhui
42. Gray, op. cit. p. 7.
43. Gray, op. cit. p. 7.
44. Joan Grant, Far Memory, Corgi, 1975, p. 170.
45. Grant, op. cit. p. 170-171
46. Mark Chorvinsky et al, 'The Search for the Thunderbird Photo', *Strange Magazine* no. 19, Spring 1998, p. 26-28.
47. Gray, op. cit. p. 13-14.
48. Marc Alexander, Phantom Britain, Muller, London, 1975, p. 204, for example. Most other BGM references consider this as a possibility.
49. Ronald J. Willis, 'Ben Macdhui - the Haunted Mountain', *Info Journal* no. 15, 2 May, 1975, p. 5. For

example.

50. Rennie, op. cit.
51. Rennie, op. cit.
52. Mike Dash, The Devil's Hoofmarks in Fortean Studies, JBP, London 1994, p. 71- 150.
53. Rennie, op. cit.
54. Rennie, op. cit.
55. Gray, op. cit., p.61-68.
56. 'Mountain Climbers and the 'ghost' of Ben Mac dhui', Aberdeen Press & Journal, 12 December 1925.
57. Email, 6 July, 1998.
58. Interview with Clive Elliot, 3 September 1996.
59. Letter from Brian Miller, 4 February, 1998.
60. Miller, 1998.
61. Otta F. Swire, Skye: The Island and its Legends, Blackie, London, 1961, p. 45-46.
62. Letter from J. Craig, September, 1997.
63. Chris Townsend, Walking the Munros and Tops, Mainstream, Edinburgh, 1997, p. 153.
64. Email, 6 August, 1998.
65. R. Thurston Hopkins, Adventures With Phantoms, Quality Press, London, 1946, p. 68.
66. *Pembrokeshire Folk Tales*, p.111.
67. Interview, 1994. Witness does not want his name used. He is known to my colleague David Clarke and myself.
68. Interview, 1994.
69. Interview, 1994.
70. Letter from Bill Steele, 17 March, 1997
71. Colin Wilson, 'A Seeker After Truth', *The Unexplained*, p. 566-569.
72. Michael Cook, 'Road Story' *Northern Earth* no. 74 (Summer 1998) p. 24.
73. John Keel, *Visitors From Space*, Panther. St Albans, 1976, p. 79-80.
74. Paul Devereux, *Places of Power*, Blandford, London, 1990. All Devereux's books are worth reading for details of 'earth energies'.
75. Albert Budden, *Electric UFOs*, Blandford, London, 1998.
76. Jim Crumley, *Gulfs of Blue Air*, Mainstream, Edinburgh, 1997, p. 191.
77. Nan Shepherd, *The Living Mountain*. Aberdeen University Press, 1981.
78. Alexander S. Murray, *Who's Who In Mythology*, Studio Editions, London, 1992, p. 136-137.
79. Tom Graves, *Needles Of Stone Revisited*, Gothic Image, Glastonbury, 1986, p. 162.
80. James Hillman, *Pan and the Nightmare*, Dallas, 1972, p. 54.
81. Gray, op. cit. p. 17.
82. Rt. Hon. Lord Tweedsmuir, 'Pan', *Scottish Mountaineering Club Journal*, vol. 22 (April 1939), no. 127. p. 41-43.
83. Tweedsmuir, op. cit. p.135-136.
84. Tweedsmuir, op. cit., p. 140.
85. Gray, op. cit., p. 102
86. Gray, op. cit., p. 143.

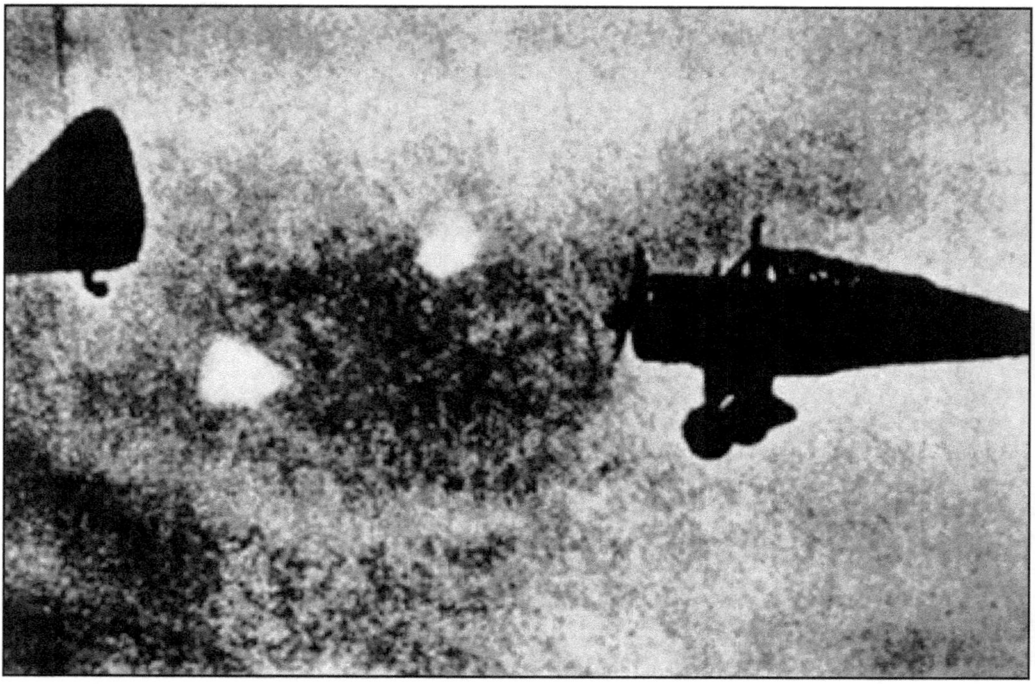

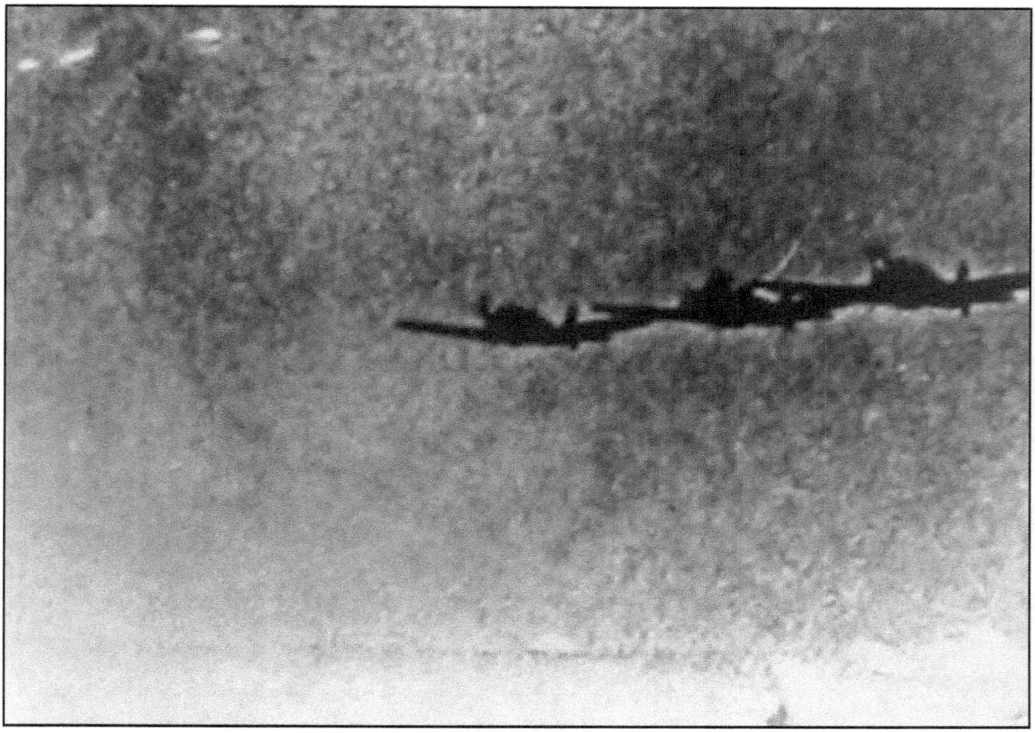

Alleged foo fighter images

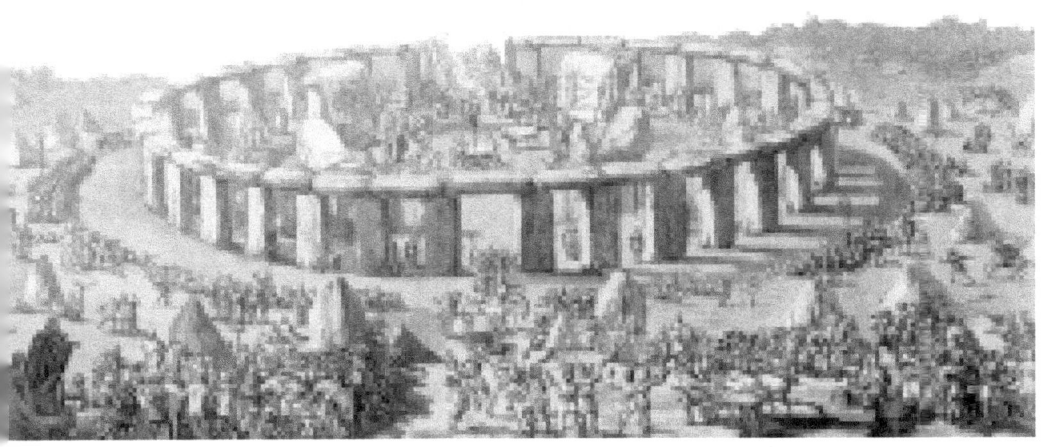

WWII DOCUMENT RESEARCH

UFO BRIGANTIA SUMMER 1990
Double Issue 44/45.
Page 14-17.

E very student of the history of UFOs knows of the phenomenon seen during WWII and known as ' foo fighters' , 'Kraut fireballs' or a variety of other names. Basically they were balls of light which followed and hovered around 'planes of all nationalities both in daylight and after dark. Research into this subject was undertaken by me on behalf of the Fund for UFO Research .

Foo fighter research shows the genesis of the modern UFO age and during my research I came across the old chestnut of the dreaded government 'cover-ups'. For many ufologists WWII is the time when the cover-up really began and there are intimations in many UFO writer's books (Keel, Fawcett, Good, for example) that both the US and UK governments were secretly involved in separate studies of the foo fighter phenomenon. These subjects are several articles long in themselves and we won't go into them here, but for the record so far there is no *documentary* evidence of a cover-up of WWII UFO sightings, or even much interest on any government's part.

No, what we are trying to get to here, are the facts surrounding one particular case of a WWII foo fighter sighting, the cover-up implications and how ufology has dealt with it. So, as the walls melt and voices become fuzzy, let me take you back, back, back .....

OK. It's October 14th 1943 and you're a bomb aimer in a B-17 going in amongst the flak for the final run over the ball-bearing factories at Schweinfurt in Germany, a trouser filling experience which us young folk can't even begin to imagine, but for this particular bomber wave they had more than flak to contend with. According to Martin Caidin who wrote *Black Thursday* (1960) which deals exclusively with the Schweinfurt raid:

> "During the bomb run of several groups, starting at about the time the Fortresses approached the Initial Point, there occurred one of the most baffling incidents of World War II, and an enigma that to this day defies all explanation. As the bombers of the 384th Group swung into the final bomb run after passing the Initial Point, the fighter attacks fell off.

This point is vital, and pilots were queried 'extensively, as were other crew members, as to the position at that time of the German fighter planes. Every man interrogated was firm in his statement that "at the time there were no enemy aircraft above"

At this moment the pilots and top turret gunners, as well as several crewmen in the Plexiglas noses of the bombers, reported a cluster of discs in the path of the 384th's formation and closing with the bombers. The startled exclamations focused attention on the phenomenon and the crews talked back and forth, discussing and confirming the astonishing sight before them.

The discs in the cluster were agreed upon as being silver coloured, about one inch thick and three inches in diameter. They were easily seen by the B-17 crewmen, gliding down slowly in a very uniform cluster.

And then the 'impossible' happened. B-17 Number 026 closed rapidly with a number of discs; the pilot attempted to evade an imminent collision with the objects, but was unsuccessful in his manoeuvre. He reported at the intelligence debriefing that his right wing "went directly through a cluster with absolutely no effect on engines or plane surface,"

The intelligence officers pressed their questioning, and the pilot stated further that one of the discs was heard to strike the tail assembly of his B-17, but that neither he nor any member of the crew heard or witnessed an explosion.

He further explained that about twenty feet from the discs the pilots sighted a mass of black debris of varying sizes of clusters of three by four feet. The SECRET report added: "Also observed two other A/C flying through silver discs with no apparent damage. Observed discs and debris two other times but could not determine where it came from."

No further information on this baffling incident has been uncovered, with the exception that such discs were observed by pilots and crew on missions prior to, and after, Mission 115 of October 14, 1943."

Caidin's account of the events of 14/10/43 has since been cited, quoted from and faithfully reproduced with not the slightest hint of analysis in over 20 UFO books. Tim Good's *Above Top Secret* uses the case to back up an as yet fictional WWII study of UFOs by one General Massey, and it is used both to support the 'UFOs were around in WWII' school of thought but more so to hint at the birth of official cover -ups. Why? Well because in Caidin's book the account is footnoted "1 Memorandum of October 24, 1943, from Major E.R.T. Holmes, F.L.O., 1st Bombardment Division, Reference FLO/IBW/REP/126, to MI-15, War Office, Whitehall, London, SW (copy to Colonel E.W. Thomson, A-2, Pinetree)", leaving us in no doubt that 'they' knew all about this UFO sighting and had full documentation (at least two copies, not to mention any subsequent memoranda).

But did they really? In fact, did the event ever really happen at all? I'm not so sure it did. When I first discovered the account I began to see what could be found out about it- it's obviously well-referenced and so should be easy to check out.......

A letter to the M.O.D at their Air Historical Branch 5 came to nothing, which suggests that either of the documents may be held at the Public Records Office at Kew, London. A professional researcher was despatched to try to find the document. She searched all relevant Air Force records available (some are still-bound by various 'rules' with embargos on viewing of up to a century) but could still find nothing, despite the help of the staff there and noting that "the reference FLO etc does not correspond with any references at the record office".

In the USA, Dennis Stacy (MUFON Journal editor) had taken an interest in the case and followed up several leads, aided by the Freedom of Information Act. Firstly the A.F. Historical Research centre at Maxwell AFB searched their 8th A.F. files but could come across no documentary record of the event (interestingly enough I tried the same source and whilst they gave me squadron histories of the 415th Night Fighter squadron and their documented foo fighter sightings, they could provide nothing on the Schweinfurt raid - odd if the Schweinfurt events were real).

The National Archives (Washington) searched their files but drew a blank. A letter written to French researcher J. M. Bigorne from the National Archives stated:

> "A search in records of the United States Strategic Bombing Survey
> (USSBS), European War, Target Damage File, 11a (2606), Schweinfurt,
> failed to disclose any documentation or information regarding little flying
> discs by B-17 pilots."

All this presents us with a quandary. If the Archives are quite free about some foo fighter info, why - if it even exists at all - should they be that bothered about concealing the Schweinfurt material? So far three independent researchers over the past ten years have had the same answer - none of the flight records for that day record the event in Caidin's book. As I have seen other pilot's logs which mention unusual UFO-type sightings during missions, it would be inconceivable for at least a few aircrew on that raid not to have mentioned it even in passing - especially as in this case it was obviously something of an item at de-briefing.

Letters in numerous aircrew magazines (UK & US) requesting info on the raid were placed and despite many replies no-one knew anything. Aviation writers Martin Middlebrook and Chaz Bowyer who have written many highly detailed books about the air war, and have interviewed thousands of aircrew, wrote to say they had never heard of the incident, despite having had foo fighters mentioned to them in other contexts.

If the account wasn't a hoax and the government archives (all of them) were either lying - or hiding - material pertaining to the event the only way of proving it seemed to be getting a fresh first-hand report of the incident. Dennis Stacy contacted the 384th Bombing Group survivors association and with no account of the UFO sighting forthcoming from them (even stranger - perhaps survivors associations are in on the cover-up too), was put onto General Theodore Ross Milton who led the raid that day and went in first with the 91st Group Formation. He wrote; "I don't recall seeing black discs or hearing about any strange phenomena from any of my group", was his reply to the questions Stacy posed him. Are we really to believe that the guy who led the raid didn't hear anything about the phenomenon? Or is he part of the cover up too?

Martin Caidin, the originator of the rumour also presents problems. His book *Black Thursday* was first published in 1960 and yet quotes an alleged SECRET report. How did he get hold of it then and why has it not been seen since?

As for Caidin himself, several people have tried to get in touch with him without success. Both myself and MUFON Journal editor Dennis Stacy have tried to track him down via his publishers and a UFO magazine that he has written for, but to no avail. He last appeared in the dodgy US UFO magazine *UFO Universe* in which he was featured on the front page as having 'chased bogies at 20,000 feet', (which was an astonishing spectacle no doubt!), but whilst the article gave details of UFOs he'd seen post WWII, government film of UFOs, cover-ups and you name it (along with mucho promotion for his many books, including UFO based novels) the Schweinfurt raid was never mentioned. Funny that, really.

So unless and until Caidin himself comes out of the woodwork with the original document to which he refers or until someone who was on the raid can verify the sighting or until other evidence about the event comes out, the discs mentioned by Martin Caidin seem to be nothing but a rumour - a rumour which like so many others has distorted UFO literature for many years.

On a more hopeful note, if the sightings did indeed take place, the event still has no real place in ufology, especially in the way it has been used. Remember from the original account the objects were only one inch by three inches which is stretching the small alien interpretation somewhat. In an air war context I would suggest that anything which is small and metallic and in clusters is some kind of 'window' or radar deflecting device, or some other war related artefact. Caidin's account also mentions that pilots saw "a mass of debris of varying sizes" in conjunction with the discs, suggesting that they had come from some explosive shell casing or damaged airplane. Note also that at least one plane was alleged to have flown through clusters of the discs "with absolutely no effect", suggesting that, like radar deflecting strips and their ilk, there was very little weight or mass to them. All this is pure speculation however. Finally, whilst this case is often included in foo fighter round-ups it really has no business there being atypical of the general foo fighter morphology and behaviour.

You may think I've been a bit pedantic here with this case but, it is very significant and the available facts need to be made known. If people are going to talk about sightings then let's at least be certain they happened. If 'cover-ups' are to be invoked, let's see some non-anecdotal evidence. As with the other foo fighter cover-up case from Germany (Project Uranus - a hoax which was generated by French ufologist Henry Durrant to see how far it would go - and it went all over the place!) the Caidin account has been repeated *ad nauseum* by UFO writers each trying to use the material for their own ends without looking into the source material - crap researchers the lot of 'em! If the document Caidin alludes to turns up - fair enough - but until then I am afraid that the case which launched the WWII cover-up idea seems to be on very shaky ground indeed.

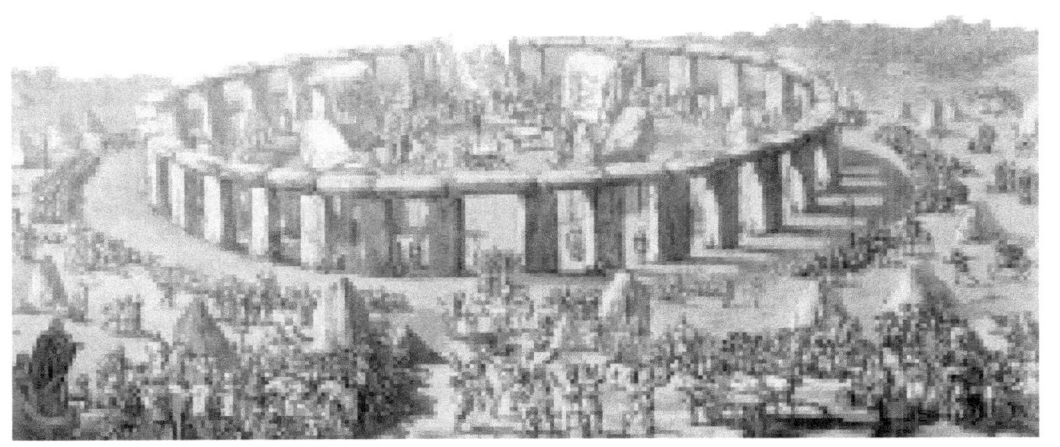

BETWEEN A ROCK AND A HARD PLACE
The Cracoe UFO photograph
From: *The UFOs That Never Were*, 1992

Or, how a rock became a UFO and then a rock once again . As Donovan
would have it , ' first there is a mountain, then there is no mountain, then there is.'

A BUFORA investigator has stated that the Cracoe photograph is 'light reflection.'
What UTTER RUBBISH!"-
Mark Birdsall *YUFOS Journal*, November 1983

"The Aliens Have Landed" screamed the *Daily Mirror* for Tuesday, August 23, 1983.

The headline was unequivocal, the accompanying photograph strange. It showed a bright, apparently luminescent, phenomenon against a rock face in the Yorkshire Dales Journalist John Gapper was impressed, writing, "This is the picture that UFO spotters claim is 'definite proof' that alien beings have ended on earth," before going on to reveal how two policemen had watched the UFO "hovering above the ground for an hour. The late Graham Birdsall, then the president of the Yorkshire UFO Society YUFOS, was noted as saying: "This is definite proof of the existence of UFOs. I am very excited about the photograph. It has convinced me that this is an area which they visit regularly. Something mysterious is happening out there, but I don't know what it is.

This newspaper article was the first major revelation to the British public of what came to be known as the 'Cracoe UFO Photographic Case'. The photograph was already two years old in 1983, but the case was to rumble on for another four years before it was finally laid to rest. And repercussions from the investigation are reverberating through the British UFO research community to this day.

Most photographs of alleged UFOs can usually be dismissed after analysis as obvious hoaxes, or camera or film-processing faults. UFO huffs place great ore in any photographs which elude explanation. Belief is strong that if a UFO is captured on film, it is somehow representative of the subject's reality status, elevating it from the shady realms of misperception or fantasy into those of scientific proof. However, less than critical UFO investigators are often quick to seize an unexplained UFO photograph in order to back up their particular beliefs and theories, ' The camera cannot lie," being their argument. The reality is usually somewhat different. A far more apt quote when one is dealing with UFO photographs is not "The camera cannot lie," but "Every picture tells a story." That the perception of unexplained photographic cases frequently leads to confusion and controversy is exemplified by the story which unfolded in the wake of the Cracoe Fell photographs.

The hamlet of Cracoe is situated just to the north of Skipton in the Yorkshire Dales National Park. It is a small place, with only a few hundred inhabitants, boasting a scattering of farms, houses, a pub and at one time a police house where the local constable lived. This police house and its occupants were the focus for the initial events of the Cracoe sighting on March 16, 1981.

At 10.55 that morning, Police Constable Steve Guest's wife was in the kitchen preparing a cup of tea for her husband and a visitor, PC Derek Ingram. The kitchen window overlooked a wide sweep of farm and moorland, which rises steeply to the summit of Cracoe Fell. As she gazed out across a landscape she and her husband must have seen many times each day, Mrs. Guest's attention was drawn to an amazing sight. According to the YUFOS file on the matter:

> "her eyes locked on to a most incredible sight. Suspended around the central rocks at the top of Cracoe Fell a series of five brightly lit spheres were shining. The glowing orbs hurt the witness's eyes. For two minutes, she remained at the window trying desperately to solve this most puzzling sight. She could not."

Mrs. Guest immediately called her husband into the kitchen to witness the puzzle. His official statement bears close scrutiny:

> "On Monday 16th March, 1981, I was in the kitchen of my house when I saw three bright lights on the rock face. I looked at the lights with my binoculars, but was unable to get a clear view, as if I was looking straight at bright car headlights.
>
> The lights were in a line, but there appeared to be a smaller light just to the side of the main light source. I saw a shape at the back of the lights, but was unable to make it out.
>
> "Sometime around 11.30, two RAF jets flew over the area. First one, then another, they were flying very slowly. There is no water on the rock face to give such a reflection, and to the best of my knowledge no metallic deposits. At about 11.55, the lights dimmed and became bright on several occasions, before disappearing. I have observed the fell every day at the same time. The light source has not reappeared. I have also spoken to several village residents who state they have no knowledge as to what could have caused the lights."

PC Ingram was called into the kitchen to witness the amazing sight. His account amplifies PC Guest's:

> "Please see account of Officer Guest, which I totally agree with. I remained

in the house during the entire incident until the lights disappeared. I am a keen amateur photographer and took the pictures between 11.15 am and 11.40 am. The lights appeared just below the top of the fell: they were hovering. The array of lights varied in intensity, and after one hour they vanished. There was no concrete shape yet the colour was the same as magnesium lights; they were brilliant. I found the lights unusual because on the fell (which is very steep) there is nothing to stand the lights on. The terrain makes it impossible to duplicate such an event."

That these witnesses to the Cracoe Fell 'UFO' were insincere in any way was never an issue. Nor was there any dispute about the veracity of the photographs which were taken. They were emphatically not hoaxed. But neither witness testimony nor photographic imagery is real proof of any objective reality. However, it was clear that these two police officers, trained in observational techniques and familiar with the local terrain, were spellbound by what they saw. There can be no doubt from both their statements and photographs that they believed *something* strange was taking place in Cracoe that day.

The phenomenon was clearly dramatic and memorable. So much so that when Derek Ingram recalled the event for a 1996 Discovery Channel TV documentary it was still vivid in his mind - "I saw a very intense bright light, a big band of light on the rock face of the fell".

At 11.15 am on March 16, partway through the sighting, the officers telephoned their sergeant, Tony Dodd, who was based in nearby Skipton. Dodd was a keen UFO buff and editor of YUFOS' Journal, *Quest*. He assured the officers that he was on his way, but that they should take no action as yet. At any time during the sighting, it would have been a relatively simple matter for the officers to drive halfway up the fell and walk the rest of the way to determine the cause of the phenomenon. People often query why they did not. But the witnesses had no idea how long the sighting would last, or how important it was going to become for believers in Unidentified Flying Objects.

At 11.20 am, one of the officers made a "vital discovery," seeing a "triangular fin" behind the central light. A 'fin' seemed to imply attachment to an object. What - or who - on earth could be responsible for a brightly lit object hovering against the side of a sheer rock face?' This was the first hint that the Cracoe UFO may have been an artificial construction.

At 11.55 am, the UFO was still being observed by the police officers. Then its lights began to pulsate in unison, dimming and brightening several times until, one by one, they went out, and the UFO vanished. Shortly afterwards, the astonished officers watched as two military jets "crossed right over the spot where the unknown targets had hovered ... The officers were puzzled by this.'" The bizarre sighting had lasted almost an hour. During that time six colour transparency pictures were taken of the phenomena. Unfortunately, both police officers were off-duty. Had they not been, an official police enquiry into the matter may have solved the case before it assumed mythic proportions. But clues as to the true nature of the case were seeded very early on in the investigation. On the first day, in fact.

Local farmer Derek Carlisle had been outside the police house during some part of the sighting. He told the officers the phenomenon was not a UFO, but a bright rock reflection, one he had seen many times before. The police witnesses dismissed his claims out of hand. YUFOS claimed they had evidence which "negated" Carlisle as a "vital observer," but agreed that as he had been looking at the same phenomena as the police; his theory should be taken into account.

The police officers made statements shortly after the UFO had disappeared and the slide film was passed on to a YUFOS investigator for processing at a "confidential address in Hull."

In the weeks following the sighting, YUFOS investigators did an excellent job in determining what the UFO could not have been. The area was examined in detail. Nothing could be found to account for the phenomenon. Environmental factors such as snow, ice and running water as a possible cause for the sighting were also ruled out. YUFOS enquiries revealed there had been no helicopters in the area, but they considered the overflight of military jets at the conclusion of sighting to be "most interesting," and "more than coincidence." As there had been a major NATO exercise on March 16, it was at first thought that the lights may have been some form of target or marker. The RAF verified they had fighter jets on low-flying practice in that area, but the "object," as they put it, had nothing to do with them. In any case, PCs Ingram and Guest had gone to the top of the fell as soon as the sighting was over and they found no evidence of any military hardware. YUFOS therefore concluded that "The military aircraft overflights had, in fact, seen the light formation and made a pass."

YUFOS were rightly puzzled by both sighting and photographs. But rather than releasing the information to the media immediately, they sensibly decided to spend the next two years investigating the case in some considerable depth before releasing their findings.

But for the inexplicable photographs, this event would probably have just gone down in history as yet another lights-in--the-sky-case, intriguing at the time, but impossible to verify or investigate. However photographic evidence is rare and valuable. YUFOS had the pictures analysed at four establishments, the now defunct Ground Saucer Watch (GSW) in the USA. Klaus Webner, a UFO investigator in Germany, a "police source," and at Leeds University.

Full results of the lengthy analysis from the first two were released in 1985 by YUFOS. Like the farmer's claims, this analysis flagged up points which should have been taken more seriously at the time.

Ground Saucer Watch concluded that whilst they were convinced the photographs were genuine, "there is no evidence that the anomalous images are 'objects' hovering between the witnesses and the distant mountain's hills." Klaus Webner's conclusions included the statement, "I have found no evidence that there was anything in the air between Cracoe Fell and the eye-witnesses." Webner also believed that the photographs were genuine, not hoaxed, and they mooted the possibility that they were lights used by mountaineers. Neither report could positively identify the phenomenon. Nor did they mention a 'fin' or craft of any kind. Far more interesting were the comments made by the analyst at Leeds University. Due to his position as head of a science department, he requested anonymity in YUFOS' published reports.

After studying the photographs in depth, he called the YUFOS investigative team together and then he astonished them with his conclusions. He was convinced the photographs showed something above the lights and said:

> "What you probably have is a most unusual structure which looks oval to the eye, yet is perhaps round. Beneath the structure (or craft) appear to be three almost circular globes ... You have an object which is tilted back towards the fell face ... It is displaying three remarkable and very luminous lights. I do not think it is natural."

The pseudonymous 'Mulligan' drew a picture to illustrate what he meant. The drawing was of a classic Adamski-type flying saucer.

YUFOS were "both delighted and bemused." "What," they mused, "was the scientist trying to tell us?"

Whereas the GSW and Webner's analyses were open to interpretation, Mulligan's was not. Here YUFOS had a qualified scientist, working at one of the country's finest universities, effectively claiming that a flying saucer had been captured on film. The three Cracoe Reports (published between 1985 and 1986) contained a vast amount of investigative data concerning the initial sighting, photographic analysis and theories pertaining to the case, both for - and against – the phenomenon being a structured object. But by far the most significant evidence in favour that it was came when Mrs. and Mrs. John Ackroyd related their sighting from March 16, 1981.

From South Yorkshire, the Ackroyds were on an excursion to the Yorkshire Dales, driving past Cracoe at around 3.45 pm when they saw three glowing spheres high over the fell. They initially believed them to be aircraft lights, but the apparent speed and height were not consistent with any aircraft with which they were familiar. After stopping their car and observing them for a while, it became clear there was a "dark shape" above the lights. Now they were certain it was not an aircraft. Puzzled, the couple drove off, and did not mention the incident until they attended a YUFOS lecture in 1985 in which the Cracoe case was featured heavily. At the end of the meeting, Mr. Ackroyd approached YUFOS officials, saying simply, "My wife and I saw that thing over Cracoe."

The implication was potentially earth-shattering. Given that the phenomenon the police officers and the Ackroyds saw was the same, a "structured craft of unknown origin" was indeed seen in the skies above Cracoe. What's more, it must have been in the area, if not constantly in the air, for over four hours on that fateful day in 1981.

YUFOS came to no firm conclusions as to the specific nature or origin of the 'UFO', but had already publicly stated in 1983 that "an unknown structure lies behind the lights - this is covered by a stream of white lights;" and "for the record, the Cracoe UFO is undoubtedly solid". I recall querying the nature of the phenomenon at a 1986 YUFOS lecture in Burnley and being told it depicted a "structured craft of unknown origin." It was clear that they believed it was solid, and capable of flight and light emission.

Throughout the Cracoe reports, YUFOS had often referred to and carefully considered Farmer Carlisle's contention that the UFO had its origins in reflected sunlight. By the end of the third edition of Cracoe: The *Evidence,* their research teams had narrowed this possibility down to zero, saying:

> "YUFOS research conjectured that the three almost circular spheres of dazzling light were not caused by sunlight reflection. The photographic content confirms this, as does *scientific* evidence."

Until YUFOS released the photographs to the media in 1983, the Cracoe case was virtually unknown both to the public and within the UK's tightly-knit UFO research community. No ufologists from other research groups had been involved in the initial investigations, and YUFOS chose to share their evidence with only a few trusted colleagues. Once the case became public knowledge, other ufologists began to scrutinise the case.

The popular perception of UFO investigation is that Ufologists share one goal, that of solving the UFO mystery, and will happily assist each other where necessary. This is a completely erroneous view of the subject. In reality, the UFO community is comprised of many small, warring factions, each driven more by belief than fact. UFO groups rarely share their information, especially *if* one group is likely to take a different view from another.

On the surface, this may appear counter-productive, but it is actually a positive state *of* affairs because it is only from these frequently intense disputes and re-evaluations of evidence that the truth of a case often emerges. Had no other investigators become involved in the Cracoe case, it would probably still be listed as 'unknown' and the photographs now elevated to classic status. YUFOS investigation of the Cracoe photograph is only half the story. The denouement comes in the aftermath of the case being made public and its subsequent re-investigation.

YUFOS released the photographs to the media in August 1983. Newspapers and TV immediately seized on the images, which were featured widely in the national Press. The *Daily Mirror,* whose headline opened this chapter, faithfully promised YUFOS they would not hype the alien angle, but went ahead and did it anyway. To their credit, YUFOS had never actually overtly claimed the Cracoe UFO was alien in origin and demanded an apology. But it was too late: the damage had been done. Whatever anyone thought of the Cracoe UFO, in the eyes of the public it was extraterrestrial in origin.

Local newspapers played their part in spreading the Cracoe myth, too. The *Yorkshire Post's* front page offered "UFO Over Yorks" whilst the Skipton based *Craven Herald,* Cracoe's local paper, ran a sensible piece entitled "UFO Siting (sic) Confirmed." They quoted YUFOS Graham Birdsall as saying:

> "We have kept this under wraps for two years because we wanted to be absolutely certain the photograph could not be knocked down when we released it. During that time, we have covered the area with a small tooth-comb, and it has left us in no doubt that no natural phenomenon could have caused this to hover there for just under an hour."

It took six days before the *Herald* was running a piece which effectively 'knocked' both the photograph and Graham's certainties for a six. The article was headed "UFO Rubbish!" and read:

> "Reports that a shiny object seen on Cracoe Fell were conclusive proof of alien visitors to the earth have been dismissed as "rubbish" by a local farmer.
>
> Hetton farmer Mr. D. Carlisle said the phenomenon often occurred on dull days when the sun caught rocks on the fell. 'It's quite spectacular, but that's all there is to it,' he explained. He was present on the morning two years ago when two policemen photographed the shining fell, and recognised it as the same optical illusion he had seen there before."

This account of the Cracoe UFO's origins did not fit in with the media's fondness for stories about aliens and was soon forgotten. But experienced UFO researcher Nigel Mortimer saw it. Had it not been for his vigilance, the outcome of the Cracoe case may have been entirely different. Nigel lived quite near Cracoe and decided to investigate the case on behalf of BUFORA. After seeing the media furore surrounding the Cracoe case and specifically Farmer Carlisle's statement, Nigel concluded eventually that there could well be a prosaic solution to the case and began to visit the area regularly, confident the rock reflection hypothesis was valid. Although he saw many rock reflections, none was anything like the Cracoe 'UFO' Nor could he identify the exact location of the phenomena captured on film by the police officers. But serious doubts had now been raised about the case - and they spread like wildfire through the British UFO community.

Meanwhile *Quest,* the YUFOS journal, which regularly featured updates concerning the on-going Cracoe investigation. One such piece about the photographic analysis was immediately followed by an article titled: "Just Coincidence? The Cracoe Connection." This dealt with several sightings of flying discs with three bright balls on the underside, all of them from the Cracoe area. Was this what the scientist at Leeds University was trying to tell YUFOS? Writer Mark Birdsall concluded,

> "We have already had a tantalising glimpse of something very similar in relation to the argument for one particular type of unknown vehicle ... The Cracoe UFO."

In March 1986, I was asked by Paul Devereux, author and then editor of *The Ley Hunter* magazine, to write a piece about the Cracoe UFO as a possible example of earthlight phenomena. I had been interested in the Cracoe area for several years as a focus for earthlight activity and agreed carefully to analyse both the YUFOS data and Nigel Mortimer's speculations before coming to any conclusion. Problems were immediately encountered in obtaining a copy of the YUFOS report for research purposes.

These were advertised in YUFOS' journal as being available to anyone, but my request was refused.

The reason given was because "you would not agree with YUFOS' conclusions." The case was getting interesting already! Nigel Mortimer was digging deep into the case, too, and facing similar obstructions. In a heated telephone conversation with YUFOS' Director of Research, Mark Birdsall, Nigel was told he had no business investigating a case which "wasn't his." "How can anyone 'own' a UFO case?" Nigel wondered. The situation deteriorated further when YUFOS' Executive Committee issued a statement in which they disassociated themselves from national investigations co-coordinator Jenny Randles, Nigel Mortimer and the British UFO Research Association (BUFORA), saying they did not regard them as serious investigators. This followed BUFORA's open support of the "light reflection theory." It was clear that sceptics were not going to enjoy any co-operation with YUFOS, as they clearly regarded the Cracoe case as 'theirs'.

This was just the motivation we needed to persist in cracking the case wide open. I and other researchers from the West Yorkshire UFO Research Group (WYUFORG) began to visit the Cracoe area frequently, searching for clues to the mystery. But we were in a difficult position. Unable to obtain access either to the original photographs or to the main witnesses, we only had YUFOS reports to go on. And YUFOS would not move from their certainty that the Cracoe UFO photographs represented a "structured craft of unknown origin."

Intrigued by YUFOS' continual refusal even to consider, never mind actually to discuss, an alternative explanation for the Cracoe 'UFO,' we decided to contact the farmer, Derek Carlisle, ourselves. He was only too pleased to be interviewed. In September 1986, we spoke to him for an hour at his farm in the village of Cracoe. Mr. Carlisle stood by his 1981 comments to the local newspaper saying:

> "I was present outside Cracoe police station on the 16th of March 1981. I observed the lights for not more than 15 minutes. The lights were on Rylestone Fell ... The weather conditions were overcast with outbreaks of sun. The lights I observed were as portrayed in the photograph and in that location. I have seen these lights both before and after on many occasions, as have my wife and son. The lights appear when the rocks are wet ... and when the sun shines on the wet surfaces ... My attitude towards the UFO phenomenon is one of an open mind. In my opinion, the lights I saw were nothing else other than the sun shining on the rocks. On the day in question, the lights were brighter than I've seen before. I did not notice any structure whatsoever behind the rocks."

Mr. Carlisle also noted that he, like many other Cracoe villagers, thought there was - and is - "something" unusual going on in the area, adding that a few weeks before our interview, bright lights were seen at night high on Cracoe Fell. The fact that he was not totally sceptical *of* the UFO phenomenon as a whole gave further credence to his story, even though YUFOS, who had spent hundreds *of* man hours and thousands of pounds on the case, still vehemently disagreed with him.

If Mr. Carlisle's version of the sighting was correct, the phenomenon could theoretically at least, be treated scientifically and replicated. Replication of the original photograph would be proof positive of the true nature of the Cracoe UFO. The only problem was just how to catch the phenomenon in action. I and other WYUFORG members literally 'stalked' the fell, visiting it several times a month at all hours and in all weathers throughout the autumn of 1986.

During this period, YUFOS published an issue of *Quest* which reviewed the evidence to date and railed against those investigators who had dared to voice an alternative opinion about the case. It highlighted a letter from one of the original witnesses, PC Derek Ingram, in which he reiterated his beliefs about the sighting, claiming, "In my opinion there was an unexplained object on the fell on the day in question, and how anybody can put it down to mere reflection is beyond me."

November 1986 finally brought a breakthrough. On a family day out in the Yorkshire Dales, I stopped in Cracoe as usual in order to look up at the fell, more out of habit than hope. The weather was cloudy with occasional shafts of sunlight. I stared at the distant rocky ridge, yet again pondering just what could have been so dramatic enough to enchant two police officers for almost an hour. As I mused, my attention was caught by a glint of light. Attention slowly turned to interest and then quite rapidly to astonishment as I realised I was looking at the Cracoe UFO! Just below the ridge of the fell, some two miles away, was a narrow strip of brilliant light, interspersed with bright 'blobs'. I grabbed the binoculars from the car and studied the light closely. There was no doubt about it: this was the Cracoe 'UFO'. Had the "structured object of unknown origin" returned five-and-a-half years on especially for my benefit, or was I looking at the elusive rock reflection seen by Derek Carlisle and speculated on by Nigel Mortimer? Was I looking at the *real* Cracoe UFO?

I returned to Cracoe a week later. Now I knew exactly where to look, the 'UFO' was instantly visible, albeit again not as bright as the 1981 police photographs. Several shots were taken with and without a zoom lens. When these pictures were processed and the image enlarged, the true nature of the Cracoe 'UFO' was apparent.

Comparison done by Mike Wootten for BUFORA showed that the two images - the police officers' from 1981 and mine from 1986 - were of *exactly* the same phenomena. Now that I had identified the correct area on the fell, I visited the site to see the now-landed Cracoe 'UFO' at first hand. As Farmer Carlisle correctly believed, the 'UFO' was due to an optical illusion. The cause of all the fuss was a rock surface just below the ridge of the fell, easily accessible by foot and about a forty-five-minute walk from the roadside. Water draining from the moor combined with lichen and produced three vague marks on the angled rocks. This combination of circumstances, coupled with tiny quartz crystals embedded in the gritstone rock, gave off a reflection which appeared as a strip of white, with three or more circles in it. The reflection could only be seen from specific locations and under certain light conditions, although once the visitor knows where to look it can be identified at any time in daylight hours.

But why had no-one cracked the case before? YUFOS unwittingly obfuscated independent researchers by printing the police officer's photographs the wrong way round. This made it extremely difficult to locate the exact area of fell amongst the tumult of rocks on Cracoe Fell. In addition, the photographs used by the media and in YUFOS publications and lectures were enlargements. This made the 'UFO' appear considerably larger than it actually was. To the naked eye, the phenomenon, no matter how bright, is quite small and distant when it is seen from Cracoe village. This was never actually made clear by the YUFOS investigators, who had also insisted their calculations gave the length of the 'UFO' as over ten metres. In fact, the entire rock on which the 'Cracoe UFO' appears is barely five metres long. YUFOS investigators must have walked past, if not actually over, the 'UFO' on several occasions!

Several UFO researchers from other groups were shown the photographs and taken to the fell to see the phenomenon at first hand. All agreed that the 'Cracoe UFO', the "structured object of unknown origin," was nothing more than an unusual rock reflection. I then contacted one of the original YUFOS analysts, Klaus Webner, and sent him copies of my photographs for his comment. He replied:

> "The 'Cracoe UFO' is unmasked. Your slides show the same phenomena under controlled conditions. The intensity of the light is not the same as it is on the Cracoe photos, but the position of the reflection is absolutely the same. Your slide is evidence that a harmless reflection on this sloping area of rock is responsible for the huge UFO headlines in the newspapers."

Now completely certain I had caught the Cracoe 'UFO' on film, the most logical course of action was to inform YUFOS, in order to give them the opportunity to examine the evidence and retract their grandiose statements about the photographs. Despite their reluctance to share the information, WYUFORG and I had consistently operated a policy of informing YUFOS officials of our every move in attempting to solve this case. Philip Mantle, their Overseas Liaison Officer and "team leader on ground research" in the Cracoe investigation, was apprised of the situation and invited to view the proof. He declined, saying that the next issue of *Quest* would "leave you and your colleagues in no doubt that the Cracoe photographs do not depict light reflection." It did not!

YUFOS punctuated their head-in-the-sand attitude by issuing yet another edition of the Cracoe report.

Hoping this might at least shed new light on their reluctance to accept alternative evidence, I attempted to obtain the report, only to be told,

> "As you are probably aware, liaison with WYFORG does not exist, and to allow reports which are for the benefits of serious researchers to be sent to your group at this time will conflict with our current attitude towards your group."

YUFOS might not have been interested in the reality of the Cracoe 'UFO', but the *Yorkshire Post*, which had broken the story in 1983, was. Journalist Tim Zillessen was fascinated by the twists and turns of the case and quoted me as saying:

> "We believe we have incontrovertible proof that it is nothing more than a complex light reflection. Undoubtedly, a lot of people saw something that day, but unfortunately they do not accept a rational explanation for it and still refuse to do so. We did not set out deliberately to dispel or to disprove the sighting: we simply set out to investigate it. We are open-minded enough to accept a UFO sighting when it happens, but not in this case."

In the interests of balance Zillessen contacted YUFOS for their comments. Mark Birdsall, still refusing to accept the case was solved, opined: "We absolutely reject any suggestion that the sighting was a light reflection. We are convinced something was seen on that day on the fell." Birdsall attempted to divert

Post readers from the facts by making:

> "a stinging attack on the research group and the photographic analyst. He said the group had only been in existence for three years and did not have enough information to make any positive claims. He dismissed the analyst as a great sceptic who had no scientific authority to make any judgments."

Obviously the scientific replication of the exact phenomena did not actually count as "enough evidence" for YUFOS to retract their claims!"

Mark Birdsall claimed he had again visited the officers who witnessed and photographed the 'UFO' and they still stuck to their accounts. Whether the original witnesses stuck to their accounts or not was yet another red herring and never an issue. It was the interpretation of the phenomenon caught on film which had been under scrutiny. In a final attempt to convince YUFOS, Graham and Mark Birdsall, together with Philip Mantle, were invited to see the photographs I had taken of the Cracoe 'UFO'. The meeting was not a success. It appeared that YUFOS could not - or would not - accept the factual evidence before them.

However, the majority of ufologists chose to believe the scientific interpretation: which was that the police had photographed and misperceived a rock reflection. The only alternative explanation, if the 1981 police photographs *did* depict a "structured craft of unknown origin," was that this particular 'UFO' enjoyed the ability to replicate the exact size, shape and position of a naturally occurring light reflection. What are the chances of that happening?

Although the case was now solved, huge question marks still hung over the whole affair. Why did two police officers become transfixed for almost an hour by a tiny natural phenomenon? Why did the case attain the status of a cause celebre for YUFOS, being featured heavily in their magazine and becoming a centrepiece of their lectures? Why did a scientist at Leeds University claim the photographs depicted a flying disc? Why did the Ackroyd family believe that their aerial sighting later that day was the same phenomenon as shown on the Cracoe 'UFO' photograph? These are just a few of the questions raised by the Cracoe case. The answer to them all can be summed up in two words - expectation and misperception The misperception in the Cracoe case was truly dramatic. The police officer who lived in the police house at Cracoe had done so for quite some time.

According to their sergeant, Tony Dodd, "his knowledge of the location is second to none." Both he and his wife must have looked across at the fell from their kitchen on numerous occasions without seeing the 'UFO'. Yet the combination of environmental phenomena which comprise the Cracoe 'UFO' is visible to some degree or other *every single day*.

Why - and how - on the morning of March 16, 1981, did the natural become the supernatural?

Unusual and unidentified lights *had* been seen in the Cracoe region for a number of years prior to 1981, possibly for centuries if folklore is to be believed. Some locals apparently even referred to the area as "flying saucer alley," so it could be said there was a long-standing *tradition* of UFOs in the area. Since the late 1970s, the Yorkshire UFO Society had been quite active in the area, interviewing witnesses and holding skywatches. Their presence and beliefs were reported by the media, so the UFO myth was fed back into the community, and so on. UFO sightings were part and parcel of the contemporary living folklore of the area in the 1970s and '80s.

This tradition was well known to the police witnesses involved through their sergeant in Skipton, Tony Dodd. In his book *Alien Investigator,* Dodd recounts how he saw many UFOs in the Cracoe area from

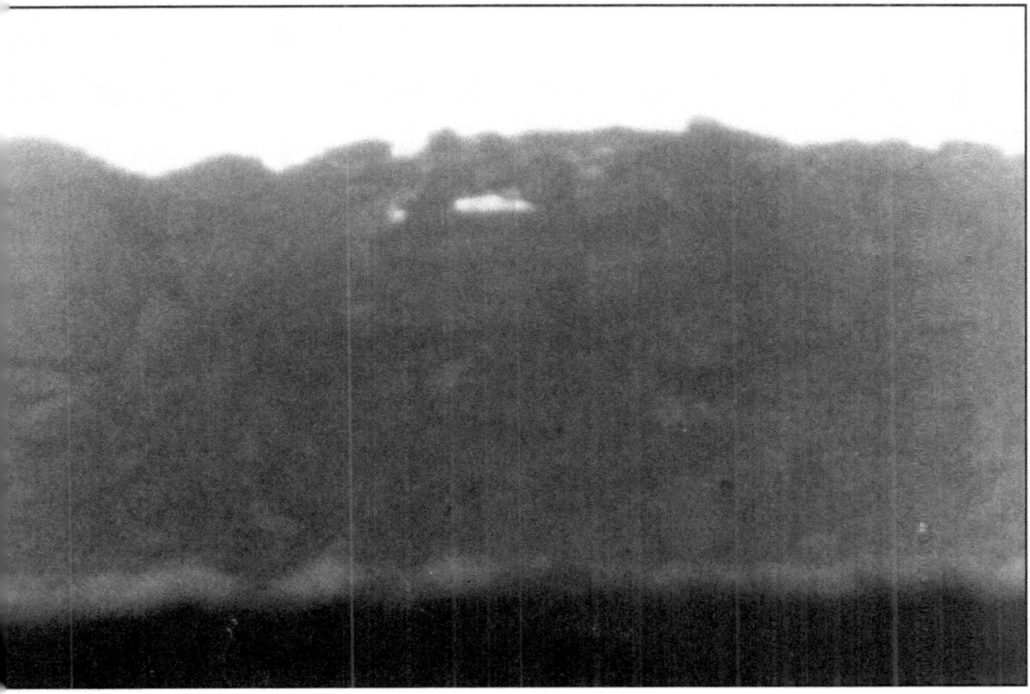

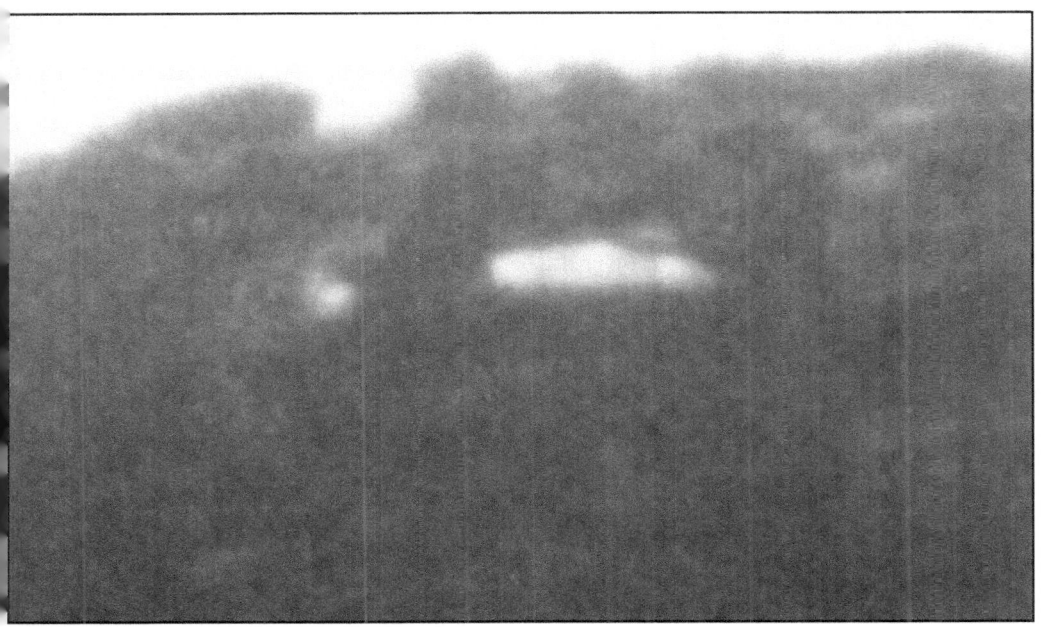

Above: Cracoe 'UFO' as photographed by police officers and published in the *Yorkshire Post*
Below: Cracoe 'UFO' - in fact a rock reflection- as photographed by Andy Roberts

1978 onwards. Several of these were witnessed whilst in the company of other police officers. Many were of quite dramatic craft. One which Dodd saw only miles away from Cracoe was a "large object, dome shaped, with white light coming from what looked like windows," whilst another from the same area was "a massive disc, with a dome shape on top."

Dodd's belief was that these craft were alien in origin and that his sightings were "an education I was being *given* by the aliens." It is likely that Dodd's interest in UFOs, if not his belief in aliens, was widely known throughout the police force in the Cracoe area, and that this led to a cross-contamination of belief and expectation. Because of this climate of expectation, a lump of shiny rock became misperceived as a UFO.

The subject of misperception is central to any understanding of the UFO enigma. But it is a subject that is widely misunderstood. Most people cannot comprehend how even the most highly trained observers can misinterpret mundane objects as UFOs. But they do. Each year thousands of people see birds, planes, and meteorological and astronomical phenomena as 'UFOs'. The current cultural template and active folklore regarding anything strange seen in the sky is automatically to dub it a 'UFO', whilst the media automatically associates the acronym with 'aliens' or 'extraterrestrials'. As Jenny Randles has said about the interaction between witness and media, "Woman sees spaceship" is news, whereas "Woman sees spaceship, but was probably mistake" is not. It does not matter if the witness is from a background of trained observation, such as a policeman or pilot.

There is never any such individual as the totally credible witness. *Everyone is* equally susceptible to misperception in that magic moment when they see something unknown. If a witness already has a belief system to fit a 'UFO' sighting into, or a predisposition to 'believe' in any aspect of the supernatural, the situation is further exacerbated. Tony Dodd said of his increasing sightings in the Cracoe area during the 1970s and '80s that "the extraordinary was becoming the ordinary." The sighting by the police officers at Cracoe was a case of the reverse of this - the moment the ordinary becomes the extraordinary.

This moment, the transition from 'ordinary consciousness' to 'UFO consciousness', is at the very core of the UFO mystery.

Unfortunately, UFO buffs fail to learn from the significant lessons taught by cases such as Cracoe and others like them. They soon forget the wild claims, the 'scientific' analyses, and the far-out theories. Instead of applying the principles learned to other cases, they move on to the next 'unexplained' case in the hope it will be the 'big one'. Eventually, in the face of overwhelming evidence, YUFOS underwent a paradigm change. In 1987, by which time no one now believed in the 'structured craft' interpretation of the Cracoe photographs, Tony Dodd wrote a piece for *Quest* magazine in which he re-framed the Cracoe photographs as being a rock reflection. There was no mention of the dramatic struggles between rival viewpoints about the nature of evidence which had been necessary to get to this point.

By 1997, Graham and Mark Birdsall, later editors and owners of the hugely successful *UFO Magazine (UK)* and *The Unopened Files*, felt able to use the Cracoe case in a round-up of sightings for the 40th anniversary of Kenneth Arnold's sighting. This time around the photograph was merely captioned: "Lights photographed on Cracoe Fell, near Skipton, North Yorkshire on 16 March, 1981. The 'UFO' is in fact simply sun rays striking the rock surface."

The extraordinary had become the ordinary once again.

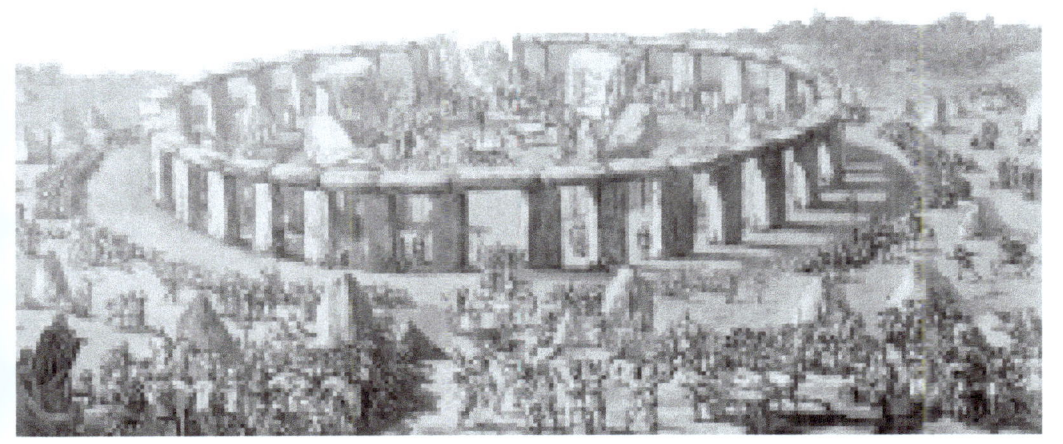

THE ACID TEST FOR LSD

A little known ESP experiment involving the Grateful Dead *and LSD*

In December 2000 parapsychologist Richard Wiseman announced he was going to conduct the "world's largest telepathy experiment" in London [FT143:24]. Unfortunately, however, Wiseman's experiment, using up to 100 telepathic 'senders', fell well short of the far more Fortean approach taken by a group of parapsychologists and musicians towards the end of the psychedelic era in America.

The real 'world's largest telepathy experiment' actually took place in February 1971 at Port Chester in New York State. Far from being conducted in the psychically arid test conditions of a laboratory, it was hosted by the world's strangest rock and roll band, the *Grateful Dead*. The Dead themselves are no strangers to Fortean phenomena, and the synchronicities surrounding their gigs at the Great Pyramid of Giza and percussionist Micky Hart's encounter with a cursed human skull drum are the stuff of legend [see FT88:34-38, FT164:24-25]. Unarguably at the cutting edge of genuinely psychedelic music, and all that entails, the *Grateful Dead* were forged in the crucible of 1960s American West Coast acid culture, playing to huge crowds where band and audience were under the influence of the strongest psychedelics.

Their music to this day both encompasses and surpasses all contemporary and historical forms, leading one critic to define their oeuvre as "music beyond idiom". Accounts of the sheer power generated at a *Grateful Dead* gig are legion, band and followers believing that when they are playing at full throttle a temporary psychedelic psychic 'church' is created in which musicians and celebrants are joined in a sort of 'wholly communion', becoming a single entity with one mind.

Micky Hart puts this succinctly:

> "Our main focus was the idea of group mind. We saw the *Grateful Dead* as a group mind and one in which we were able to share with the audience. We were able to take an image and project it into the audience and send it to receptive receivers." With this kind of belief it was only a matter of time before the parapsychological fraternity became seriously interested in the *Grateful Dead*.

The link came in the form of parapsychologist and author Stanley Krippner, at that time director of the Maimonides Dream Laboratory in Brooklyn, New York. Krippner had been working at the far edges of parapsychology for several years and since 1964 had been involved in experiments testing the hypothesis "that sleeping subjects are able to incorporate aspects of randomly selected target stimuli into their dreams". Krippner was also a Dead fan and had used their music in previous ESP experiments. The *Grateful Dead*'s biographer, Dennis McNally, described, in *A Long Strange Trip: The Inside History of the Grateful Dead* (Bantam, NY, 2002), Krippner's entry into the Dead's world:

> "Krippner was yet another of the fascinating people the Dead had attracted, a distinguished psychologist who was comfortable with the rational study of 'fuzzy' things like ESP, or psychedelics, or both together."

Jerry Garcia, the Dead's lead guitarist, and Micky Hart first met Stanley Krippner at a party in 1970. McNally recalls,

> "Eventually Krippner found himself in conversation with Garcia, who wondered about the potential interaction of various altered states of consciousness, for instance sleep and the psychedelic state, and whether or not that could aid sensitivity to ESP. Their conversation eventually yielded the Dream Experiment, which was deemed worthy of publication in a formal, academically refereed journal of psychology."

Krippner initially conducted a smaller version of the Port Chester experiments, in which ESP, hundreds of people, rock music and psychedelics were brought together. This took place at a *Holy Modal Rounders* concert on 15 March 1970 where five volunteer telepathy 'receivers' were selected for the experiment. Each receiver was told the geographical location of the concert and asked to 'tune in' at midnight, when certain images would be telepathically projected by the audience. The receivers were situated at random locations within a 100-mile (160km) radius of the concert venue. The target image chosen to be projected was 'birds', and a sequence of appropriate moving images and transparencies was prepared by the psychedelic light show operator Jean Mayo. These consisted of a film about eagles and a number of slides depicting photographs of various birds, together with key symbols such as the Egyptian hieroglyph for bird and phrases such as 'Think birds' and 'fly high'. One crucial slide sequence showed a mythological phoenix appearing and disappearing in flames.

The audience were informed verbally that when these images appeared they were to concentrate on them and 'send' them telepathically. To create the strongest link between the target images, the power of the music and the audience, the images were projected during the band's performance of *If You Want to Be a Bird*. This song was already fixed in the audience's minds as it had been featured in the 1969 cult film *Easy Rider*, during a sequence in which Jack Nicholson looned around on the back of a motorcycle.

Midnight duly passed and the audience, high on music and drugs and open to the potential of telepathic contact, did their best to project the chosen images into the collective unconscious. The five receivers reported variously, 'something mythological, like a Griffin or a Phoenix', 'a snake', 'grapes', 'an embryo in flames growing into a tree'. The fifth receiver was singer Richie Havens, who also reported seeing a mythological creature like a phoenix.

Was this experiment successful? Maybe. Interpreting a telepathy experiment can be difficult because, unless the images received are exactly the same as the ones sent, the results are open to scepticism at best, ridicule at worst. However, at least two of the images received appeared to be within acceptable parameters and Krippner felt that with some important changes to the methodology of the experiment, he could improve the results.

Buoyed up by the apparent success of the *Holy Modal Rounders* experiment, Krippner decided to plan something much more ambitious involving the *Grateful Dead*. This was to take place at each gig of the Dead's six-night run at the Capitol Theatre in Port Chester, New York State, during February 1971. The Port Chester shows themselves have become legendary in 'Deadhead' circles as being fantastic examples of the transformative and redemptive power of music. Listening to them you are aware of a music being created which is truly 'out there', an ideal backdrop against which to conduct a telepathy experiment.

Contrary to the somewhat shambolic psychedelic milieu in which the *Grateful Dead* existed, the Port Chester experiments were planned in some detail. In attempting to refine the methodology used at the *Holy Modal Rounders* experiment, Krippner's team made some radical changes. It was decided to make the instructions to the senders (the audience) much more specific, and also to make them aware of the physical location of one of the receivers. To insure against the possibility of the target images being leaked, either consciously or unconsciously, they were to be selected at random immediately prior to being shown to the senders.

For the Port Chester experiments just two receivers, Malcolm Bessent and Felicia Parise, were chosen.

Both were experienced 'psychic sensitives'. During the experiment Bessent was to be observed whilst under laboratory conditions, sleeping at the Maimonides Dream Laboratory, 45 miles (72km) away. Parise was to sleep in her flat where she would be telephoned several times during the night and asked to describe the content of her dreams.

The audiences on each night were told only about Bessent's involvement in the experiment. This was so the Dream Laboratory staff could monitor 'intentionality', i.e. whether or not the senders' knowledge of who was taking part and where they were could affect results. In this case, if intentionality was relevant it would be expected that Bessent would have more success in receiving the images than would Parise. Conversely, if it were the receiver whose subconscious mind reached out and located the target images, both senders could be expected to score equally well.

Krippner's assistant, Ronnie Mastrian, was in the audience at the Capitol Theatre and immediately prior to each gig selected one of two envelopes by the flipping of a coin. Each envelope contained a series of slides containing images to be the focus of the evening's experiment. The selected transparencies were loaded into a projector and shown on the stage backdrop. At 11.30pm when the concert was well under way, the bemused and excited audience read the instruction slides;:

> "1) You are about to participate in an ESP experiment,
> 2) In a few seconds you will see a picture,
> 3) Try using your ESP to 'send' this picture to Malcolm Bessent,
> 4) He will try to dream about the picture. Try to send it to him,
> 5) Malcolm Bessent is now at the Maimonides dream laboratory in Brooklyn".

One of six randomly selected pictures was then projected onto the stage backdrop for 15 minutes whilst the *Grateful Dead* played. Unusually for the Dead, there was no psychedelic light show at any of the Port Chester gigs, thus making the projected images the visual focus of the concert.

When Malcolm Bessent had been observed to be engaged in REM (Rapid Eye Movement) activity for 10 minutes, he was woken and asked what he was dreaming. This took place several times throughout the night. Felicia Parise was contacted by 'phone at 90 minute intervals and her dreams recorded. On the following morning, both subjects were asked to add any details that they had missed, together with any associations they attached to their dreams. Their recollections were tape-recorded and transcribed for use by the evaluators.

At the end of the six-show run, the two evaluators were each given the full receivers' transcripts together with copies of the images used. The evaluators, working independently of each other, or the telepathy receivers or Dream Laboratory staff, were asked to read the tape transcripts. They then recorded on a 100-point scale any correspondences between the dream recollections and the images projected during the experiment.

As with the *Holy Modal Rounders* experiment, the results were encouraging, but were open to a wide spectrum of interpretation.

One example of this dichotomy can be seen from the 19 February gig where a painting called *The Seven Spinal Chakras* was projected. This showed a male in the yogic full lotus position, deep in meditation, each chakra vividly illuminated. When Bessent was awakened during this specific run of the experiment he remembered dreaming he was, "very interested in... using natural energy... thinking about rocket ships... an energy box and... a spinal column". This correspondence was classed as a success, although sceptics will have their doubts.

Another debatable success came from the night of 20 February when the surrealist painter Magritte's *Philosophy in the Boudoir* was selected and projected. The painting is of a headless woman wearing a transparent robe. Bessent dreamed about a "little girl's doll" which Krippner believed demonstrated "a degree of correspondence".

The Dream Laboratory's report on the experiment noted:

> "The average evaluation of the two judges was computed for each pair of dream transcripts and target pictures. If coincidence, rather than ESP, had been operating, the judges' evaluation of the correct transcript/target pairs would have been higher than all other pairs one time out of six. For Miss Parise, one correct pair obtained the highest rating. In the case of Mr Bessent, the judges gave the highest score to the correct pairs four times out of six... Thus, for MrBessent, the ESP hypothesis is supported. Further, some support is given to the position that the agents must know who the target is to be transmitted to and where he is located for telepathy to occur."

So, were the experiments a success? Krippner and his team certainly thought so, although sceptics and debunkers will snort derisively at the lack of rigour in parts of the experiment's design. And, of course, the results were open to interpretation and raised many questions, such as: how clearly and exactly does a received image have to correspond with the image projected? Does the whole dream have to correspond with the target image? – and so on. No-one said parapsychology was easy!

Other rock commentators doubted the psychedelic component of the experiment. Former band manager (and not entirely reliable commentator) Rock Scully, in his book *Living With The Dead* (Little, Brown, 1995), expressed a jaundiced view of the event:

"The results turned out to be shady... the Port Chester audience is 18- and 19-year-old kids who've hopped over the border from Connecticut to get drunk and are all screwed up on beer and hard liquor."

Hardly the blessed-out psychonauts of mid-60s San Francisco's Haight Ashbury who were the Dead's original constituency.

In both design terms and organisational terms, the *Holy Modal Rounders* and *Grateful Dead* telepathy experiments probably weren't as rigorous as the parapsychological establishment would have liked. But from a Fortean angle the results are not really the point. The point is that all concerned had the courage of their convictions and strength of belief to attempt the manifestation of a wild talent, involving over 6,000 people. These experiments were, to date, the largest telepathy tests that have ever been conducted outside of laboratory conditions, with over 2,000 people being involved at each concert. They reflected a zeitgeist, rapidly fading from our memories, in which it was believed that the human subconscious had limitless potential and could be accessed and directed by drugs, music and intent. Contrast that with the general drabness of psychical research in the early 21st Century!

Now largely forgotten, the world's biggest telepathy experiment has become just another footnote in the annals of both parapsychology and rock and roll. Ah well, I guess you had to be there!

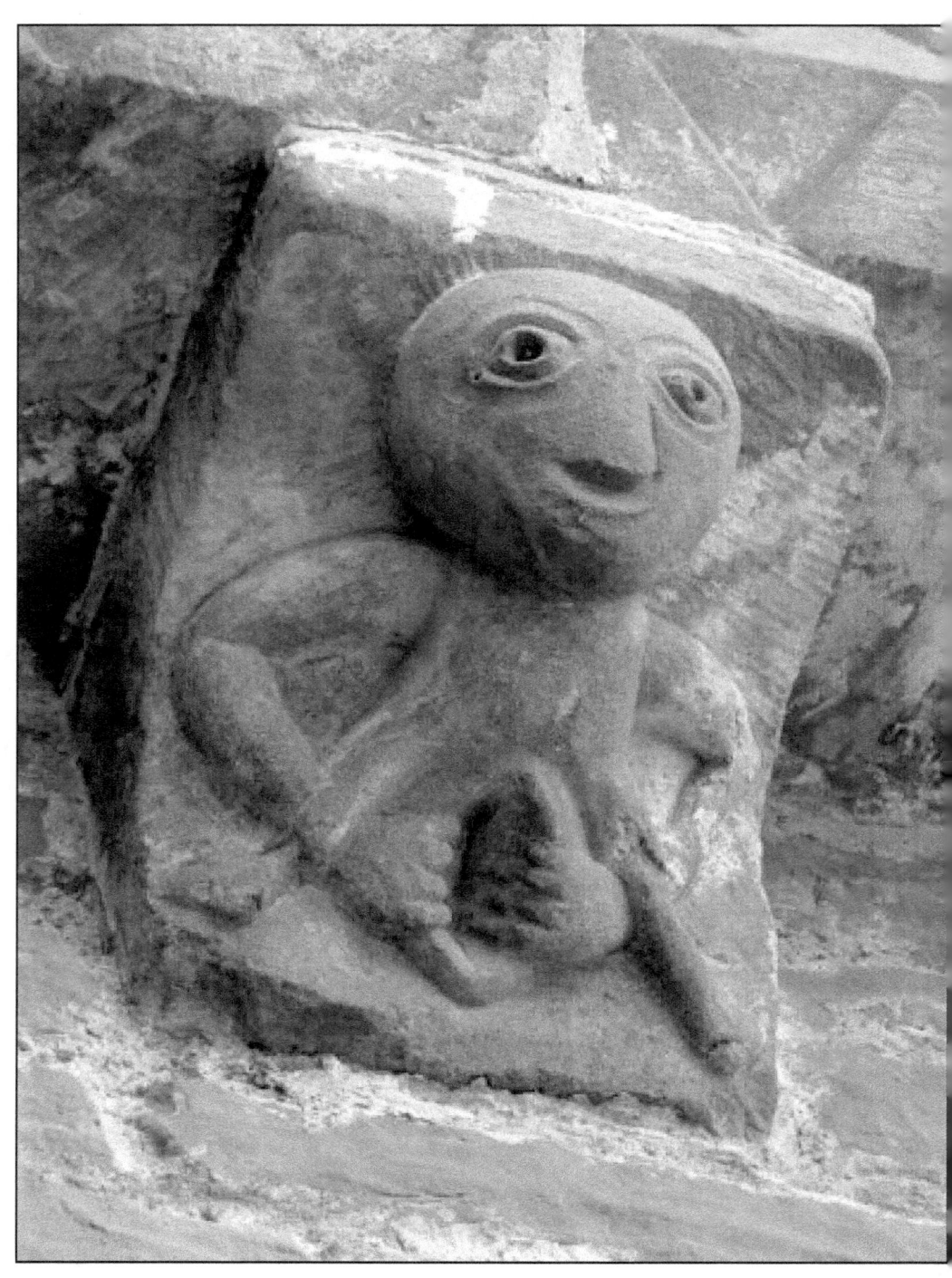

The famous *Sheela na Gig* at Kilpeck, in Herefordshire

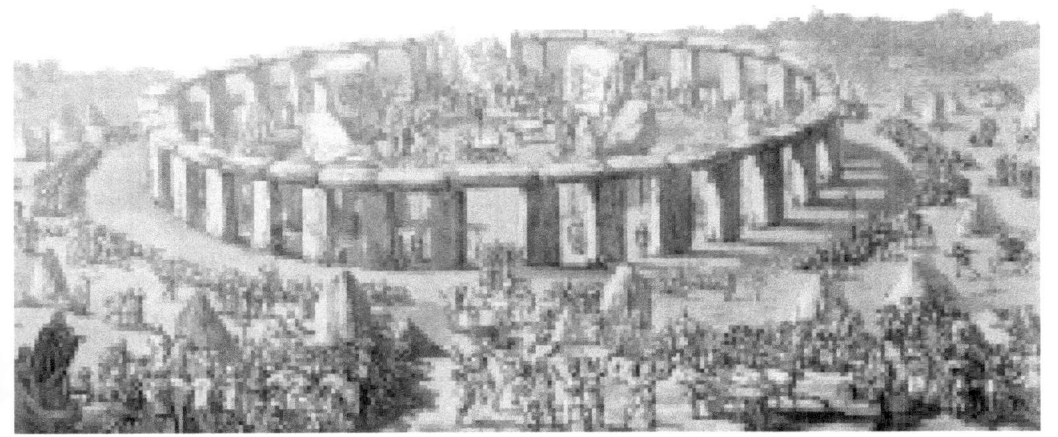

AN ENCOUNTER WITH FREYA

L ooking for interesting things to visit on a holiday in the Lake District last summer, I chanced on a book entitled *The Companion to the Lake District*, by Frank Welsh. On page 171 I found, to my delight, this short paragraph:

Pennington Church has a real *Sheela-na-gig*, a medieval fertility figure, an unusual figure anywhere, but even rarer in the Puritan parts. She owes her survival to having been buried in the east wall, and only revealed during the rebuilding of 1925, the last in a series since the church's establishment. The workmen were understandably embarrassed. They 'would not like the parson to see it and wanted to smash it up.

But, happily, she survived, and is shown triumphantly in the porch.

Great, I thought; an interesting carving with a bit of history and lore thrown in – well worth a visit. So I cycled the fifteen miles or so from where I was staying and located the tiny village of Pennington in the hills about two miles south of Ulverston. Riding toward the village down the hill I could immediately tell that the church, dedicated to St Michael and the Holy Angels, was old from the raised circular churchyard.

As I dragged the bike through the gate in the churchyard, disappointment struck – the porch was of the enclosed type, with a large closed and locked door.

If the Sheela was in there I probably wasn't going to be able to get in to see it, but just as I was beginning to consider the ride wasted, an old be-hatted villager came out of the door and locked it behind him. The dialogue which then took place is recreated as close to the original as I can:

Q: Excuse me, is the church locked?
A: Yes
Q: That's a pity; I've ridden a long way. You've got a carving?
A: No, that's gone. It used to be in the porch, but it's gone now, gone to Kendal museum
Q: What a shame. I'm interested in these things from an archaeological and folkloric point of view, and I really would have liked to have seen it. Do you know if it's on display at Kendal?

A: (after long pause) It's not gone, it's still here.
Q: Oh! Where is it then?
A: It's in the cellar. Current Parson's superstitious, thinks it's a bad influence. Old Parson used to have it in the porch. It were taken out of the church wall and must be 1000 years old...

The old man led me down into the cellar and opened an old ammunition case under a petrol can and some rags, to reveal a wonderful Sheela-na-gig, a full female figure carved onto an block of stone about 2.5 feet long by 1 foot wide. The vulva was a deep incision which looked as though it had been well rubbed, either by human hand or perhaps farm implements. As I looked and photographed the carving the old man went on to say:

'Some local folk didn't like the old Parson. It were terrible what they did and he left'.

He wouldn't expand on what had been done to him, but only that it was 'terrible' and resulted in him leaving, to be replaced by the 'new Parson'. I enquired as to the new parson's views and was told: 'The new Parson thinks Freya might have put a curse on people and that's why she's going'.

As soon as I heard the word 'Freya', I interrupted and asked if he meant the carving.

'Aye, lad.'

'Have you always called it that?'

'Aye, all the time.'

It transpired that he had always called the figure 'Freya' and many other local people did too. As for why, he didn't know, or wasn't saying. The carving was apparently going to be transported to Kendal museum, the church deeds having been altered to accommodate such a move, but when this was he couldn't say. Giving him my profuse good wishes, I rode off, glad that I'd chanced upon the caretaker rather than the 'new parson', who probably wouldn't have shown me the carving.

I later obtained the first available record of the carving, from the *Barrow News* of 14 September, 1929, and discovered that as the old gentleman had said, the carving was found in 1925, built into the east wall of the church. The article reported that the vicar of the day had specifically asked the workmen to look out for strange carvings during their alterations, but when they found the Sheela they were about to smash it, thinking it was crude and that 'the parson would not like to see it'. Luckily, the parson retrieved it at the last minute.

Later in the same piece, it is noted the stone was 'deliberately and secretly built into the church beside the altar – thus propitiating both old and new gods.'

This is all very intriguing and raises quite a few questions. Why did he know the figure as 'Freya'? In northern mythology she was, as we all know, a fertility goddess, and the Furness area in the Pennington is situated was heavily settled by people from Norse and Germanic tribes. Was his calling it Freya a folk memory, or was it instead something he had heard as a child when the carving was unearthed (It was called 'Freya' in the newspaper article)?

Just what did happen to the 'old parson' and was it connected with the Sheela? The whole episode was just like something you read in a book and then say, 'nah, sort of thing that never happens'. Well, it did, and to cap it all the photographs didn't come out!

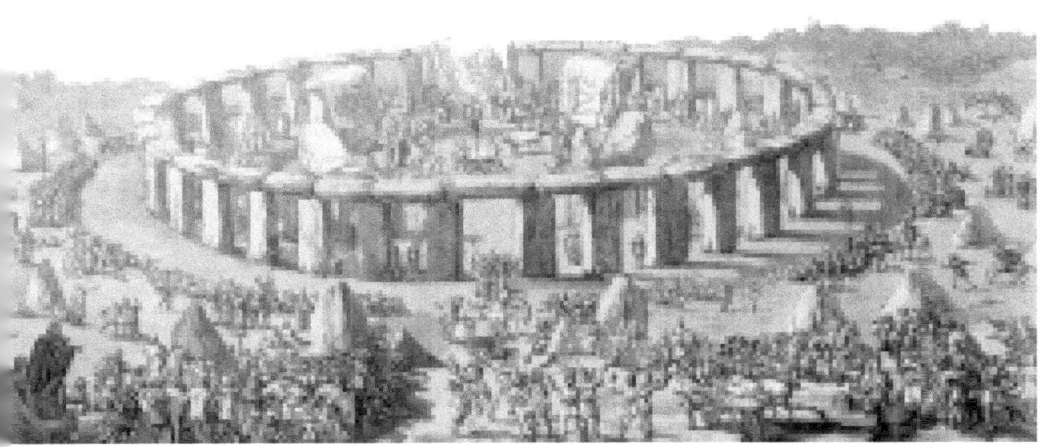

DEATH RAY MATTHEWS

They called him 'Death Ray Matthews'. It wasn't a name he chose for himself, but of all the inventions Harry Grindell Matthews was known for, it was the death ray for which he was both feted and vilified. Was he a charismatic mixture of visionary and charlatan, or an ignored and embittered inventor who could have shortened both World Wars? Whatever the answer, his story is a fascinating one, not least because it brings into sharp focus how the British Government viewed Fortean ideas in the early years of the 20th Century.

By any standards Harry Grindell Matthews led a remarkable life. Born in 1880 at Winterbourne in Gloucestershire, he was educated at the Merchant Venturer's School in Bristol before he trained as an electrical engineer. During the Boer War he enlisted in the Baden-Powell South African Constabulary and was wounded twice. On his return to Britain he pursued his keen interest in the burgeoning electrical sciences on the estate of Lord de la Warr at Bexhill-on-Sea. There he displayed a natural aptitude for 'thinking outside the box' and began to first visualise and later to actually produce a remarkable series of inventions. For years Matthews had been fascinated by the idea of communication over distances without the use of wires and, following in Marconi's footsteps, in 1911 he went on to stage a demonstration of radio telephony, transmitting a message from the ground to B C Hucks flying two miles (3.2km) away and at 600 ft (183m). Hucks himself deserves a footnote in the annals of history as being the maverick flier who was sent out to search the Scottish lowlands for alleged German bases during the phantom Zeppelin scares of the First World War. His wireless telephone experiments attracted a great deal of attention in high places and the Court Circular of 5 July 1912 edition of *The Times* boldly stated, "Buckingham Palace, July 4th. Her Majesty this afternoon inspected the wireless telephone invented by Mr. Grindell Matthews." Contemporary photographs depict him chatting with the likes of future Prime Minister Lloyd George. These early forays into the world of invention were soon noticed by the War Office and the Admiralty, forerunners of today's Ministry of Defence.

Fame and fortune awaited those who could successfully develop inventions that could be useful to the armed forces and Matthews saw a gap in the market through which he could become wealthy and serve his country. How he went about that process, however, does cast doubt upon his real motives and the authenticity of all his inventions, most notably the death ray.

But to understand both Matthews' relationship with officialdom and the ultimate failure of the death ray we need first to trace his steps between 1911 and 1924.

In the run-up to the First World War, the Admiralty took a real interest in his Aerophone device and Matthews was invited to give a demonstration. As his patents at that time were sadly only provisional he demanded that no 'experts' be present. The Admiralty agreed and the demonstration went ahead. But before it was completed, Matthews' assistant discovered that four of the invited observers had taken advantage of his absence from the room to dismantle the apparatus, taking notes and sketches. In a rage, Matthews cancelled the demonstration immediately and sent everyone away, despite the protests of the Admiralty officials.

The press scented a scandal and was immediately on Matthews' side, national and provincial papers trumpeting his cause, outraged at the intransigence of the Admiralty. Public opinion was whipped into such frenzy that the War Office had no option but to face up publicly both to the press and the upstart who challenged them. A statement was issued via *The Daily Telegraph* in which the War Office denied any tampering and insisted that the Aerophone experiment had been a failure. As the experiment had not even begun before the men from the ministry began their tampering, Matthews sensed jealousy, if not a cover up, was at work. Faced with an official denial, he had a change of mind and in turn he issued a statement retracting his claims and downsizing the affair to a 'misunderstanding'. This bizarre incident was one of many where Matthews would announce an invention only for it to fail at the last minute, for whatever reason, to demonstrate it working successfully. It was also the genesis of the media's ardent love affair with Matthews and his inventions. More importantly it marked the drawing of a line in the sand between Matthews' essentially Fortean ideas and the staid mechanistic and unimaginative traditions of the British scientific establishment. Matthews then faded from the public gaze until the war.

Now, in 1914 and faced with the prospect of a lengthy conflict, the British government was desperate for innovations which would help them wage war against Germany. Two inventions interested them greatly. The first was a ray which would disable the Zeppelins, and the second was a ray which could control unmanned craft. A reward of £25,000 was offered to the person who came up with either. Matthews was convinced he could provide the latter and claimed he had developed a remote control system using cells containing selenium. After testing his invention on Edgbaston Reservoir, he demonstrated it to Admiralty officials at Richmond Park's Penn Pond. They were so impressed that Matthews received his cheque for £25,000 the following morning, a not inconsiderable sum of money in 1915.

Yet there was something not quite right about this event. Although the remote control boat had been proven to the Admiralty officials and a vast sum of money paid, the idea never manifested as workable in practice. The Admiralty, for whatever reason, chose not to pursue Matthews' selenium control system which, besides operating boats remotely, was claimed to be able to detonate explosives at a distance. Was this ignorance and jealousy on behalf of the War Office or the first hints that Matthews wasn't quite as genuine as he appeared? Again Matthews lapsed back into obscurity. He re-appeared briefly, yet rather significantly, in 1921, breaking new ground by producing the world's first talking picture. This was a short interview with the explorer Ernest Shackleton prior to his fatal attempt at circumnavigating the Antarctic. This film is important because it proves that Matthews, despite the hype and ambiguity which often attended his inventions, was not a charlatan, and was in many ways years ahead of his time.

Unfortunately, the British film industry told Matthews that 'talkies' would never catch on. Just a few years later, the Americans embraced the talking film and revolutionised the movie industry for ever. Why was Grindell Matthews' invention not taken up? Why indeed? The static carnage of World War One had set inventors thinking about how the impasse of trench warfare could be broken. All the talk was of some kind of 'ray' which could disable men and machines at great distances. Both H G Wells and H Rider Haggard had produced fictional accounts of such a 'death ray' years earlier and as Forteans know, whatever can be imagined can be invented.

Matthews turned his mind to the idea of a possible death ray in the autumn of 1923. After reading news reports of French airplanes dropping out of the sky over Germany, he said: "I realised that the Germans had found an invisible ray that put the magnetos of the aircraft out of action. I concentrated on efforts to discover what it was, and with the electric ray now at my command I think I have succeeded." Select journalists were given a demonstration of Matthews' 'ray' stopping a motor cycle engine at 50 ft (15m). "I am confident," Matthews announced, "that if I have facilities for developing it I can stop aeroplanes in flight - indeed I believe the ray is sufficiently powerful to destroy the air, to explode powder magazines, and destroy anything on which it rests."

Thus the death ray was born in the mind of the popular press. Matthews capitalised on his new-found fame, being well aware that his stock was not particularly high with the British government. So, rather than approach them directly, he went to his old friends the press. They were only too happy to help, and fanciful accounts of the death ray and what it could do began to have appeared by late 1923. Bemused by Matthew's sudden re-appearance but fearful that the publicity he was enjoying would lead to another nation bidding for the notorious death ray, the War Office was forced to act. Swallowing their pride and suspending their disbelief, in February 1924 the Air Ministry offered Matthews the opportunity to be able to demonstrate his death ray to them. Matthews at first ignored their advances, perhaps hoping the government would simply accept his assertion that the ray did as he said.

When no such offer was forthcoming, Matthews contacted the press with further dramatic claims and by April 1924 the death ray – or more properly the idea of the death ray – was world news. *The London Star* announced the invention as a "wonderful invisible ray which has turned into fact the dreams of Wells' fiction." And they hadn't even seen it yet! A wide-eyed Star reporter was ushered into Matthews' London laboratory and shown a bowl of gunpowder being ignited by the ray. Matthews was at pains to explain that this was only the beginning, a small scale demonstration of what could easily be the destruction of ammunition dumps at huge distances or the destruction of aeroplane engines in flight.

The scientific principles on which the 'ray' worked were glossed over by everyone concerned. Ionised air carrying an electrical current was mentioned by some commentators, others talked of exceptionally short radio waves. Matthews wasn't saying and sadly no-one appeared to be asking the right questions, certainly not the press. To them the idea of a death ray was enough. But still the government wouldn't commit itself and now Matthews was receiving offers from other countries, most notably big business concerns in France. By mid-May 1924 the press was reporting,

> "...while the British government is interested it is not willing to assist him
> in perfecting his experiments and he is unable to resist the princely offer
> made by the Lyons firm."

Despite their initial interest, strong doubts were beginning to be expressed by the Air Ministry. They had been duped or conned many times before by 'inventors' who made great claims but failed to deliver the promised inventions. They may even have been duped by Matthews himself. An internal government memo coyly suggested that Matthews' 1915 payment of £25,000 was largely due to the influence of one particular lord and was not entirely deserved. Worryingly, it also suggested that enquiries should be "instituted with the Birmingham Police records as to Mr G Matthews' past history." A top secret report looking into Matthews' claims and history had been apparently generated by the Intelligence Services, but appears not to survive in the Public Record Office at Kew. The old rivalries were at work again. But Matthews had some support in the British government, notably from Admiral Kerr who persuaded him not to sell his invention to another power. Kerr claimed that Matthews "had given his word of honour not to divulge the secret of the ray until I confer with members of the British cabinet."

Matthews, now in negotiations to sell his invention in France, was persuaded to return to England to demonstrate his 'death ray' to the three armed forces on 26 April at noon, one o'clock and 1.30pm. But the much vaunted 'death ray' demonstration was something of an anti-climax. After being ushered into Matthews' laboratory various leading government officials were shown just two examples of the ray's efficacy. An Osglim light bulb was held in the path of the 'ray'. When the ray was switched on the bulb lit. A small motor mounted on a bench was then started and immediately brought to a halt by the 'ray'.

From these experiments – which were both easily carried out using scientific techniques available at the time – Matthews expected the full confidence of the British government. He would be disappointed. Immediately following the demonstration, a meeting was convened by the Air Ministry at 4.00pm to discuss the death ray. Those present at the demonstration were now joined by representatives from each of the armed forces. Each commented on what they had seen in Matthews' laboratory. The reports were not positive. Major Wimperis from the Air Ministry stated: "I was rather surprised to find the inventor should imagine that one would be impressed." The Admiralty's F Smith, also doubted what he had seen, adding that Matthews' assistants even appeared ignorant of how the 'ray' was operated. Smith was also concerned that when he suggested that Matthews move the cycle motor down from the lab bench to the floor, Matthews "did not like this suggestion and explained further that he was in a great hurry."

Odd behaviour from a man who dearly wished to convince the British Government of one of the greatest inventions yet seen. Smith sensed trickery was afoot, adding that he had been visited by the mysterious 'Appleton' – possibly an MI5 agent – who claimed that Matthews had no scientific knowledge as such but liked to experiment with "all sorts of gadgets". This source suggested that Matthews "brought things up to a certain stage and no further, he would then raise money on what he had achieved". In short, a scientific confidence trickster.

Furthermore, Appleton claimed Matthews was "working the press, but had now lost control of it." The explicit conclusion of this meeting was that the government did not trust Matthews. Yet they were loathe to dismiss him completely as long as even a small chance remained that he could be onto something. No government wanted to turn down the death ray only for it to turn up later in the arsenal of an enemy. Air Vice Marshal Salmond wrote immediately to Matthews suggesting details of some further, more detailed demonstrations. Matthews replied that he could not understand why the government would not accept the evidence he had presented to them.

He had now lost patience with England and was now offering the 'ray' to the French. Following this breakdown of communications, events took a turn that was both dramatic and ludicrous. Tuesday 27 May 1924 saw scenes which could have come straight from an Ealing Comedy.

The Daily Express summed up the farce perfectly a day later with its front page headline "Melodramatic Death Ray Episodes". Their lead article opined:

> "Melodrama has seldom surpassed the heights which were reached in yes-
> terday's 'Death Ray' episodes. Hurried legal action in the High Court was
> followed by an unsuccessful motor-car chase, an air journey by Mr. Grin-
> dell Matthews to Paris, a belated renewal of conversations on this side of
> the channel, a reopening of negotiations in France and a deluge of claims
> by rival inventors. Beneath all was the undertone of tragedy suggested by
> the terrible powers which are attributed to the ray."

At 10.40 that morning, the High Court in London granted an injunction to Matthews' financial backers, restraining him from selling the rights to the death ray. At 10.45 am a blissfully unaware Matthews set off for Croydon aerodrome and the lunchtime flight to Paris. Three minutes later, Major H Wimperis arrived at Grindell Matthews' laboratory, in an attempt to further broker a deal. As they were leaving, Matthews' financial backers and their solicitor arrived bearing the recently issued injunction. Finding Matthews gone, they hired the fastest car available and sped to Croydon in order to prevent him leaving for France. They roared on to the runway seconds too late and could only watch in dismay as the small mail plane headed towards the Channel.

Questioned later, E Gubbins, one of Matthews' investors, remained still utterly persuaded of the ray's potency, saying, "I am convinced that the ray is the most terrible invention which has been created in recent years. It is of such a nature that it will make wars impossible if held by Britain. Other countries could not hope to combat a power armed with such a weapon." Matthews, meanwhile, was once again negotiating terms with the French and was met at Le Bourget airfield by Eugene Royer prior to a meeting that evening with the director of the Chantier du Rhône, an important Lyons steel firm.

Meanwhile the deluge of publicity which had attended Grindell Matthews' stand-off with the British government brought a flood of other death ray inventors out of the woodwork. At least 10 people, it seemed, had been harbouring death rays in their private laboratories and sheds, and the War Office was inundated with claimants. Several of these inventors were also investigated by the War Office but, as with Matthews, none could back their claims with meaningful demonstrations. The press were incensed when they discovered Matthews was dealing with the French, and wouldn't let the matter drop.

Once again, the government was forced by popular opinion to make official statements and on 28 May questions were asked in the House of Commons. Mr Leach, Under Secretary for Air, was questioned by Commander Kenworthy, who demanded to know what steps were being taken to prevent an invention of the death ray's magnitude from leaving the country. Leach reiterated the government's position:

> "We are not in a position to pass judgment on the value of this ray, because we have not been allowed to make proper tests. Therefore whether there is anything in it or not still remains unexplored. The Departments have been placed in a difficult position in dealing with the matter partly because of the vigorous Press campaign conducted on behalf of this gentleman, and partly because this is not the first occasion on which the inventor has put forward a scheme for which extravagant claims have been made. The result is the Departments are not able to accept Mr Grindell Matthews' statement about this invention without a scrutiny which he is not prepared to face."

Unpicking this carefully-worded statement laid bare the government's inherent scepticism regarding Matthews' claims. Yes, government officials had seen a demonstration of the alleged death ray – but they were keen to point out that the circumstances of demonstration were of Matthews' choosing, at his laboratory with all equipment being provided and set up by him. In government speak:

> "The departmental representatives were shown nothing which would lead them to credit the statements which have appeared in the Press as to the possibilities of the invention."

Furthermore, His Majesty's Government believed that "the conditions under which the demonstrations were made by Mr Matthews were such that it was not possible to form any opinion as to the value of the device." Carefully worded or not, the implication seemed to be that Grindell Matthews at best may have not demonstrated his invention under correct laboratory conditions, and at worst had brazenly attempted to defraud the British Government. The statement went on to stress that the government had been at pains to be scrupulously fair with Matthews, offering him the chance to repeat the demonstration. All they required to be convinced was that he use his ray to stop the engine of a petrol driven motorcycle engine provided by them. On successful completion of this test, Matthews would then be given £1,000 as a retainer for 14 days whilst the government considered "the basis of further financial negotiations for the purchase or development of his invention." As yet, the government didn't even want to know how the ray worked, just for it to be demonstrated to their satisfaction using their own laboratory conditions.

Not an unreasonable request.

The statement ended somewhat tersely:

> "Mr Grindell Matthews has refused this offer and it is clear he has left the country." Unfazed by this scepticism, Grindell Matthews, still in France, announced he now had eight bids under consideration. Charles Dick of the British Consulate in Paris met with Matthews. Dick had investigated Matthews' French backer, Eugene Royer, and found him to be untrustworthy and on the point of bankruptcy. Matthews seemed unconcerned by this news, happy to work for Royer seemingly to spite the British government for daring to ask for that most vulgar of displays, 'proof'. Dick's subsequent letter to the Air Ministry contained a stark character sketch of Matthews, observing: "It would certainly be advisable to recommend the very greatest caution in dealing with Mr Matthews if he is in any way connected with Royer. If such a connection comes about after the warning I gave Mr. Matthews, I should feel obliged to consider that the latter was as unworthy of confidence as the former."

The British government wasn't the only party in the country that was interested in the death ray. Sir Samuel Instone and his brother offered Matthews a substantial cash payment plus a salary of several thousand pounds a year if he would only keep the invention in the UK. "Our offer still stands. It is made on purely patriotic grounds. Mr Grindell Matthews can have all the money he needs," said Theodore Instone. Yet Matthews refused this offer too. Perhaps it had something to do with the concluding part of Instone's statement which read,

> "...providing he satisfies our scientific advisors that the ray has serious possibilities."

There it was again. The small, but significantly unavoidable matter of conclusive proof that the alleged death ray worked as its inventor claimed. Even the loftiest Fortean ideas begin to crumble when they are revealed to be empty promises. And by now, to all but the most gullible observer, the 'death ray' was looking very much like an empty promise. An Air Ministry official summed up the problem succinctly, saying:

> "This invention is either worth a large sum of money or it is worth nothing. No inventor could reasonably expect the government to pay a large sum of money for a patent until it had been fully tested. If the invention fulfils all that is claimed for it, the inventor has nothing to fear from official sources."

Quite so. But neither Matthews nor any of his imitators could provide the vital proof needed. The death ray, upon which thousands of pounds, hundreds of hours and millions of column inches had been spent, was worth nothing to anyone as an idea alone.

The 1st of June 1924 saw Matthews returning to London, and he was angry. In an interview with the *Sunday Express* he defended his life's work even to the point of raging at those who had referred to his notorious invention as a 'ray'. It was, he claimed, a 'beam', not a ray, although quite what the difference was he failed to say. Matthews still believed he had a deal with Royer and was insistent his death ray was all packed and ready to be shipped to France for further development.

Once again the press took up Matthews' cause and allowed him space to rail against those who doubted him. In response to Lord Birkenhead who had written to *The Times* criticising his 'ray', Matthews argued that it was this attitude which had lost Britain the advantage in many other areas of scientific warfare such as aeronautics and torpedo development. Despite all the talk of ideas and possibilities, as yet few people outside Grindell Matthews' intimate circle had actually seen his death ray apparatus. This was rectified in the summer of 1924 with the release of the film *The Death Ray*. Made by Pathé, the 25-minute film was basically a drama-documentary, an advertisement for Harry Grindell Matthews and all his works.

From an entertainment perspective, however, the film made great viewing, coming as it did in the wake of the massive publicity given the death ray furore. Yet there was no evidence that the subject matter of the film had any basis in reality. Stills show fantastic apparatus, claimed to be the death ray, but which bear no relation to the small Heath Robinson-like machine demonstrated to the government inspectors weeks earlier. Poetic license was clearly at work and S R Littlewood, in *The Sphere*, made perceptive observations relevant to the whole affair:

> "...The Death Ray in which Mr Grindell Matthews is shown pulling levers of his machine and a rat is shown falling dead in its cage, a bicycle stopping and aeroplanes galore falling down in flames from the sky. From the scientific point of view – that is to say as a proof that it was the ray that killed the rat – I do not suppose that The Death Ray is intended to be regarded as of any value at all. One does not for a moment disbelieve Mr Grindell Matthews. At the same time a film which could have been so obviously 'faked' leaves one simply with the same amount of information as one had before save, perhaps, as to the shape of the machine, which is a sort of searchlight with three megaphone-like ears attached to it.

> There remains, however, the remarkable personality of Mr Grindell Matthews himself. One cannot help being at least bewildered by the psychology of a scientist who can enter into the spirit of a piece of mummery like this so completely that it is quite clear he was acting for all he was worth. In view of his many experiments it can evidently have been no great emotional strain to Mr Grindell Matthews to pull a lever with the intention of doing nothing worse than stopping a bicycle-wheel. Yet he pulls that lever with as much impressive gravity as if he were about some operation upon which life and death depended."

This seemingly trivial excursion into film may have been a shrewd move by Matthews. The blanket press coverage of the death ray story had captured the public imagination. Now the death ray film allowed them to 'see' it with their own eyes, and was a perfect visual advertisement for Matthews, one which was shown widely across Britain and America. It comes as no surprise therefore that following Matthews' inability to conclusively demonstrate the death ray he eventually abandoned the long quest to sell his invention to European governments and in July departed to America. Once again he set about publicising the death ray, announcing that he would develop a higher-powered version of the machine that would convince the world his "beam deserves a place among the great inventions of history". But there were immediate problems when he was offered $25,000 to demonstrate the ray to the Radio World Fair at Madison Square Garden in December.

Matthews once again declined the offer of easy money, this time claiming that he was not permitted to demonstrate his invention outside England. This is a curious statement as there is no evidence he was under any such constraint, legal or political. Once again, Matthews the showman was taking his game to the brink. He tantalised the American public, telling how he would return to Britain and set up a research station on an island in the Bristol Channel to continue his work so that, "in eighteen months I can perfect my apparatus so that it will be the most formidable war weapon of the future".

Somewhat predictably, his assertions drew some criticism from the American scientific establishment. Professor R Woods was scornful of the death ray and even offered to stand in front of it for an indefinite period, confident it would do him no harm. "Nothing", he said, "has been done that could lead a scientist or engineer to place the slightest credence in the death ray." Criticism not-withstanding, on his return to Britain Matthews later claimed that 'America' (he was vague) had snapped up his death ray invention. Quite where this left his claim that he was not permitted to demonstrate the ray outside England was unclear. Nor was it stated to whom he had sold his ray.

The Observer seized on these contradictions, noting how: "Many people in this country will be curious to know the terms and conditions on which the United States have obtained a monopoly of Mr Grindell-Matthews' 'Ray'". Matthews himself was tight-lipped, refusing to say who or how much. All he would say was that he had returned merely to collect everything he owned before returning to America.

There the saga of the death ray ends. Matthews never managed to successfully demonstrate his invention to anyone's satisfaction. Whether this was because it was a complex money-making scam or whether the world's governments were just incapable of grasping the enormity of his ideas is unclear. We do know however that no-one ever developed a death ray, nor did Matthews pursue the invention further. Instead he went back to America where he worked as a consultant for Warner Brothers, putting his genuine skills in sound and vision technology to good use.

By the late 1920s, Matthews was back in Britain with a series of new, bold inventions which actually worked. His *piece de resistance* was a device to project advertisements on clouds. On Christmas Eve 1930 he stunned London by projecting the image of an angel onto clouds above Hampstead Heath. The apparition was so realistic that people miles away apparently fell to their knees in worship, believing the Second Coming was at hand! He followed this with demonstrations in New York, where he projected the Stars and Stripes 10,000ft (3,000m) above the city (see below).

This invention clearly worked, yet once again Matthews was beset by problems. Although the invention could have revolutionised the emerging advertising industry, no-one seemed interested. Matthews had little time to reflect on this new failure as darker clouds were gathering and in 1931 he faced bankruptcy.

His bankruptcy papers make interesting reading.

Question: "What is your full name?"
Answer: "Harry Grindell Grindell."

Grindell Matthews, it seems, wasn't even his real name. The bankruptcy enquiry laid bare his financial and personal affairs, reducing his claims and inventions to mere transactions in a ledger book, profit and loss. The papers reveal a series of loans and investments made to Matthews, none of which made money, but which had allowed him to live in hotels and luxury rented accommodation whilst he developed his various inventions. Undeterred, Matthews' bounced back from bankruptcy and by 1934 he had raised sufficient funds from a new generation of financial backers to relocate to South Wales. There he became a semi-recluse, building a fortified laboratory with its own private airfield on the summit of Tor Cloud near Swansea. He soon became the subject of local lore and legend, with the police arriving in response to claims that his 'rays' were causing illness among the local population. Other stories spread that car engines would stop if they drove too near Matthews' mountain fastness.

Financially secure again, he embarked on another series of inventions. Seeing that the Second World War was on the horizon, he began to develop the idea of aerial mines fired by rockets or suspended by barrage balloons. These, he claimed, could create an effective aerial ring of defence round cities such as London. This idea was discussed seriously by the government but never taken up as a practical proposal. Matthews' mind, never still, then came up with the idea of the 'stratoplane' – a "plane which could fly on the edges of space." He became a member of the British Interplanetary Society and actively pushed forward ideas which led eventually to the development of rocket technology.

There were many more inventions, including a system for detecting submarines. Matthews hauled these around government departments but as war clouds gathered people had less and less time for Matthews' speculations. The death ray had proved the death knell for his reputation.

When war finally arrived, Matthews noted that had his inventions such as the aerial mines been taken up, London would not have suffered as much as it did in the Blitz. He could now also see how useful his submarine detector would have been against the U-Boats stalking the Atlantic. But it was to no avail. Time had passed him by and on 11 September 1941 Death Ray Matthews died of a massive heart attack.

Genius or charlatan, probably a little of both, Grindell Matthews inspired intense debate and massive publicity. Some of his inventions such as the talking films, aerophone and sky-projector certainly worked and were years ahead of their time. Other ideas such as his theories of space travel were to eventually come to fruition later in the 20th Century. But it was for the death ray he was best known and it was his eventual failure to deliver the goods which was his eventual downfall, leading the scientific and political establishments of the era to overlook his other inventions.

It would be charitable to speculate that his flirtation with the death ray was mere showmanship to attract money for his more conventional ideas, much in the same way that the SETI programme continues to maintain interest in more mundane aspects of space exploration. If so, it was a gamble which didn't pay off.

We will probably never know.

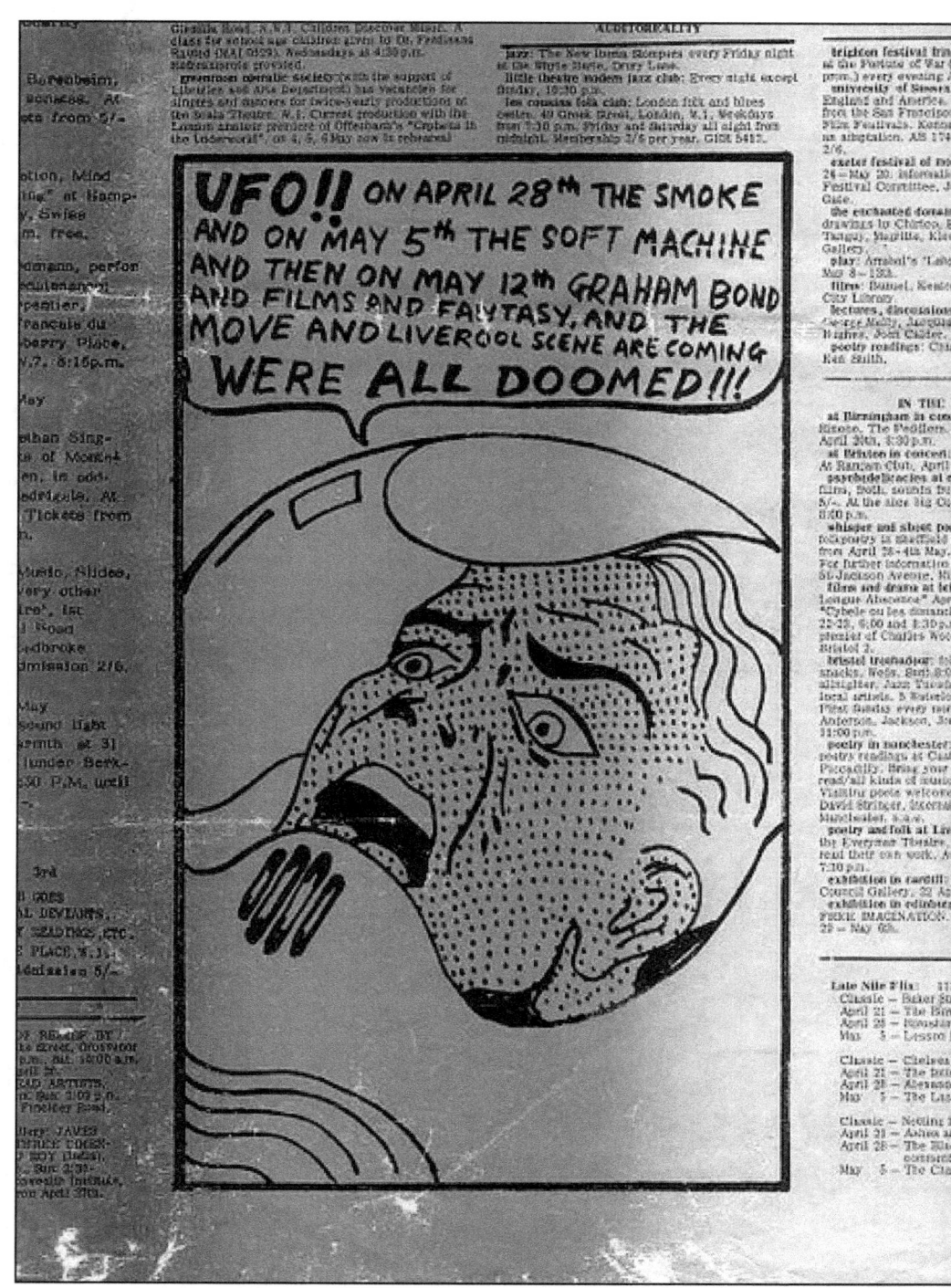

Advert from *International Times* April 1967 for the *UFO Club*

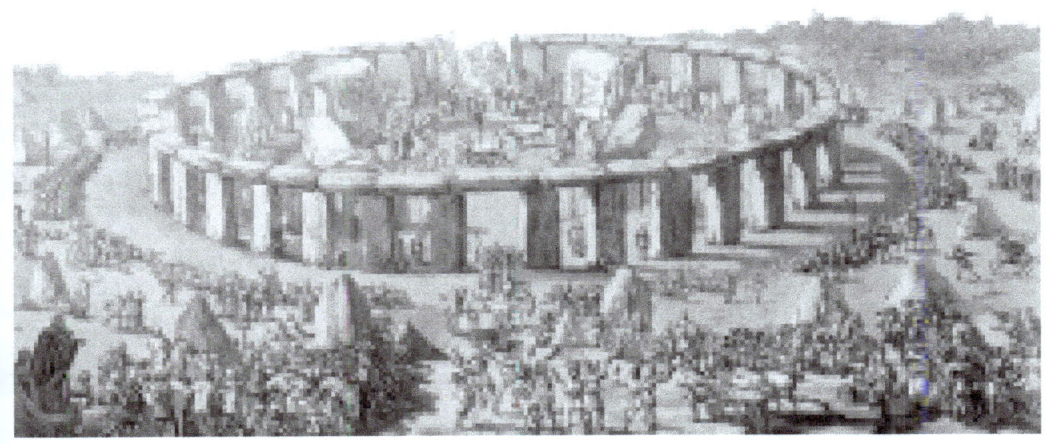

ROCKING THE ALIEN

First published n *Fortean Times*, July 1996

Good rock music pushes the limits, dealing with the outlands of sound, toying with the news and interesting ideas and reflecting the essence of the times it is played in. Its performers are often 'out there' on the edge too, sonic shamen mediating between the ether and the ordinary, and so it should come as no surprise that rock'n'roll is littered with references to UFOs. Think about it: all those pre-pubescent rockers growing up through the great UFO waves of the Fifties and Sixties, the explosion in books on the subject and then the omnipresent psychedelic drugs which brought the truth from 'out there' to 'in here'. There was no way UFOs were going to pass rock'n'roll by.

Exactly *why* rock'n'rollers chose to take UFO imagery to their hearts is hard to pin down, but from what they say, the implication seems to be that UFO represent the *ultimate* non-hierarchical power. accessible to all. No money down and no priesthood necessary. *They* were out there, just waiting, pregnant with the knowledge of the ages. To interpret it according to Floydian analysis, all and everything as contained in the great *Saucerful of Secrets*. UFOs were the ultimate light shows, and they represented the highest consciousness, the most arcane knowledge.

The UFO experience, like psychedelic drugs, offered immediate and direct connection to the power from which good rock music comes, a source more than adequately summed up in beat poet and proto-rocker Allen Ginsberg's *Howl*, as the 'ancient heavenly connection to the starry dynamo in the machinery of the night.' The first direct UFO reference in rock music was the long forgotten *Flying Saucer Rock'n'Roll* by *Billy Lee Riley and the Little Green Men*, but before that, before rock music *per se* even existed, UFOs and alien imagery were being incorporated into jazz by the famous experimentalist Sun Ra, who claimed to have come from outer space and to be in regular communication with extraterrestrials. Album titles such as *Space is the Place* reflected this obsession and, garbed in flowing robes decorated with UFOs and galaxies, *Sun Ra and his Intergalactic Research Arkestra* pave the way for the next generation of cosmic rockers.

As befits a royal entrance to the world, the birth of the King, Elvis Presley, was attended by UFO-like phenomena. His father later recalled, in conversation with his son: "We were waiting round and thinking,

'When is that baby comin?' Well, I remember walkin' outside and all around that li'l house there seemed to be this blue light, a strange blue light that lit up the house…and you were born, Elvis." Perhaps 'they' were watching him, because Elvis himself later had a UFO sighting when he observed an unidentified light flying low over the roof of his Bel Air mansions during 1966. Presley told the two friends who also witnessed the UFO that he firmly believed it was a flying saucer driven by benevolent aliens who would one day make contact with Earth people.

The heady years of the late 1960s inspired some pretty strange beliefs among rock musicians and UFOs cropped up everywhere. Even the title of *Pink Floyd's* second album, *Saucerful of Secrets*, captured the zeitgeist perfectly. Everyone now knew about UFOs and they represented just what the hippies wanted; strangeness, the antidote to the tedium of everyday life, and the possibility of communication with other species, other worlds.

Cosmic fun, in short. It was no accident that John 'Hoppy' Hopkins' psychedelic London club was called UFO and one nickname for LSD during that period was 'flying saucers'. Over in the USA, *Jefferson Airplane* were already enquiring, *Have you seen the saucers?* and the singer Grace Slick's lyric railed clumsily against materialism – *Do you know the people out there who aren't happy with the way they care about here?* – before going on to talk of brotherhood with the space people.

The drug culture, dissatisfied with the state of things material and its emphasis on 'higher' consciousness and environmental concerns, offered images aplenty of redemption by religion, ufonauts or, preferably, a combination of both. This was a theme taken up (dare we say exploited?) by many musicians of the day. Neil Young gave us *After the Goldrush* with its plangent image of a post-holocaust society being whisked away to pastures new by 'silver spaceships' who would take us to 'new homes in the sun'. These themes continue and eventually developed the contactee philosophy of the Fifties and Sixties when silver-suited Venusians warned mankind that it was going down the wrong path and needed to change direction to avoid nuclear annihilation.

Young's erstwhile partners, Crosby, Stills and Nash covered the same area of thought in *Wooden Ships*. Young later qualified his views in an interview, saying 'If anyone wants to take me to space, I'm ready to go. I'd like to take my family too,' and adding hopefully, although not entirely convincingly, 'I think there'll be rock and roll on other planets' And the rock'n'roll based film *Easy Rider* also contained a sequence in which Dennis Hopper (Billy the Kid) and Jack Nicholson (George) espoused their (and a million other hippies') beliefs about UFOs and their colonisation of Earth to a stoned and incredulous Peter Fonda. George: 'That was UFO beaming' back at ya. They've got bases all over the world now, you know.' UFOs were everywhere.

This viewpoint crystalised itself for the hippy movement with the Jimi Hendrix film *Rainbow Bridge*. Director Chuck Wein said the film was about 'removing the mass paranoia against the arrival of the Space Brothers'. Hendrix himself was an avid UFO buff who read all the available literature. No doubt it was this barrage of information, taken in tandem with his prodigious consumption of LSD, which led him to believe he had actually been born in outer space and had been sent to earth on a divine mission. He told Wein he believed he came from 'an asteroid belt off the coast of Mars'.

But perhaps it wasn't all imagination because, following the *Rainbow Bridge* concert on the Hawaiian island of Maui, local residents reported UFOs and strange noises from the rocks. Prior to the film, Hendrix's album *Axis, Bold as Love*, began with the part-spoken track *EXP*, which featured an interview with a man claiming to be an extraterrestrial. Hendrix's fascination with UFOs continued to his death.

Among the writings completed on the day of his death was a poem containing the words "Angels of heaven, flying saucers to some".

The early Seventies were a fertile time for rock and UFOs. Ideas promulgated in required counter-culture reading such as John Michell's *View Over Atlantis* and *The Flying Saucer Vision* were taken up by bands such as *Gong* and *Hawkwind* who embraced the mythology with open minds. Even the more whimsical groups such as the *Incredible String Band* were seeing strange lights in the sky above their west Wales commune and attendees at the first Glastonbury Festival, held in 1970, were so certain that UFOs were out there just waiting to make contact that they built a UFO landing platform at the site.

It was around this time, the early Seventies, when rock music's interest in UFOs began to grow more diffuse. Bands and fans, following the example set by their American spiritual cousins, were moving out from the towns to less populated areas; 'getting it together in the country' became a cliché. Michell's books, and a growing sense of environmentalism, led to the fairly straightforward message of the UFO blending with native British mysticism in what has since become known as Earth Mysteries.

The West Country was a focus for these mystic types, and ex-Gongster Steve Hillage made his home in Great Bedwyn. Taking a walk there with music scribe Chris Salewicz, Hillage points out a fighter plane on manoeuvres. "Chasing UFOs, I expect", Hillage comments, fairly bluntly, making one the first rock and roll allegations of Government knowledge of UFOs.

Some bands, whose origins lay in the Sixties, could never quite shake off their UFO fixations and in 1977, when the *Grateful Dead* played a momentous gig at the Great Pyramid in Egypt, guitarist Jerry Garcia belied his expectations when he said: "the fact that the Pyramid didn't open up and flying saucers pour out didn't make it less of an experience." David Bowie was a one-time UFO buff who achieved his ambition to play an alien in Nick Roeg's film *The Man Who Fell to Earth*. In an interview revealing his UFO past, he admitted:

> "I used to work for two guys who put out a UFO magazine in England about six years ago (1969) and I made sightings six, seven times a night for about a year when I was in the observatory. We had regular cruises that came over. We knew the 6:15pm was coming in and would meet up with another one. And they would be stationary for about half an hour and then, after verifying what they had done that day, they'd shoot off."

That a regular 6;15pm UFO could possibly have been an aircraft is a thought that might have occurred to Mr. Bowie but, when we remember that "there's a Starman waiting in the sky; he'd like to come and meet us but he thinks he'd blow our minds"", it hardly seems to matter does it?

The list of rock luminaries who were actively involved in UFO investigation is as long as it is strange. For instance, cosmic crooner Kate Bush was once the head of a local UFO investigation group, while *Rolling Stone* Mick Jagger and his former guitar-slinging sidekick Mick Taylor both had an interest in the phenomenon. One of Jagger's houses housed a UFO detector which apparently always went off when he was out, and Taylor was a regular visitor to the UFO-haunted hills of Warminster.

Even guitarist Dave Davies of the *Kinks* (Ray's brother) once appeared on a TV programme about UFOs, wandering around Warminster with a UFO detector and extolling the virtues of our interplanetary guests. It was hip to be hip to UFOs and even hipper to let your public know about it.

Another musician who dabbled in UFO investigation before fame took over was *Talking Heads* front man David Byrne, whose abiding interest in the subject led him at one point to attempt to teach an art history class about the subject. He would also quiz people about their attitudes to UFO experiences and at one time issued a 14-point questionnaire soliciting their views about flying saucers and extraterrestrial visitors.

And who can forget, or remember, the band *Klaatu*, once thought to be *The Beatles* under a pseudonym, whose song *Calling Occupants Of Interplanetary Craft* (more famously covered by *The Carpenters*) speculated wildly about those who watched over us. If *Klaatu* weren't *The Beatles* who were they? Well, numerologist John Squires studied the hieroglyphics on their *Hope* album and determined that the band were in fact extraterrestrials! Readers of a sceptical bent should bear in mind that this was an era when divination by album sleeve was all the rage - an era when a casual misinterpretation of the cover of the *Beatles'* 1969 *Abbey Road* album indicated to the best minds of the generation that Paul was dead.

There are no recorded instances of any of the Fab Four seeing UFOs during their days together, eastern religions being more to their taste. In his post-Beatle years, however, John Lennon saw a cigar-shaped object zoom over the Hudson River and later wrote about it on his *Milk and Honey* album, where the track *Nobody Told Me* informed us all that "There's UFOs over New York and I ain't too surprised". Leading ufologist Jenny Randles has often on the connection between childhood experiences of balls of light in the bedroom and adult UFO events. One personality from the world of rock music who had such an experience was *Echo and The Bunnymen's* Ian McCulloch, who recalled in a *New Musical Express* interview that "the room was always filled with these lights that went all round the walls. Even when I was ten I knew I had to make sense of all that had to use it poetically. '*Flickering Lights*, the first song on the new album is all about that." Food for thought for those who speculate that the UFO experience often accompanies or manifests itself as a form of creativity in later life. Even the hard edge of the punk era couldn't stop its practitioners being fascinated by UFOs. Lene Lovich famous for *My Lucky Number*) was unsure as to whether she was an alien or not. "I've never felt at ease in this world," she was quoted as saying. "When I was a little kid, I was from another planet. When I was seven or eight, I was obsessed with space stories. I thought I was an experiment, a visitor sent from another planet to try living on earth. I'd hang out of the window every night, searching the sky, looking for the aliens to come down and take me back home."

Post-punkstress Debbie Harry believed in much the same idea and another punk princess, Poly Styrene of *X-Ray Spex* (*Oh Bondage up Yours*, anyone?) experienced a UFO sighting which changed her life completely. The Spex had been treading the boards at Doncaster's Outlook Club and were leaving the venue when Ms Styrene saw her UFO. Her reaction was simple, clear and prophetic: "I just need to go on searching for more knowledge. Inevitably it's going to lead to religion in the end. Lead to religion it surely did, and subsequently Poly renounced her name, her band, her music and her hair for the rigid devotions of the Hare Krishna sect. Rock'n'punk hard men, *The Stranglers*, delved into the more arcane regions of ufology when they titled an album *Themeninblack* after the fashion dissonants who cruise the highways in out-of-date but perfect black Cadillacs, harassing witnesses and investigators who get too close to the 'truth'. Coincidentally (or was it?), after the release of this album, the band were plagued by a chain of misfortunes. That's what you get for messing with those unknown forces, I guess. Germany's disco diva, Nina Hagen, held a flying saucer fixation so deep it antagonised people.

She became the focus of attacks by fundamentalist Christians, both verbal and physical. On the rear of her album *Fearless,* she is depicted standing in the vapour trail of a UFO. The lyrics of the song *Flying Saucers* demonstrate her belief:

> "Flying saucers everywhere, For flying saucers are unbelievably important,
> because they know the secret of life. And we are observed in the name of
> the light."

Her song *UFO* goes on to tell us that "You are not alone. The UFOs are picking us up". Eventually they came to Nina in the shape of a sighting at her Malibu home.

Rock singers may have translated their personal and heartfelt UFO beliefs and experiences into their songs but the marketing men in rock long since realised that the 'flying saucer' was a potent image for inclusion on album sleeves, Roger Dean's early Seventies artwork drew heavily on the UFO mythos for its inspiration. Other album sleeves, which feature UFOs of one sort or another, include: *Wishbone Ash's Argus* (Adamski-type saucer on rear), *Led Zeppelin's Third* (small UFOs on cover), *Grateful Dead's Mars Hotel* (large disc seen through a window on rear of sleeve), *Jefferson Airplane's After Bathing At Baxter's* (Adamski type craft), *Barclay James Harvest's Eyes of The Universe* and albums by the *Electric Light Orchestra*.

Even without the direct connection of belief or experience in the subject by the artist, UFO connections crept into songs and lyrics. Stories gleaned from the media and the UFO literature was reflected back in song lyrics.

The list is a long one, but how about *Purple Saucers over Yatton* by *Stackridge* or that ancient astronaut fancier's, perennial favourite *A Spaceman Came Travelling* by Chris de Burgh, or even the unlikely sounding *A UFO has Landed in the Ghetto* by Ry Cooder? There is now a small but rapidly developing niche in the record collecting market for albums and singles by artists who either sing about UFOs or feature them on the cover. Jenny Randles proposes that writing lyrics about the UFO experience may be part of the UFO phenomenon as a whole, the experience, in these cases, occurring on a psychic level. But to most people it's just fun!

Personal experience of a UFO informed the song by pop funsters *Hot Chocolate*, entitled *No Doubt About it*, which is all about strange lights and a craft they had seen while returning from a gig in London: it glided down so silently. It wasn't an illusion."

Try telling them about misperception! A similar event happened to 1980s Liverpool band *A Flock of Seagulls* who were buzzed by a UFO in a forest near Southport following a gig in the area. Band member Ari opined that it apparently it happens quite often in that region. They fly in from the coast and go there because it's a forested area and there aren't many people." Their interest piqued by the sighting, the band pursued the subject and later claimed to have contacted aliens by telepathy. As they vanished from the public eye shortly afterwards, it's quite conceivable they were abducted!

The crop circle phenomenon, although now largely credited as the work of enterprising landscape artists - led to one of the more spectacular formations appearing on the front cover of *Led Zeppelin's Remasters* album. Reg Presley, the leader of vintage rockers *The Troggs*, who hails from the centre of crop circle country, now spends much of his time investigating both the not-so-enigmatic circles and the broader UFO phenomenon. Reg was one of the first to see the infamous Santilli 'Roswell autopsy' film.

The explosion in ufology over the past 10 years or so has brought a whole new generation of rocksters, weaned on Close *Encounters of the Third Kind* and *ET*. Dance music in all its forms has also taken the UFO scene to its heart.

Clubs such as Pete Avila's *Osmosis*, whose fliers were in the shape of flying saucers, featured the classic 'grey' head and advertised the experience as being "99% pure euforia", Many dance artists, particularly of the ambient persuasion, have used the iconography of UFOs to grace their album sleeves, posters and fliers for events. The fact that this resurgence of interest in UFOs among the young groovers has arisen at the same time as a huge upsurge in the usage of LSD and Ecstasy may help shed some little light on the connection between UFO experiences and altered states of consciousness. Dancing under the influence can create trancelike states and this may well be the window through which UFO imagery shines.

Famed ambient experimenters *The Orb* have long been into the UFO mythos. Their third album was entitled *UFOrb*. Orbmeister Dr Alex Patterson himself is a firm believer. He has to be, because he saw a UFO in 1987. "It was in a valley just outside Turin. I saw this red disc moving slowly away from me, then it suddenly picked up speed and disappeared." Tracks on *UFOrb* with names such as *Operation Majestic*, *Blue Room* and *Close Encounters* speak for themselves, and increasing numbers of people at their gigs can be seen sporting the 'grey head' logo on their clothes and bags.

Ozric Tentacles's techno offshoot band, *Eat Static*, released an album called *Abduction*, the cover of which featuring a classic UFO beaming a ray down onto a stone circle, effectively combining today's alternative youth's two fascinations: earth mysteries and ufology. Another old rocker who has recently reinvented himself for today's market is Julian Cope, who blends earth mysteries, crop circles and UFOs together in one potent brew. Cope, a fervent believer in ET and author of a book about stone circles which includes UFO accounts, has mentioned the subject on many occasions in interviews and his song *Upwards At Forty Five degrees* from the *Jehovakill* album speaks of a craft "400 metres across, hanging like a football field, over the valley of the stone circle, for the mothership has come, who's she gonna take this time". *EMF*, best remembered for their chart topping single *Unbelievable*, on their tour of America took in several *UFO Parties* which at the time were all the rage with the youth of California. Singer Derry said "The kids hand around details of all the latest UFO sightings. They all know where the craft have landed and how long the aliens were incubated for." These dance parties are held in remote desert areas where ravers can, er, 'rave' and watch out for the craft they just know, like the truth, are out there somewhere. Terry Vickers, of *Levitation*, was quoted in the *New Musical Express* (16 May 1992) as saying:

> "If *Levitation* make money, I'm going to set up a platform for extraterrestri-
> als to land on." Vickers went on to say that he hoped "the ancient South
> American prophecy will come true and we're going to be revisited by
> extraterrestrials."

One of the first home-grown UK heavy metal groups, UFO, naturally sported UFO iconography on their album sleeves. 1974's *Phenomenon* and the collection *Essential UFO* are the two best examples, while the album *Making Contact* (1983) also hinted at communion with the space brothers. Dave Grohl from *Nirvana* reinvented himself under the nom-de-musique *Foo-Fighters*, the name given by World War II aircrew to the balls of light, precursors to modern day UFOs, which buzzed them on missions across Europe. And will we ever be able to forget *Babylon Zoo's* karaoke-Bowie chart-topper *Spaceman?* UFOs and rock'n'roll are here to stay, it seems, and I've only scratched the surface of the connections between UFOs and rock music. Trivial pursuit or not, this aspect of the wonderful world of ufology is just another one of many where the basic precepts of the late 20th Century UFO mythos is subliminally spread through popular culture.

As we neared the Millennium, there are bound to be more and more references to UFOs by rock 'n' roll-ers; more spotty string-strokers who will report their abduction experiences in song and interview; but I'll leave you with *Happy Mondays'* and *Black Grape's* Shaun Ryder's unequivocal views on the subject.

You ever seen any UFOs Shaun? "I have yeah, a few times. I've seen fookin' hundreds and hundreds of spacecraft flying across the sky over Salford. I mean hundreds of them. Hundreds!"

It's great when you're straight. Yeah!

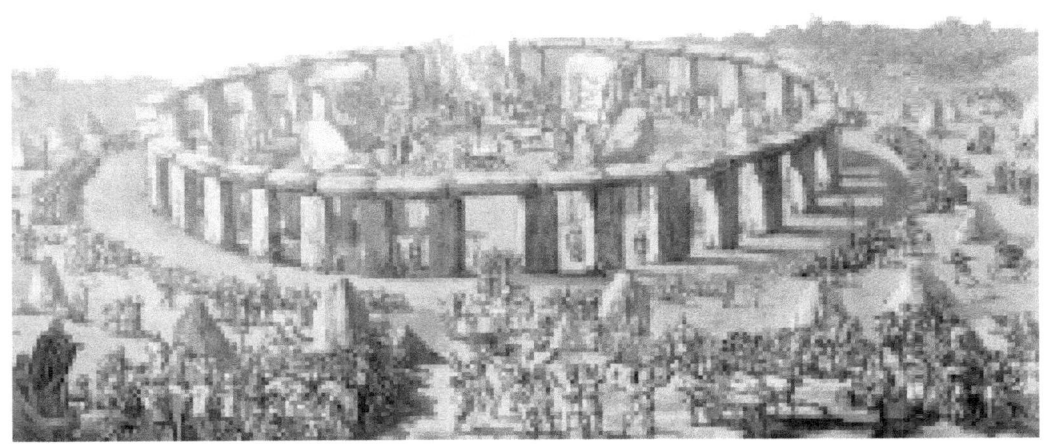

FOO FIGHTERS: THE STORY SO FAR

The subject of foo fighters, the mysterious aerial phenomenon seen by aircrew during WWII, is probably the most neglected area of study in the field of ufology. Once ufologists realised that their world did not in fact begin on June 24th 1947 with Arnold's infamous sighting, it has become fashionable to conduct research into "historical" UFO's which has led to some useful insights into the nature of the UFO phenomenon as a whole.

IGNORED

The pre-Great War Airship, and between-the-wars Mystery Flier Waves, plus the post-war Mystery Rocket waves have all been admirably covered by researchers in the UK, USA and Sweden, but foo fighters have been virtually ignored. With this in mind I began in 1987 to seek out all material extant relating to foo fighters to try and put the subject into a much-needed perspective and with the hopeful intention of publishing the end results in book form as a reference tool for other ufologists. This is some way off yet and I think it may be worthwhile detailing the progress made, and the problems encountered so far.

Sadly neglected as an area of study they may be, but every ufologist has at least *heard* of foo fighters and almost every writer on the subject has mentioned them. So you would think that a mass of information would exist on the subject. Unfortunately this is just not the case. Look in any UFO book and you will find that foo fighters are just given a few lines, at most in some rare cases a few pages and in only one or two instances a whole chapter.

This is pathetic really for an area of UFO activity which immediately proceeded the modern era and one which, if we are to believe the more "enthusiastic" ufologists, was the start of the so-called "Government Cover-Up". The history of foo fighters as represented within the subject of ufology is sadly riddled with problems which have put foo fighters in the historical niche they occupy today. These problems need stating and dealing with before the foo fighter phenomenon can be seen in anything approaching a clear perspective.

For a start even the name 'foo fighter' is problematic; did it come from the old Smokey Stover cartoon character saying "Where there's foo there's fire"; or was it from the French word *feu*, meaning fire, or was it, according to one ex-B17 waist gunner I spoke to, from "phooey".

Needless to say, he didn't believe they existed! Also, what exactly is the definition of a "foo fighter"? It usually depends on what obscure theory a particular writer is trying to prove. For the purposes of my study I have used the criteria of any unexplained light source seen in conjunction with an aircraft either from the air or from the ground. This is deliberately descriptive as to include all war-time UFO's, which are as diverse as the ones we report nowadays, would need many years research itself.

RE-ARRANGED

Firstly, when considering the written sources in the literature, it should be made known that almost every author who has mentioned the subject, in a book or a magazine article, has quite literally stolen his or her material from someone else and invariably left it unreferenced to create, no doubt, the illusion that the author in question discovered the facts themselves. Furthermore even the copied facts are often woefully misquoted or conveniently "rearranged" to suit the author's particular argument and all obviously done without checking the salient facts at source.

For instance, if we constructed a "family tram" of foo fighter material we would find, almost without exception, that the "grandpappy of them all" is the 1945 *American Legion Magazine* article, written by Jo Chamberlin. This article forms the substance of almost every piece written on the subject of foo fighters.

Fortunately this article is based on accounts which can be (has been) checked with squadron records and appears largely correct but its incessant copying has precluded any original work actually being done on the subject and has subsequently led to many writers extrapolating generalisations about the foo subject as a whole, most of which are demonstrably untrue. Examples of this armchair theorising are legion but for instance; many items dealing with foo fighters state almost as an article of faith that foo fighters only appeared in the later stages of the war, specifically around the winter of 1944-5.

SECRET WEAPON

This is a direct result of Chamberlin's article, and has led to further speculation that perhaps they were Nazi secret weapons which were pulled out of the hat at the last minute, or even perhaps that the foo were extraterrestrials keeping an eye on us before we used the atomic bomb. This time scaling is false and the first record I have of a foo fighter comes from 1940 and they were seen often throughout all the war years. Another false fact of the foo fanciers faith is that the phenomena were mainly seen over the European theatre of war and just occasionally over the Pacific. This is again false and the product of sloppy research.

So far I have accounts of foo fighters having been seen over Norway, Germany, France, Italy, Sicily, The Pacific, Burma, Tunisia, and all of the sea areas adjoining these countries. They were very clearly an international phenomenon.

Still another mistake is the statement made by many authors that the axis pilots also were seeing the phenomena and that they thought, just as our pilots did, that it was an allied secret weapon. This may yet be proved true but I have so far to find an original reference made by an axis pilot, or authority, that this was the case. The statement seems to be ufological canard employed on the basis of 'well if our boys saw them they must have too', and again has been used to support the ETH argument. The facts behind the rumour must await further verification. Axis aircrew was in fact seeing unexplained aerial phenomena but as yet most of their accounts await translation.

HOAX

We have at least one outright hoax too in foo fighter lore. For years rumours had been flying round that the Germans had been fully aware of the foo fighter phenomenon (perhaps that's where the above canard originated) and that they had a special study group formed to look into the problem under the name of "Project Uranus," backed by a shadowy group by the name of Sonderburo 13 (reminds you of Majestic 12 doesn't it?).

This was first detailed in *La Livres Noir De Soucupes Volantes* (The Black Book of Flying Saucers-1970) by French ufologist Henry Durrant. The rumour spread in Europe and eventually took physical form in the English language in Tim Good's acclaimed book *Above Top Secret* where it is used to help substantiate further vague rumours of an Anglo/American foo fighter study. Good had not checked his facts and had in fact just copied the information direct from Durrant's book. When I checked this out with Durrant he informed me that the whole "Project Uranus" affair was a hoax which he had inserted in his book precisely to see who would copy it without checking. The hoax apparently had been revealed in France some years before but hadn't percolated its way through to English speaking ufologists. Perhaps other foo hoaxes await discovery.

I could go on listing mistake after mistake and misquote after misquote from which we have drawn the current idea of foo fighters. The quality of research and writing on the subject of foo fighters has been truly appalling. Once these primary problems were realised I found that trying to research the subject from within the UFO literature was pointless and incestuous and so attempted to get back to the source material -- the pilots and crew themselves and the official records.

FRESH REPORTS

With this in mind I wrote to every air-related magazine in the UK with a request for information from ex-aircrew. To date I have had some thirty replies from pilots and crew detailing their experiences with strange balls of light (incidentally not one of them knew them by the name "foo fighters," or any other name for that matter). I will be repeating the procedure this year both in the UK and the US to draw in more fresh reports. None of these respondents connected their sighting in any way with the modern idea of UFO's and their information is so much the better and clearer for that. In many cases I have copies of entries made in log-books immediately after the flight which details what took place.

BALLS OF LIGHT

In the main, the descriptions are similar to the many already portrayed in the literature. Balls of light of varying colour (mainly orange) and number would appear from nowhere and play tag with aircraft for up to forty minutes. They were not hallucinations, being in some cases seen *en masse* by the entire crew of a Lancaster bomber, and were not reflections as they were seen from many different angles or from two 'planes at once.

Evasive action to shake them off was no use. In one case a Lancaster almost burnt its engine out, going "through the gate," a slang term used by pilots to denote pushing the engine to its limits, in an effort to lose its incandescent follower, but to no avail. One of my respondents had fired on the phenomenon, in some cases fearing it to be a secret weapon which would explode when fired upon, and in others just attempting to evade it on the basis that as long as it wasn't firing at them they weren't going to antagonise it. Having said this I have heard an unsubstantiated tape of an interview with an American gunner which cites a case in which a foo was fired on. And the shells went straight through it! Interesting and very supportive of the unexplained atmospheric phenomenon theory. Although some books note the (unreferenced!) fact that some foos appeared inside the planes or affected the electrics etc. I have found no record of that taking place. Nor is there any verified account of foo fighters showing up on ground radar. The phenomena whatever it was, is clearly distinguished by the aircrew from common natural phenomena such as St. Elmo's Fire, and was a completely separate entity from the 'plane they were in. It appears to have been totally independent and able to change shape, speed and position at will.

LACK OF INTEREST

Clearly something was being seen. A few pilots and crew chose not to report their experience at the time for fear of ridicule or for fear of being grounded for having hallucinations. Many though did record and report what they saw however and the response of the intelligence de-briefing staff varied considerably from total disinterest or hilarity to, in one case only, great interest and a further interview by intelligence officers. This apparent lack of interest on the part of the intelligence services begs the question of whether any official RAF or US 8th AF study was ever actually undertaken. It was certainly claimed to have, instigated by the untraceable Massey in the UK and Eisenhower in the US. Although my sample of respondents is small is seems odd that only one crew out of thirty or more were actually de-briefed at length specifically on the subject.

This was more than likely to be concerned with the possibility that the crew had seen one of the new German jets than anything else. In view of the amount of time, effort and expertise needed it seems unlikely that any nation during the hard pressed times of WWII took time and effort out to study what was essentially an ephemeral, elusive and ultimately harmless phenomenon. This will certainly not please cover-up aficionados but it seems to be the case on current evidence.

My research so far with the RAF/MOD/PRO in the UK has drawn a total blank regarding the official documentation and investigation of the subject, as have preliminary investigations in the USA. UFO sceptics will of course say that this is because it doesn't exist, proponents, especially cover-up buffs, will say it is because it is being kept secret.

The simple facts are that if documentation does exist in the UK I am unlikely to be able to get at it easily because of our comparatively archaic procedures for obtaining any government documents. The Freedom of Information Act has revealed that the Royal Airforce did create a number of files relating to unusual aerial activity during WWII. Unusual lights, rockets and aircraft are detailed but nowhere can I find that they are referred to as foo fighters. The flight logs of some aircrew often mention being chased by 'the thing' but if further documentation does exist in the UK it is likely to be buried in a mass of unrelated documentation.

In addition to these facts I have spoken to some ex-wartime RAF intelligence people in the UK and they claim no knowledge of the phenomena. As no photographs of foo fighters from a UK source exist we are left with the tension between them actually being genuine and unexplained aerial phenomena and the misperceptions of aircrew whose perceptions were heightened often to the point of paranoia because of the threat of imminent death, and obtaining any document depends on whether a department can actually be bothered to answer your letters or if so, and can be bothered to undertake a meaningful search of their records. The situation is further complicated by the fact that many records in our Public Records Office are hard to locate due to how it is organised and furthermore are subject to "rules" such as the 30 year rule whereby information is not available for 30 years from date of classification.

Worse still many WWII records are languishing under a 75 year rule for reasons I have not yet fathomed! In addition to these facts I have spoken to some ex-wartime RAF intelligence people in the UK and they claim no knowledge of the phenomena.

This area is clearly a matter for further study but, as with contemporary UFO research it should be borne in mind that whilst there many rumours of government interest and intervention regarding foo fighters the actual evidence cannot be found. I do not think this points to a `cover-up' in any way. The situation in the US may yet turn out to be different as regards obtaining official documentation and I would welcome help from any US readers who have an interest in the foo-phenomenon.

NOT VALID

The German secret weapon hypothesis (GSWH) promoted by such writers as Renato Vesco is unlikely to be valid. The reports are too widely spaced out throughout the war and come from too many differing theatres for them to be a secret weapon of any kind. Certainly the Germans were experimenting with saucer-shaped craft, flying wings, etc., but they had not got very far beyond the drawing board and model stage.

In addition, if foo fighters were a weapon they were clearly ineffective as one. The GSWH can be seen in the same light *vis a vis* foo fighters as the way many people relate modern UFO sightings to alien craft. It is a cultural or, in the case of foo fighters, an occupational artefact which when seen in retrospect (as will the ETH no doubt) can be identified and discounted.

CONCLUSION

Out of all this some clear facts are apparent. Hundreds of aircrew saw and recorded what we now call foo fighters during WWII There must be many thousands of ex-aircrew who have stories to tell. The problem is finding them and the odd advertisement or article is only going to draw a few out and I have yet to attempt to get to American information from squadron survivors, units etc.

The situation regarding German information is further complicated by a language barrier but it is only a matter of time.

I firmly believe that foo fighters were a real, although non-solid phenomenon and I am forced to reject the hallucination/misperception hypothesis almost entirely. These people's lives depended on being able to see and identify aerial objects extremely quickly. One mistake and it was their last. Some crew have admitted misperceiving Venus etc., but realising it in seconds, and certainly not a whole crew being fooled for any length of time.

Foo fighter reports give us a "genuine" UFO report, uncluttered by contemporary ideas about aliens, saucers and the like and which, as appear to be many 'genuine' UFO reports when they are stripped of cultural bias, consists basically of rudimentary light sources performing odd manoeuvres in the sky. My research has a long way to go yet but I would offer the suggestion that foo fighters and their pre and antecedents which are still being seen today by people both pilots and ground observers are a type of natural phenomena, possibly related to ball or bead lightning, but equally possibly not.

They may be something as yet totally undiscovered. They are also the stimulus for many of today's UFO reports which are subsequently overlaid by the prevailing cultural perceptions, i.e. alien craft. Mystery airships, ghost fliers, foo fighters, flying saucers - they may well all turn out to be different facets of the same phenomenon.

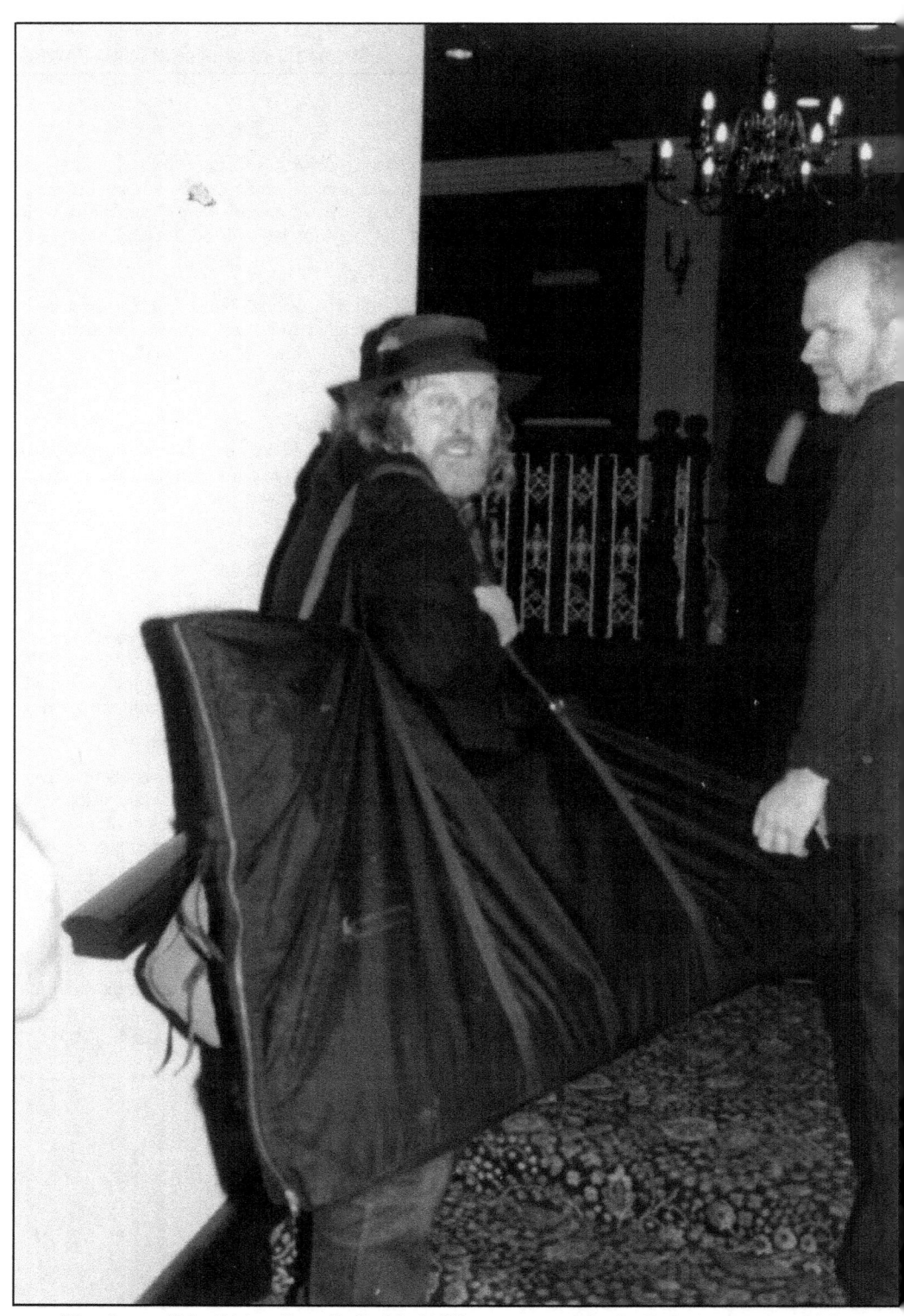

The *Incredible String Band's* Robin Williamson and Andy Roberts, at the 1994 *Incredible String Band* Convention

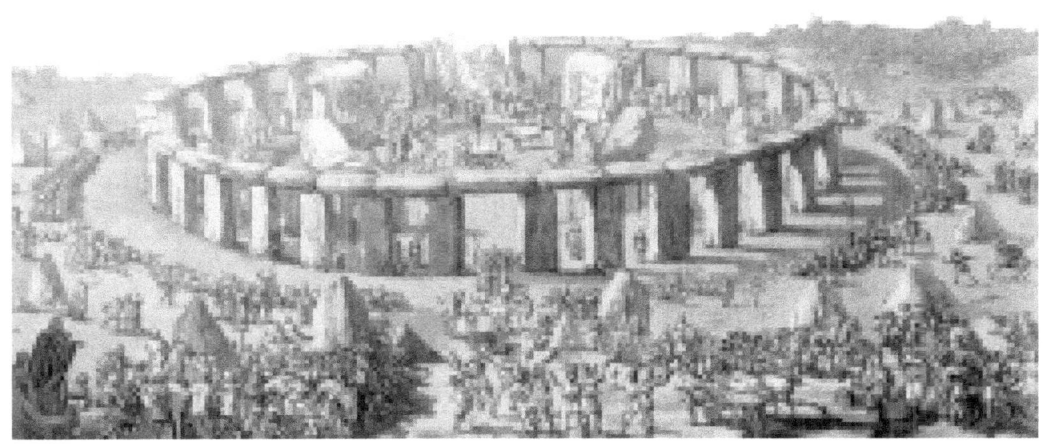

THE HANGMAN'S BEAUTIFUL DAUGHTER

In 1967 the ISB were still a bit of an inside tip for the cognoscenti (including most of the Stones and Paul McCartney), but 1968 was the year in which they started to reach a much wider public. The album which helped them make that transition had been recorded during the winter of 1967...

The *Hangman's Beautiful Daughter*: catalogue no EUK 258 to its matrix, but something vastly different to the people who know and love it for what it is, and what it has become over the years. Of all the String Band albums *Hangman* seems to give something the others don't, to touch places only hinted at elsewhere; if any album ever made you want to renounce temporal obligations and head for the wildwood this was the one. Maybe it was the times, maybe the chemicals.

Maybe it was just the right people at the right time, tuned in and turned on, waiting to receive, to receive a transmission from *something*. The zeitgeist was never ensnared better than on *Hangman*.

Hangman was the album which finally catapulted the ISB from being quirky post-Dylan folkies into psychedelic stardom, in sales, live performances and critical appraisal. Prior to its release the String Band had played a few London clubs and smaller concert venues up and down the country; their biggest gigs to date had been as support to the *Pink Floyd* and *Fairport Convention* at the Saville Theatre in October 1967 and a double bill with Shirley & Dolly Collins at the Queen Elizabeth Hall later that month. Their manager Joe Boyd had a master plan which was to change all that, involving the band's first solo tour of big halls. Joe: 'I just knew it would be fine, the tour sold out and the second week the album was out it was at number three!'

The title? Karl Dallas interviewed the band just prior to the album's release and queried the title: 'It was an interview filled with sudden, reflective silences in which I sometimes felt that my questions were like rocks being thrown into a deep, clear pool, disturbing its calm.'

Robin: 'In a way you could say the title thought of us. What does it mean? You can explain it at several levels.'
Mike: 'The hangman is death and his beautiful daughter is what comes after. Or you might say that the hangman is the past twenty years of our life and the beautiful daughter is now, what we are able to do after all these years. Or you can make up your own meaning. Your interpretation is probably just as good as ours.'

A biography of Dylan Thomas suggests another source. The young Thomas spent his childhood holidays at an aunt's house deep in the country. Local legend recounted how this house was once the dwelling place of the area's hangman. His daughter was so beautiful that he hid her away from the sight of any man lest she fall in love and leave him. She became depressed and whilst in this state took her own life - by hanging. But Robin, a big fan of Dylan Thomas, says he was unaware of this.

Robin once described *Hangman* as a 'winter album', and the original front cover finds Robin and Mike, suitably wrapped in stout winter garments, on a snowy moor near Balmore against a backdrop of icy blue sky. The rear cover photo catches them communing in a sheltered copse with Mike's new girlfriend Rose Simpson and Licorice, Robin's dog Leaf, two friends, Roger Marshall - with chain - and Nicky Walton, and a gaggle of perplexed-looking children (Mary Stewart's) in wacky hats. The picture strongly evoked the communal ethic emerging in the Sixties counter-culture; hitherto it had been usual for musicians to be portrayed in splendid isolation from their social milieu. Another novel feature of the album's original sleeve design was the total absence of credits or even a track listing. These details were included on an accompanying lyric sheet. Perhaps it was felt that the world wasn't quite ready for titles like *Koeeoaddi There* and *Three Is a Green Crown*. *Hangman* was often regarded as the acid album, though Williamson claims to have given up psychedelics by then: '...by that time I'd probably stopped taking drugs, it was very much what was going on at the time but I'd pretty much lost interest in drugs by then.' It certainly was what was going on and, drugs or not, the ISB looked to be living the psychedelic lifestyle - the time-less life. In fact, whether *Hangman* was created with or without psychedelics is largely immaterial as once that viewpoint is attained it tends to manifest itself in your life and the drugs become, to a large extent, superfluous. However, their presence and influence cannot be ignored. Many musicians whose work was grounded in psychedelics nowadays try to play this side of things down somewhat, whether through embarrassed hindsight, to hide their pasts from their offspring, or whatever. Whether listener or artist is drawn into the labyrinth that psychedelics provide is a personal choice. Humour and awe were and are the key, I suspect.

A Very Cellular Song is a case in point here. Heron has alluded to the fact that it had close connections with the LSD experience - as if we hadn't worked that one out - and told me: 'All it was, was a trip, and that was the music I was listening to, that and interspersed with Radio 4, bits of plays, people talking to each other, and I happened to be listening to the *Pindar Family* before I started.' The Bahamian *Pindar Family* did the original version of *We Bid You Goodnight* from *A Very Cellular Song* - it was also, trivia delvers, done frequently by the Grateful Dead at the end of concerts. The tune for the final 'long time sunshine' bit is from a traditional Sikh spiritual song called *On That Day*.

Contemporary reviews show the almost universal acclaim which met such a strange album - and also that critics could, when they wanted, write some pretty good descriptive stuff about music. The *Sunday Times'* Derek Jewell was well impressed, making *Hangman* Record of the Month in March 68: 'Quasi poetry and phoney mysticism now cling to the skirts of popular music, but the Incredibles are not pseudo. Their work is convincing, beautiful, idiosyncratic, and yielding more with each playing.' *The Observer's* Robin Denselow: 'Together with the *Beatles'* *Sgt. Pepper* it seems...to be the most important disc to have been produced in Britain for several years.' *Melody Maker* ran a preview, opening with:

> 'When poet Pete Brown, lyric-writer for the Cream, heard...*Hangman*, he said: 'That's what the Rolling Stones have been trying to do.' He was right, and on *Satanic Majesties Request* you can hear several *Hangman*-isms. But the Stones' media-hyped association with the dark forces (did you know Satan was originally known as just plain ol' 'Stan' until an extra 'a' was added by a mushroom-addled desert scribe?) was transparent when compared to the far deeper source that the ISB were tapping into on *Hangman*.

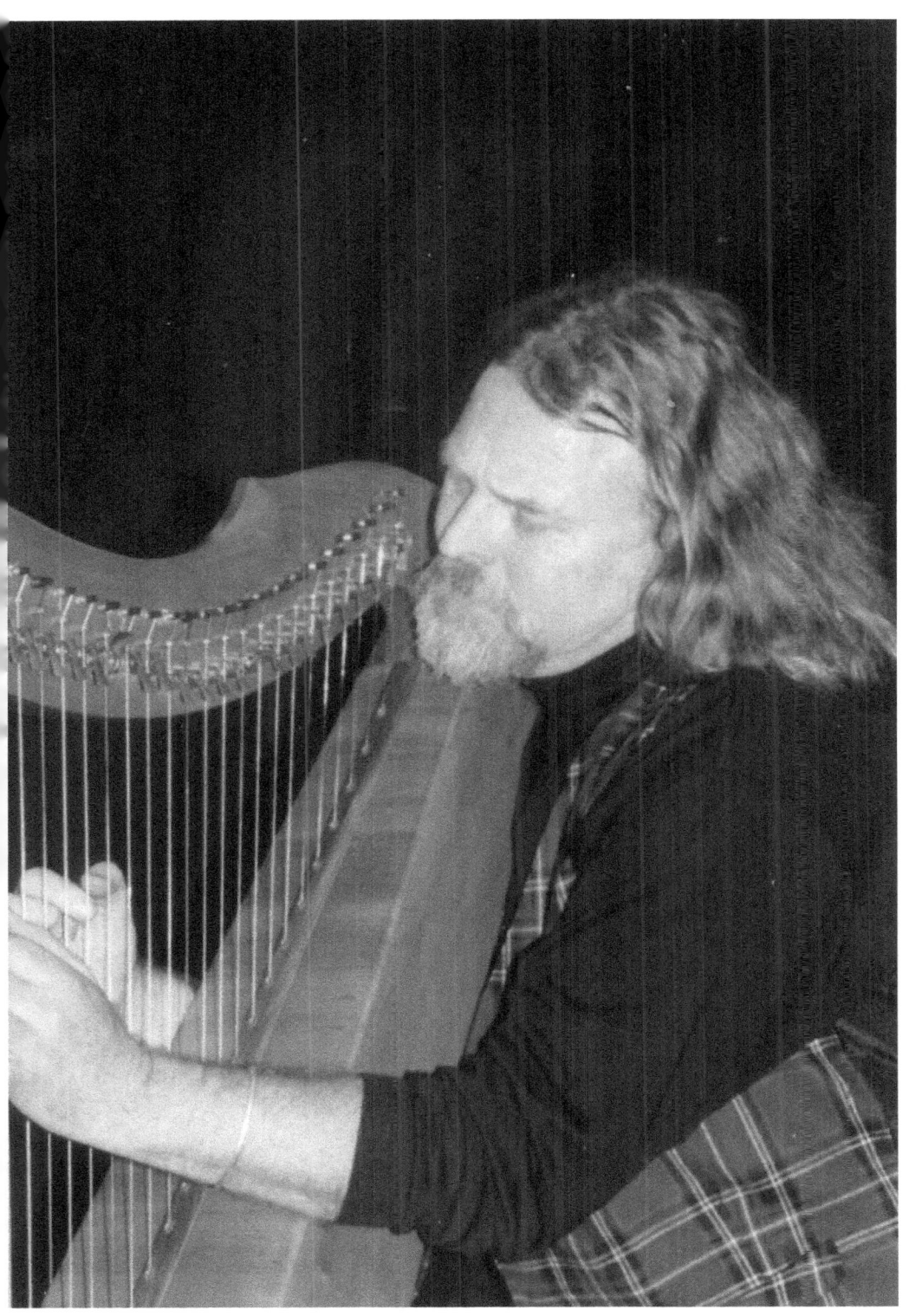

Robin Wi liamson at the harp

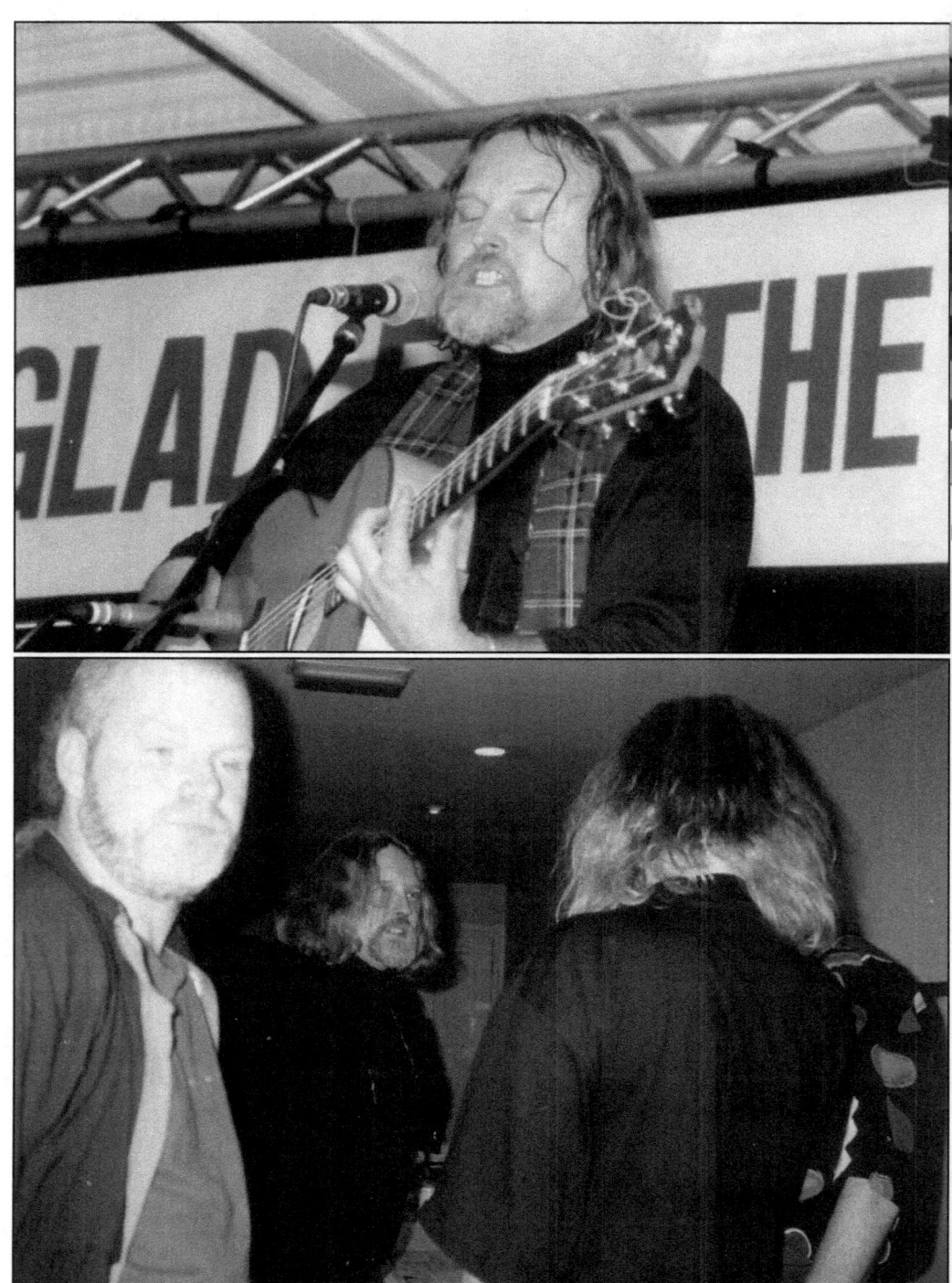

Robin Williamson and Andy Roberts, at the 1994 *Incredible String Band* Convention

Robin Denselow again:

> 'Taken as a whole, the songs are a plea for wonder at existence, a sometimes mystical, sometimes pantheistic involvement in a very live universe. In many ways it's a Wordsworthian romanticism, pro-nature, pro-imagination and anti-urban The expression of awe at being alive and the sense of organic connecting between all things comes, at times, near to religious statement.'

Praise indeed from the establishment – and more followed in the reviews of the March 1968 concert at the Festival Hall. In the *Financial Times* Anthony Thorncroft penned a perceptive piece about both the concert and band:

> 'The ISB are the nearest thing to godliness among the art school set: judging by the Establishment figures scattered among the audience they are about to be taken up by a more hard-bitten public.'

(You can just imagine Marc, Syd, Paul and the rest in the audience, furtively scribbling notes under their Afghans!)

> 'It is doubtful whether the delicate flavour of the Incredibles will make the transition. They compose their own mystical songs around melodies which ebb and flow with butterfly brittleness, and lyrics which link poetry and nonsense in an unholy marriage. The principal sources are Eastern and medieval music and, after a first hearing of disbelief, those prepared to accept the Incredibles' magical world can get on terms with the most unique talent to come out of the current song-writing revival.'

Americans were no less enthused; Richard Goldstein (*New York Magazine*) hit the nail on the head, and described Robin's voice as having a 'reedy whisper that sounds like water seeping out of ancient rocks', exhorting his readers to go out and buy *Hangman* so they could be the 'first (on your block) to worship at the universal church of magic'. Let's have some more Goldstein, it's nearly as good as the album! How about: 'Each song is a tone-poem etched in filigree; delicate yet sturdy. Each lyric is an utterly disarming cross between a hymn and a nursery rhyme.'

I couldn't find a bad review and the ones that weren't full of superlatives owed more to the reviewer's lack of imagination and skill with language rather than any dislike of the album. Everybody knew, to some degree or another that, in the words of Buffy St Marie, 'music is alive, magick is afoot' Or something like that. And so it was. Switched-on people all over the country were rushing home and turning on to *Hangman*, their minds scarred and certainly scared by its austere, cold beauty to such an extent that we have to write pieces like this decades later. The power of music eh? Critical acclaim was so great that *Hangman* was nominated for a Grammy award in the USA in 1969. *Cash Box* listed the Grammy nominees and there, in the 'Best Folk Performance' section along with Judy Collins' *Both Sides Now* and Dylan's *John Wesley Harding* is *The Hangman's Beautiful Daughter*. Strange days indeed.

Me? I love it, find it always challenging, always rewarding, always refreshing. If you haven't listened to it for a while I suggest you prime yourself by a long country walk, preferably in wild weather, slip it onto the turntable (or whatever) and connect with something.

But remember: 'The opposite is also true'.

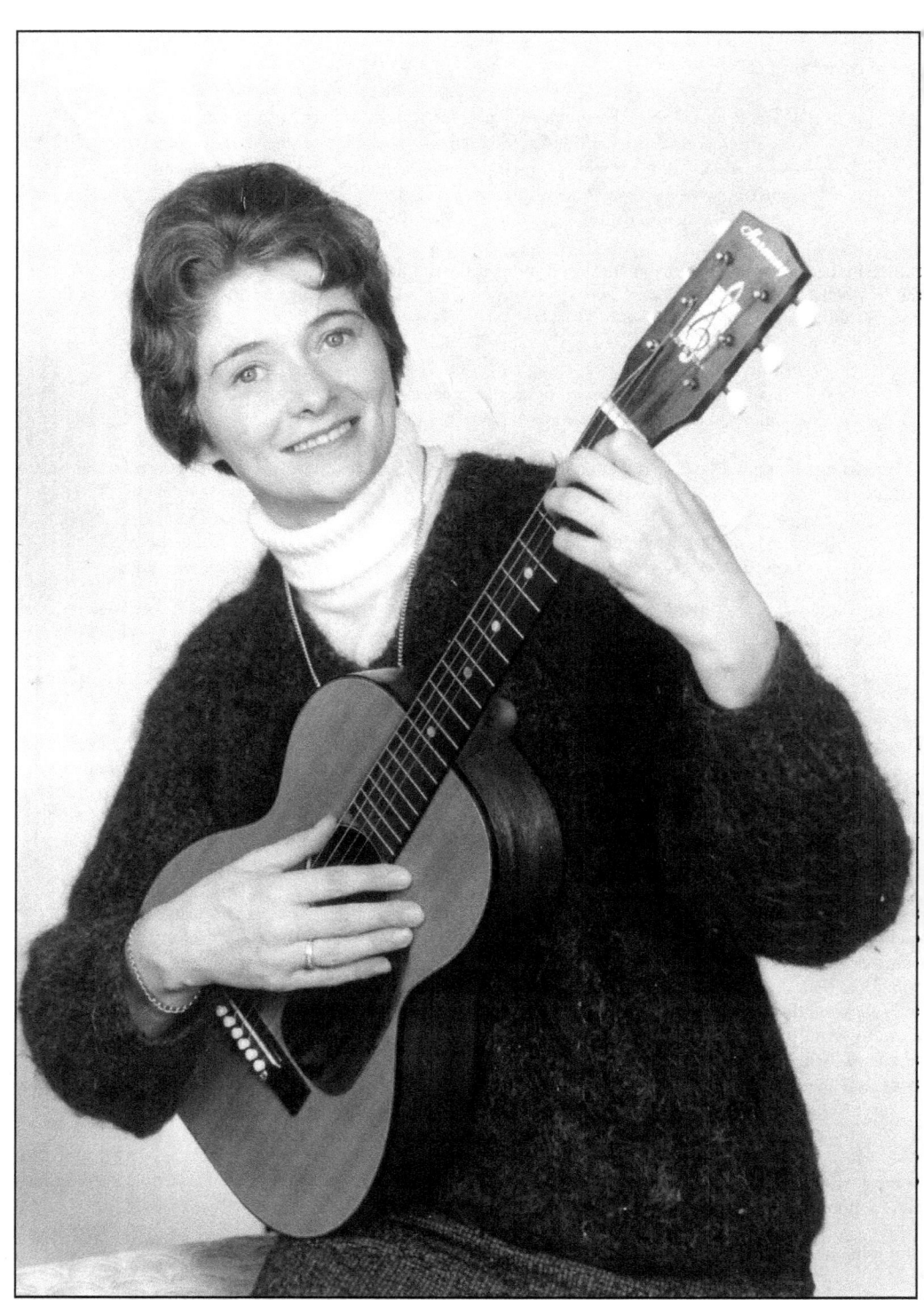

Molly Thompson, folksinger

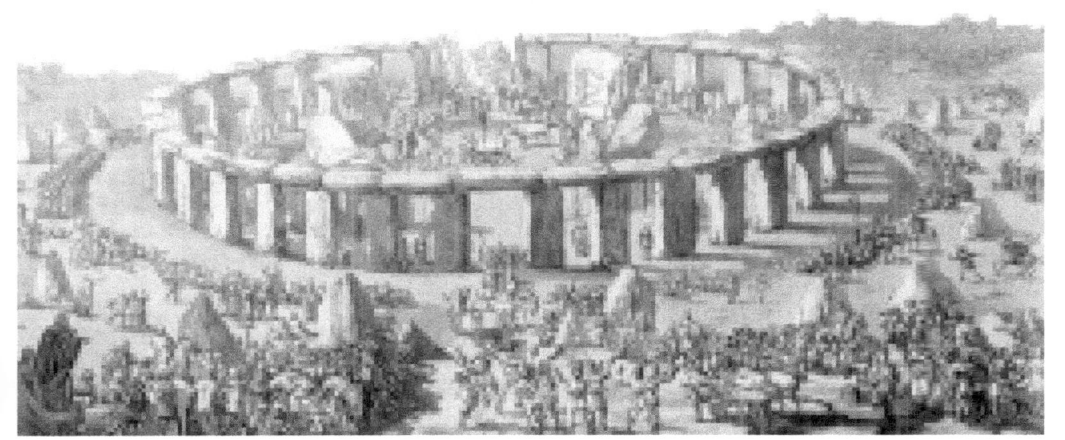

FROM WORLDS AFAR:
The Mollie Thompson Story
The story of the discovery of a long-lost British UFO contactee and songwriter

The UFO scene is vast, and many players have strutted and fretted on its stage since the modern era of the subject began in 1947. Books, magazines and TV documentaries are as yet our only, if fragmented, history of the subject but they feature only those individuals who have become 'famous' in some way, either as witnesses or as UFO researchers. This skewed version of ufological history is one written by the participants themselves and doesn't necessarily reflect the grass roots of the subject, doesn't reflect the involvement and aspirations of those who just wanted to pursue their interest and weren't unduly bothered about leaving their mark. Yet it is precisely these individuals who are the truly important people within ufology, people with no axe to grind or belief to push. Mollie Thompson will be a name unfamiliar to most readers. Unless you knew her, or are a *very* keen student of ufological history her name will mean little. She is one of the 'forgotten' ufologists. She shouldn't be because she contributed much to some of the more obscure corners of the subject and was responsible for enhancing people's lives as well as in transporting idea and philosophies within the subject.

This is a short insight into her story.

Mollie's interest in UFOs began, as did many people's, in the early 1950s after reading Leslie and Adamski's *Flying Saucers Have Landed,* "It spoke to me, it tweaked a nerve that I couldn't resist" she said. This remarkable book set her off on a journey of discovery which she is still pursuing to this day. Her interest in flying saucers grew rapidly and she started to read more, initially looking into the subject on her own. From the beginning her insights into the problem of contact with aliens were thoughtful and well in advance of much of the 'nuts and bolts' thinking of the era. She believed, "You can't expect what will be a superior intelligence to be understandable to you....you expand yourself to meet whatever is to come.". It was this point of view, which Mollie held from the start of her UFO studies, which would eventually lead her away from the 'nuts and bolts' certainties of the 1950s into the wilder fringes of the flying saucer movement and beyond, into the burgeoning new age movements of the 1960s and 70s. Initially Mollie joined the Manchester UFO Research Society, run by Harry Bunting and mixed her growing interest in flying saucers with her studies at a teacher training college, where she met another woman with whom she shared an interest in reincarnation. In the spirit of experimentation, they explored the ouija board together, making it 'work'.. Mollie is keen to stress that she prefaced her ouija sessions by "bringing in the light", but it was via the ouija board that she "Contacted something that I thought was a space entity…It had a name, it called itself Ornoor (stress on the first and last r) and it later had a friend called Lon.". She soon realised these contacts were not space people but spirits, of a sort. These contacts were followed by others with an entity called Philemon. These were telepathic contacts which enabled Mollie to ask questions and receive answers. At first she was confused as the answers didn't seem to make sense, but she slowly realised she was being 'taught', after which she was happy to accept the teachings. A four part series of her dialogues with Philemon appeared serialised in an early flying saucer magazine.

These contacts left Mollie wondering just what it was that people were contacting when they claimed to be contacting space people. She freely told her friends in the Manchester UFO Society of these contact and they, steeped in the nuts and bolts saucer lore of the 1950s thought her a little "odd". But as she says, "I was not trying to wean them away from nuts and bolts but trying to present a different picture they could take hold of if they wished."

Mollie and her friend Emily Crewe, who she met through the Manchester group, were lucky enough to meet George Adamski in person on his final visit to the UK. Hearing rumours that Adamski was staying with Desmond Leslie at his St John's Wood flat they travelled down to London on the overnight train on June 1st 1963, caught a taxi and, "I just went up and banged on the door and said we know he's here, we've come a long way and could we possibly see him?". There were several people waiting to meet Adamski at the flat but he was sequestered in another room, out of sight. Mollie recalls that Adamski specifically asked her to speak to him in the kitchen, where he told her that he and Desmond Leslie were going to visit someone who had seen a UFO and would she come too? During the course of the journey Adamski expounded his philosophy to Mollie and eventually asked her if she would go and work in the states with him. Unfortunately Mollie had only recently taken up her first teaching post so she regretfully declined the offer.

Mollie isn't entirely sure who they went to visit and it's here that the plot thickens and where we see how two people at the same event can recall things differently. Her friend, Emily Crewe, is absolutely certain that Lord Louis Mountbatten and Lord Dowding, both flying saucer aficionados were at the meeting and went in the car with Adamski and Leslie. Mollie, however, is adamant that neither of those two were present in the flat. By 1963 Mountbatten was playing down his earlier public interest in flying saucers so it would have been rather odd for him to have been mixing with people who could have exposed him. However, a clue may lie in a letter which Adamski subsequently wrote to Mollie in which he says, "…on the trip we took with Desmond to hear Mt. Batton (sic) story…". It seems probable that Mollie was taken to see a bricklayer named Briggs, who claimed to have been zapped by a flying saucer at Mountbatten's Broadlands estate in Hampshire on in February 1955.

Adamski also told Mollie, somewhat mysteriously, "The Brothers have work for you".

Besides being interested in flying saucers Mollie was also a music lover and a guitarist but not formerly trained. But in 1965 she recalls that: "words and music dropped into my mind. At first I thought it was my imagination, but I did begin to write them down. They fit together…I somehow knew they were going to be a song." And "It was as a result of these thoughts that were coming into my head, because I thought I've got to do something, they're not just given to me to play with, I've got to use them somehow, but how?"

One of the many people who got to hear Mollie's songs was Anthony Brooke. Brooke had been the last Rajah of Sarawak and closely involved in the 'new age' side of the flying saucer movement in the 1960s.

He crops up in several UFO books of the period, most notably Arthur Shuttlewood's books about the Warminster 'thing' and was a frequent visitor to the early Findhorn community. He had several of Mollie's songs on a tape recorder and played them to UFO groups across the world. Brooke decided that Mollie's songs needed a wider audience and arranged for her to make an LP. They approached Nield & Hardy Ltd of Stockport, Cheshire, who ran a small record label called Asteroid Records. The LP was duly recorded and was titled *From Worlds Afar*. The LP cover consisted of three distinctly Adamski-like saucers against an abstract backdrop of space. The rear of the sleeve had an introduction from Mollie plus brief notes for each of the ten songs. Some of the songs were about flying saucers; others had a more 'new age' tinge. All were thoughtful, heartfelt simple tunes with just Mollie and her acoustic guitar as backing and whilst Mollie tells me that a session musician filled in on some of the difficult bits you wouldn't notice. One of her earliest songs, and the first on the LP, was *The Cockeyed Ballad*, which contained these lyrics:

"Those flying saucers whisking through our skies
Must take some power to make the rise
But government departments just hide their eyes
And call them meteors
"Got brothers on Venus and Saturn it seems, fly their ships on magnetic beams
They wear one-piece suits and you can't see any seams
But apart from that they're just like us."

One night Mollie wrote three songs, complete with music, in hour and a half. This, she says, convinced her that they were not of her own doing. The LP was sold through the close knit network of flying saucer conventions, clubs and magazines. These days it is extremely rare and whilst it's occasionally possible to buy a copy for £30 or so I have seen it change hands on eBay for up to £200. Private pressings of 1960s musicians are highly sought after by collectors and *From Worlds Afar*, with its sincere but slightly naïve flying saucer/new age ambience makes it especially collectible.

Mollie made a backing track of herself singing harmony so that this could enhance her performance and a ten second video snippet of her singing *Cockeyed Ballad* at an American UFO conference exists to prove just what an accomplished performer she was.

Mollie seems to have visited almost every flying saucer group, cult or major event during the 1960s. She went to visit contactee Cynthia Appleton in Birmingham, chanted on hills with the Aetherius Society and meditated at Findhorn. Among the many ufological adventures Mollie had was a visit to Warminster at the height of 'The Thing' phenomenon. She spent an evening on Cley Hill, met Arthur Shuttlewood but saw no UFOs and was slightly disappointment there was no warm soup left for her! One visit or not she made sufficient impression on Arthur Shuttlewood to merit him giving her a short paragraph in 1968's *Warnings From Flying Friends*:

Molly Thompson is another person gifted in her liaison with space friends,
in the musical sense. She has sung her space songs by popular request in
many sectrors of the world, inspired by melodies lazily drifting through the
ether and captured by her ready consensus of their presence.

Her memories of these meetings are slowly fading now and as she said, much of it didn't really interest her and if she didn't like any aspect of saucer culture she wouldn't engage with it again. The area she was most drawn to was the new age side of things and she became increasingly involved with Liebe Pugh's Universal Link, based in the north west of England.

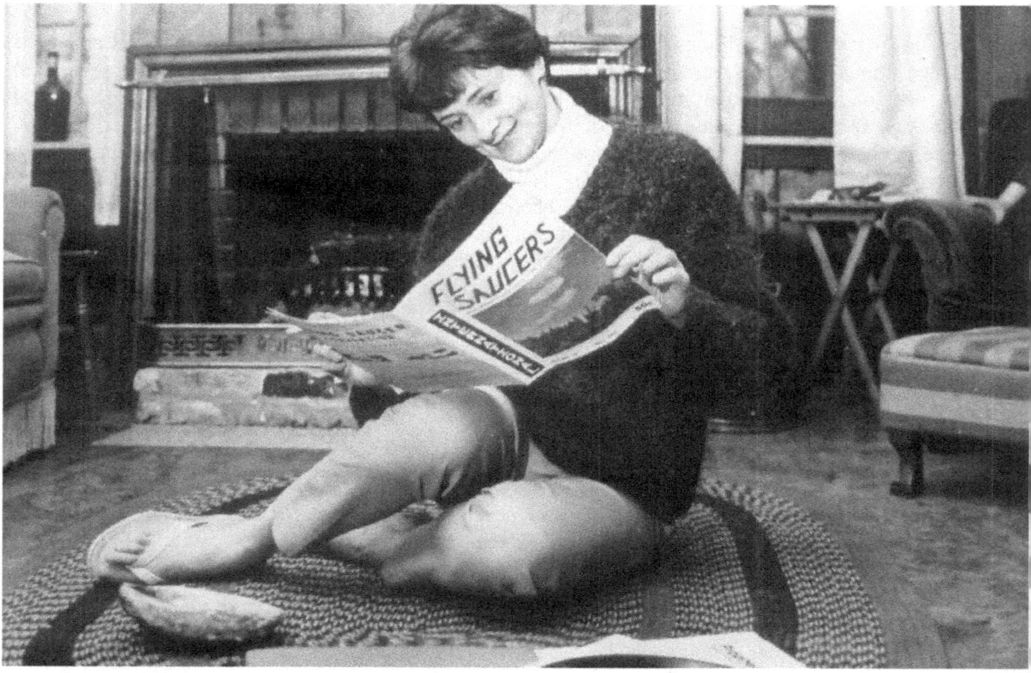

Top: Molly Thompson catches up on UFO news in 1966. Bottom: Molly Thompson, May 2005, holding a rare copy of *From Worlds Afar*

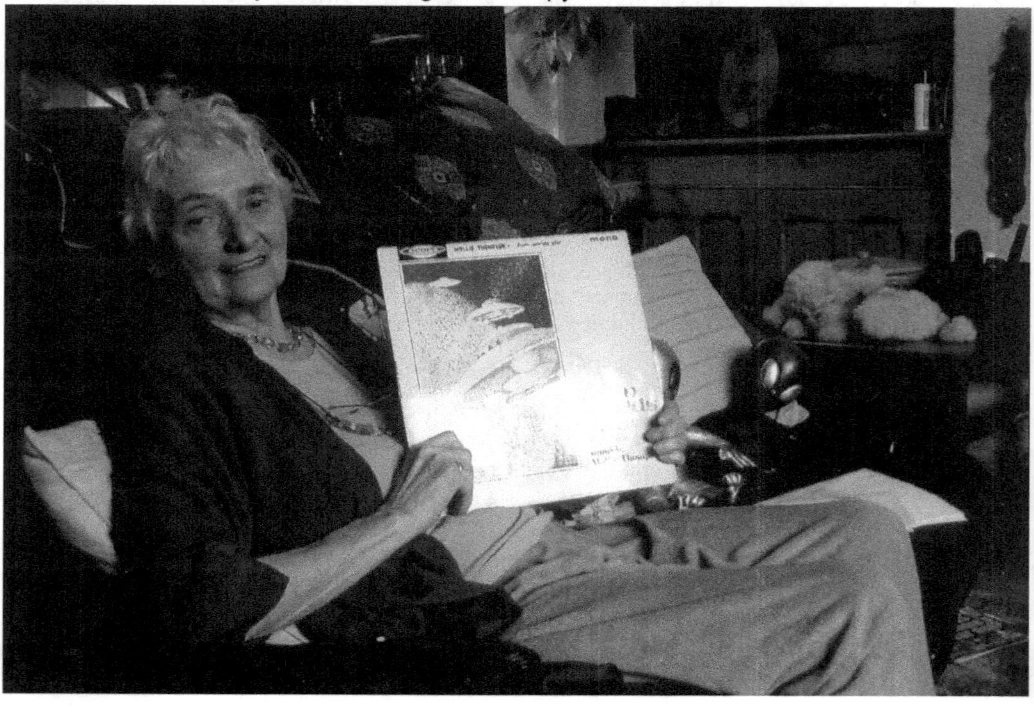

When Anthony Brooke visited America in early 1966 he played Mollie's songs to the president of the Amalgamated Flying saucers Clubs of America, in Los Angeles and they knew immediately that they wanted her to sing at their convention on 8th 9th and 10th of July. Universal Link paid for Mollie to fly to America in July and at lunchtime and in the evening on each of the three days she played a ten minute slot of her songs. Although she was due back in the UK shortly after the Convention there was a major air strike and she couldn't return. Seizing the opportunity she resigned from her job and spent several months travelling around the USA, literally singing for her supper. A Brit in the US was still a bit of a novelty in the mid 60s and more so on the saucer scene. As such she was treated very well by American ufologists who offered board and lodging as she travelled from one UFO group or convention to another, giving lectures and singing songs as she went.

During her American sojourn Mollie was lucky enough to hang out with many famous ufologists and contactees such as Mel Noel, Gabriel Green, Howard Menger and Dan Fry among a host of others.

In one interview whilst in the USA Mollie spoke about the prophecies people which those involved in the Universal Link believed. Some of this was then enshrined in her song *Three Wise Men*: 'The third wise man is a baby, the future looks bright to his eyes For his brothers will be from the planets, and his teachers will drop from the skies' And Mollie believed that 'something' was going to happen soon, 'this will all be revealed to all in 1967'. Universal Link teachings inferred that something was going to reveal itself via nuclear activity on or by Christmas Day 1967. Exactly what this revelation was going to be was unclear but it would be significant and world shattering. Mainstream ufology has always been wary of prophecies but where it interacted with contactees or the elements of the early new age prophecy abounded, and often revolved round a major earth change taking place.

When she returned from the USA in January 1967, back to life, back to reality, back to Britain, Mollie began to be disillusioned with flying saucers. There was no major world upheaval – no more than normal anyway - and Mollie began to slowly drift away from the saucer scene. However 1967 *was* a significant year for ufology though with the UK having possibly its biggest sighting wave ever, and in the US the events which John Keel wrote up as the *Mothman Prophecies* in which 38 people died when the Silver Bridge collapsed on December 15th.

But for Mollie, active participation in ufology was now over. Instead she intensified her work with the Universal Link and since then has worked 'behind the scenes' - as she puts it - in a number of new age organisations, eschewing publicity for the simple joys of service. When I first became aware of Mollie Thompson there was little information about her. The internet had no information about her at all and, other than the short paragraph in Arthur Shuttlewood's book, she had to all intents and purposes, been written out of UFO history. I was determined to find out more about her so that her imprint on ufology wasn't lost forever and I was assisted enormously by her old friend Emily Crewe.

However, Emily hadn't seen her for almost forty years and no-one had the faintest idea where she was or even if she was still alive. Among the many theories as to her whereabouts it was thought that she had emigrated to America. I asked questions, wrote letters to newspapers and trawled the internet for months, but with no luck. Eventually, one night in May 2005, I followed up a hunch based on something I'd seen on a web site unrelated to saucers or the new age. A tentative reply from the site owner gave me hope and said he would ask 'his' Mollie if she were *the* Mollie. Amazingly she was, still alive and healthy, and living in a town in the north of England. Within a couple of weeks we had spoken by telephone and I had interviewed her, the rest was history.

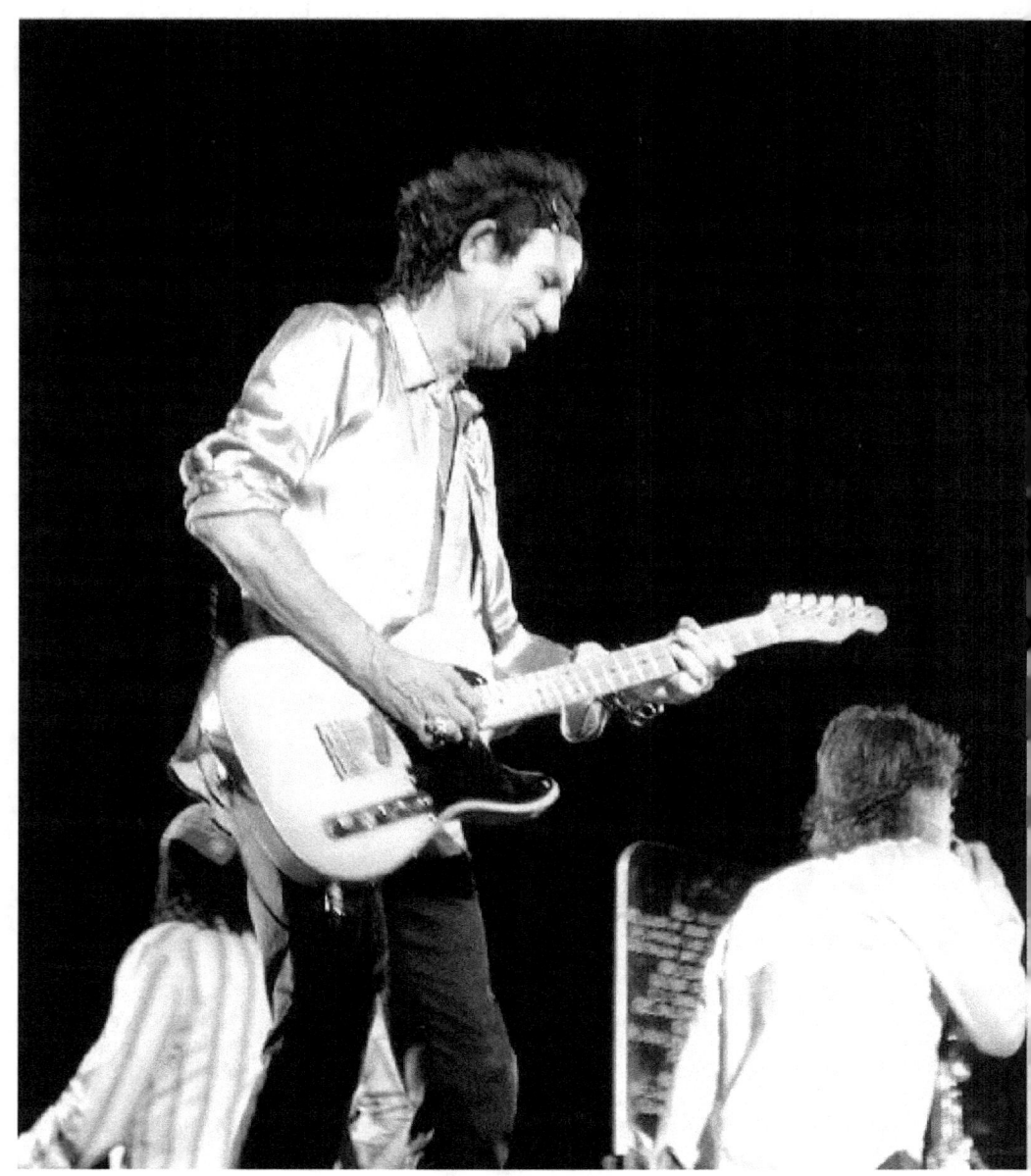

The human riff

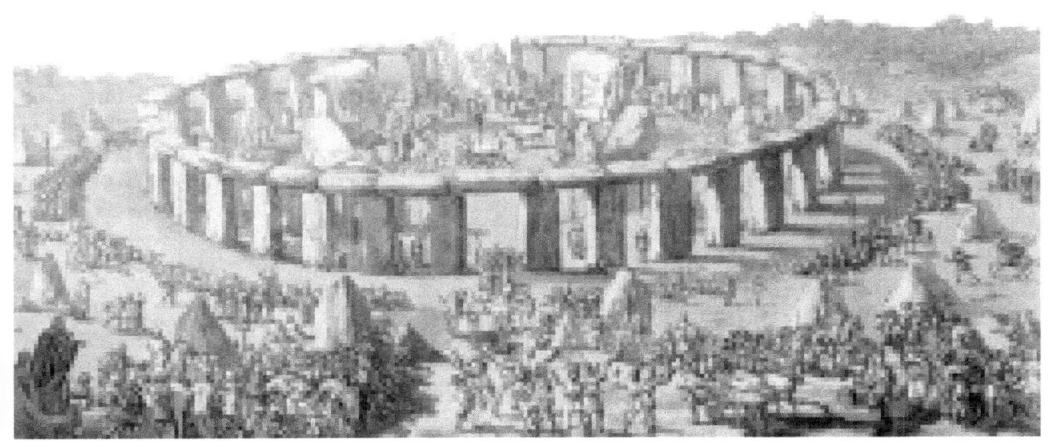

ROLLING STONES
27 AUGUST 2006, DON VALLEY STADIUM, SHEFFIELD
Written a day or so after the event and published on my website.

Any consideration of a big outdoor gig, let alone a Stones gig, has to work on many levels. My critical faculties were well attuned and is what I thought about the experience....

The venue wasn't too bad for a big place. Good sight lines. Crap toilet facilities, long queues for everything. But it was all seated and the idea of a seated audience at any gig is repulsive. Rock'n'roll should be experienced in a hot and sweaty group of people who are at liberty to dance if and when they desire. Seated, corporate shite such as the Stones' gigs are very far from the essence of rock'n'roll and are essentially pantomime, at least on one level. But as it's the only game in town it's the one we have to play and decide what to make of it.

The stage set was very good. Excellent light show and big video screen, but otherwise basic rock'n'roll stage set. Always something to look and marvel at. The big thing that moved into the audience looked like some futuristic D-Day landing craft delivering a crack troop of guitar manglers right into your face and was tippety top - even if just another panto on a smaller level to give the audience the idea they d had value for money, seeing the old gods, almost dead, at first hand.

I can't recall how much it cost to see the Stones last time I saw them, but it was less than 50 quid. 90 quid a few years later is a tad too much. However, when you are sponsored by American Express you have to have some way of explaining the high ticket prices - hence the seating, the no one allowed in the main audience area if you don't have tickets to sit there rule, the officious but entertaining stewards etc. I know, it's only rock'n'roll and we have to put up with it. VFM? We spent money, it had value. How can you quantify VFM? We wanted to see the Stones and were prepared to pay the asking price. Of course we got VFM!

If you asked the band they'd probably say their performance wasn't, musically, one of their best gigs. A few mashed lyrics, Jagger bizarrely changing the timing on some of them. Piano mixed too far back, which is a great shame because Chuck Leavell is one of rock's greatest pianists. Excellent guitar from Ronnie, standard rock'n'roll shape-throwing from Ron & Keef throughout. It's always good to see a live a horn section including the awesome Bobby Keys. One level it's a pantomime, a karaoke pantomime, in which the Stones become their own covers band and we all join in the illusion. But if you're prepared to pay 100 quid for your ticket you'll always invest in illusion. On another level if you ignore the size of the venue, the lights and corporate shite (I mean, seating above the stage for the privileged - what the fuck is that about and did you have to have a Platinum Card to get there?), it's the thrill of watching men and women doing their day job, cranking out high octane R&R in a fashion which pleases those in the cheap seats as much as those in the expensives. It's the only job these boys have done and despite all the cavils, today they had a very good day at the office.

It was a pretty standard set list; crowd-pleasing fare with a few oddities thrown in. *She's So Cold*? A ridiculous song best left in the 80s where it was conceived. Good choice in *Sway* and *Bitch*, although I thought *Bitch* was a bit messy. *Sympathy for the Devil* was entertaining - do you think every now and then Sir Mick has a moment of clarity as he's poncing about in his long red mac, making devil shapes with his arms. Do you think that, just once, when he's out on the lonely podium, old men cranking a rock'n'roll facsimile behind him that he's heard a thousand (two thousand actually), times before - do you think he occasionally thinks, 'What the fuck am I doing here trying to look like a teenager, singing about the Devil being misunderstood, when I've got a knighthood, more money than I can spell and a warm tour bus not ten minutes from my last song away?' I'd like to think not. Perhaps being on stage is like fucking and it's always good, always different, always to be looked forward to? Jagger's voice was a bit strained although he excelled himself on *You Can't Always Get What You Want* - which should have gone on much longer in my opinion. No *Midnight Rambler* though, which was a sad disappointment. Personally I think that if they ever tour again they should just go back to basics and play old blues stuff, just as they did when they started out.

And what about those who paid to see the band, the audience? Lawdy! If you're sitting you can't really be an audience, you have to be an observer. Even standing in your seats (would you really have sat down if security told you to - I think you would!) is merely being a standing observer. Rock'n'roll is all about participation first and foremost and you can't participate when sat, segregated by your ability to afford better or worse seats. You can kid yourself, but you'd be wrong. Audiences are always bizarre, Stones audiences more so than most as you get the complete spectrum of age, fashion and musical allegiance. You also get a lot of middle class twats who treated the stewards like shit, you could see thought bubbles saying, 'Don't you know who I am? I read the *Guardian*, enjoy the Sunday supplements, eat pesto and have a rather smart jumper thrown over my shoulder. My wife has actually bought trainers for this event you know, and you expect me to walk around the field rather than across it?'. They appeared to be there because it was the done thing to be there, to say they'd been there and how awful the stewards were. Fuck 'em! Then there were the housewives, singing their little hearts out to their favourite tunes. Unlike Jagger they certainly got what they wanted, as did the hardened rockers who were just rejoicing in the sheer glee of being there and part of it; the show that never ends inside their heads made real. All in all though, a very staid group of people. But just imagine what it would have been like if there were no seats and a general admissions policy? Wild scenes of rock'n'roll bacchanalia, I suspect, but there y'go.

Did I enjoy it, and would I see them again?

What a bizarre question!

I originally said 'no' this time but was seduced by the idea of the spectacle of seeing the World's Greatest Rock'n'Roll band in the flesh, at their age, at my age, just to see if the magic still worked. And yes, it did. The clattering, grinding brand of rock'n'roll the Stones can still, effortlessly, churn out is still the sound that cut through my adolescence and is still the sound that drives me. In summary I can only quote from Bill Drummond's book, *Bad Wisdom*, in which he sums up both essence of rock'n'roll and the essence of Keef, the Human Riff, The World's Most Elegantly wasted Human Being and the driving force behind the world's Greatest Rock'n'Roll Band - still!

"Keith, Keith! KEITH! What is it that we must never do? But he never tells us. So sometimes we don't keep ourselves in check and we go off and make a record with some South American rainforest people or decide that the electric guitar is too limiting in its ability to express the magnitude of our imagination. Of course, we make arseholes of ourselves and we come back and we are sorry; we pick up our guitar and some time soon see a picture of Keith, and those eyes of his tell us, 'I told you so,' and yes, he did.' "

You know what it is, you know it's 'only' that (only!) and you like it, very much indeed.

See you next time!

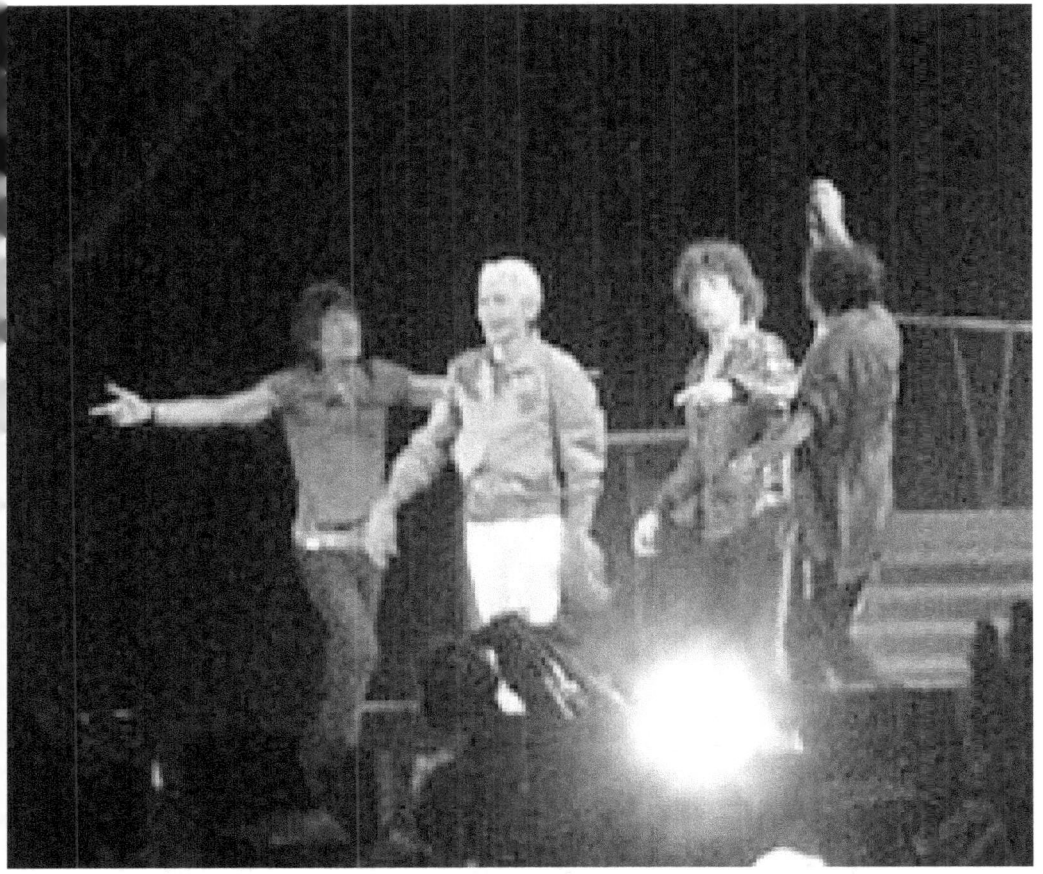

"Pictures of us show that we're all one"

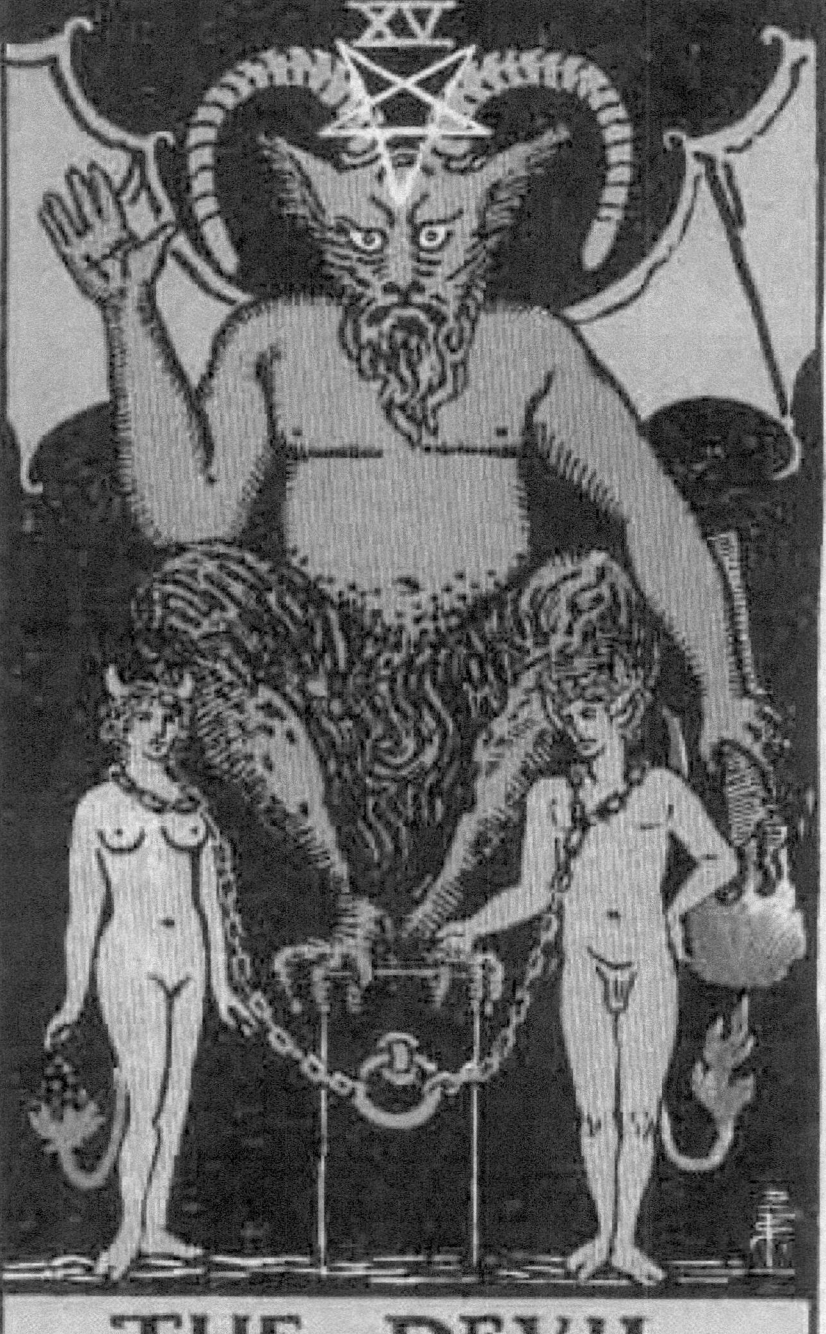

THE DEVIL .

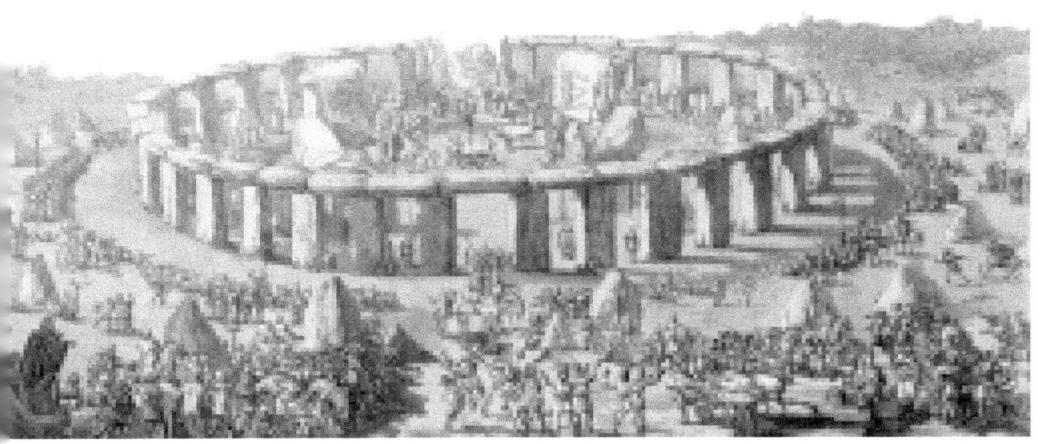

SYMPATHY FOR THE DEVIL

First published in *Uri Geller's Encounters*, August, 1997

Believe the religious hyperbole and you'll know the devil really does have all the best tunes. The big problem for rock musicians over the years has been how to relieve Old Nick of his riffs and come out of the deal smiling. And they've tried, believe me, they've tried. Let's take a magical mystery detour round the back alleyways of rock's fascination for the occult. To a place where fact and fantasy achieve union in the truly alchemical process of turning music into gold. Consider the typical big rock gig and its parallels with a magic ritual. Take a carefully laid-out stage, often with a precisely decorated stage set inscribed according to the band's particular symbolism. Add an array of lighting, appropriate to the mood and the music. Bring in worshippers... sorry, fans - many of whom are primed with, as Crowley would have it, "wine and strange drugs". Then, at the appropriate hour - and let's face it, both music and magic work best after dark - on come the magicians... erm sorry, musicians.

Dressed for the occasion in special clothes and holding their ritual instruments of guitars, drums, and microphones. You've felt that pre-gig tension, haven't you? That build-up of energy when everything seems possible, anything likely. The audience are chanting, clapping, and hanging. The lights go down. The Lizard King himself, Jim Morrison, got it spot-on when he said, "The ceremony is about to begin."

Are you ready to rock?

A KIND OF MAGIC?

Seriously though, some magicians would sacrifice their grannies for the sort of power and energy that a rock band can generate on a good night. Magic offers the musicians a chance to raise and wield power themselves and the possibility of causing change in the material world. Historically, music has always been closely tied to magic, and anthropologists are certain that at one time music was performed purely for magical purposes. Central to the link between rock and magic is rhythm and the drum beats which drive it. Whilst the examples given here are from what might be termed the 'Golden Age of Rock', the form's mutation into dance music followed pretty much the same path, with many practitioners making it perfectly clear that they want to cause a trance not only in themselves but also in their listeners.

Psychedelic indie-dancers *The Shamen* were the most vocal exponents of this idea and even called their most successful album to date, *Boss Drum*. I'm sure a time-travelling shaman, ritual magician, or witch-doctor visiting any big rave would know exactly what was going on. Furthermore, like traditional shamen, many rock musicians live apart from society, barely bound by its rules. To quote Mick Jagger, "they've been outcasts all their lives"; their *raison d'etre* is to perform, and in return to receive the adulation of their followers.

And just like shamen many of them have been to the Otherworlds, courtesy of drink, drugs, and the fleshy excesses that are so freely available, if not obligatory, to gods of the rock pantheon. So is it any surprise that some of them have pursued the left-hand path further, taken the powers and possibilities seriously? Even (gulp!) sold their soul to the devil?

I GOT THE BLUES

Everyone knows that rock music is primarily descended from the blues. But in turn the blues developed from African tribal music brought by the slave trade to the USA. These pre-blues ballads and chants were little more than spells set to music. It was here where the blues clichés of 'black cat bones' and 'mojos' first surfaced in song.

And the conceits which have become common in rock lyrics were there too. The spell-songs then, as now, were primarily concerned with the driving forces of human existence: sex and death. The problems and pleasures of the former and the certainty of the latter. One of the unwitting founders of the rock genre was Robert Johnson. Originally an undistinguished harmonica player and wannabe guitarist of the 1930s, he disappeared for a year, returning, with a mysterious ability to compose and play the blues. Son House saw the transition, noting that on his return Johnson sat down and "...starts playing, and when he got through, all our mouths was open ... He sold his soul to the devil to get to play like that."

How, exactly, does this transaction work? Simple. Just mosey on down to the crossroads at midnight with your guitar and, in Tommy Johnson's words, "A big black man will walk up there and take your guitar, and he'll time it, and then he'll play a piece and hand it back to you. That's the way I learned to play anything I want." Beats Bert Weedon's *Play in a Day* books hands down any time! This devil/crossroads combination was a certain way to get in the groove, but it had just one teensy problem. In return for guitar-prowess, the Lord of Darkness wanted our mortal soul. It's the sort of thing that slips your mind at the time. But for Johnson it was too late; the deal had been struck and it was now only a matter of time. The hellhounds were on his trail in more than just his lyrics and he ended up buried in an unmarked grave, poisoned by a cuckolded husband. The pact with the devil had been fulfilled but his musical legacy went on to form part of the essential canon of blues and rock, his compositions being interpreted by the likes of *The Rolling Stones* and *Led Zeppelin*.

WICCAN WEDDING

Fast forward. Without a doubt the 1960s and '70s were an occult time. Psychedelic experimentation and the earlier repeal of the Witchcraft Act in the '50s, combined with a general air of musical and personal freedom, led to musicians and fans alike discovering the fact behind folk singer Buffy Sainte Marie's statement that "music is alive, magic is afoot".

And so it was. Magic proliferated and the "King of the Witches", Alex Sanders, even had an initiation ceremony released on vinyl record featuring Wiccan authors Janet and Stewart Farrar being sworn in to Sanders' coven. His style of in-your-face Wiccan showmanship did much to popularise witchcraft, and his flamboyant witch-as-rock-star approach appealed to many rockers of the day - notably to an outfit by the name of *Black Widow*. In keeping with the times, *Black Widow* played up the black magic hokum and their first album, *Sacrifice*, featured tracks such as *Attack Of The Demon*, and most notably *Come To The Sabbat*, whose repeated chant of "come, come, come to the Sabbat, come to the Sabbat Satan's there" brought listeners either to a state of hysteria or hysterics depending on their particular mental ambience. For the sake of authenticity, Sanders helped the band with lyrics and wife Maxine was brought in for a spot of on-stage sacrifice for their press performances.

The Doors front man Jim Morrison also portrayed himself as a shamanic figure, sensing the power which could be raised from crowds; and Francis Ford Coppola was savvy enough to use *The End* as the sound-track to the closing death ritual of *Apocalypse Now*. In 1970 Morrison married Patricia Kenney, but instead of the traditional church service Pat 'n' Jim decided to jump the broomstick literally - in a witch-craft wedding. The Lizard King's spouse was an adherent of Wicca and one can imagine that Jim needed little encouragement to join with Patricia in a traditional Wiccan hand fasting, conducted by a High Priestess. At the conclusion of the ceremony, the pair solemnly signed a runic document in blood. It was reportedly all too much for Jim and he fainted!

SABBATH BLOODY SABBATH

With a name like *Black Sabbath* you'd really expect those precursors of heavy metal to have had some serious dealings with the devil. And they did, but seemingly entirely by accident. Guitarist Tony Iommi thought one of their early songs, the eponymous *Black Sabbath*, sounded "really strange. We couldn't explain what it was... and when we played it at gigs we'd get people coming up to us saying "That was really weird!" Little did they know it at the time but the Sabs had hit on the devil's riff itself. Better known in medieval church circles as the *Diabolis in Musica* (the Devil's chord), this particular harmonic configuration of notes has a strange and discordant air about it.

Musicians using this progression - actually a diminished fifth - were reputedly executed at one time.

Singer Ozzy Osbourne was unimpressed, saying, "It's not that we're Satanists. I wouldn't know how to conjure a rabbit out of a hat, never mind a devil." Maybe Ozzie, but where did that devil's chord come from then? Magical power, it seems, can slip through into music and musicians, whether bidden or not. *The Grateful Dead*'s drummer Mickey Hart was offered, and perhaps foolishly accepted, a Tibetan ritual drum known as a damaru. Fashioned from a human skull, the drum was a power object intended to be handled only by the most enlightened lamas. His benefactor quite obviously rated his skills as a musician because he told him, "I knew you could appreciate its power." Although entranced by the drum, Hart only played it once - and promptly threw up!

Over the following weeks Hart was apparently plagued by nausea and a series of small accidents and injuries. Eventually he remembered the power drum, made the connection, and thought it might just be a good idea to pass the gift on. Bassist Phil Lesh took it, but was soon on the phone requesting Hart to take the drum back! After some discussion they decided it would be best to return the drum to its own culture and took it to the Tibetan Buddhist centre in Berkeley.

Head lama Tarthan Tulku handled the drum carefully, saying, "So you've come home at last", before turning to Hart with the remark, "I hope you have been most careful. This is a drum of great, great power. It wakes the dead, you know."

BAD VIBRATIONS

During the recording of *Smile*, the legendary 'lost' *Beach Boys* album, Brian Wilson seemed to become the focus for some high-magnitude strangeness. About to start recording of a track called *Fire* (aka *Mrs. O'Leary's Cow*), the Beach Boy must have sensed something as he refused to enter the studio for the first sessions, claiming that perennial excuse of the zeitgeist, "bad vibes". When eventually coaxed into the studio to begin work on the track, he turned up in a red fireman's helmet! Still not happy, he outfitted the rest of the musicians with red fire hats, commenting "We've really got to get into this thing"; and, to make things complete, ordered a fire to be started up in a metal bucket. This act of sympathetic magic accomplished, he remarked that "the tone was set", and 24 takes later *Fire* was complete. Wilson knew immediately something wasn't quite right, saying, "You know, I think that music might scare a whole lot of people." It does. *Fire* is a powerful and evocative musical conflagration. Wilson believed he'd "tapped into a dark source" to unwittingly create "extremely powerful fire music that emitted bad vibrations".

The following morning matters worsened when Wilson discovered the building next door to the studio had burned down overnight; and in the days that followed, a greater than usual number of fires were reported in the LA district. Now absolutely convinced he had been "dabbling in some kind of musical witchcraft", Wilson decided that the music was too powerful to be unleashed on an unsuspecting world and as a consequence hid the recordings away. **

Arthur Brown couldn't have put it better when he sang, "Fire, I'll teach you to burn."

JAGGERY POKERY

"Please allow me to introduce myself..." The opening line to the *Rolling Stones* satanic classic *Sympathy for the Devil*; a song which for many only served to confirm that the Stones were the dark to the *Beatles'* light. Jagger, Keith Richards, and the ill-starred Brian Jones had all sojourned in Morocco, and Jones in particular hung out with the Master Musicians of Joujouka, ancient tribal exponents of hypnotic rhythms designed to alter consciousness. But the Stones' most intense involvement with the dark side came with Jagger's role in a masterwork of British cinema, the film *Performance*.

Performance is the ultimate rock'n'roll movie, riven with disturbing images, time-shifts, and hints of the heavy devil-tripping darkness which was slowly beginning to engulf the peace and love generation. The intensity with which its participants played their parts is legendary and in itself may be considered an evocation. An everyday tale of decadent rock stars and gangsters, hallucinogens, and sexual ambiguity, it featured Jagger as faded rock icon Turner alongside James Fox, Anita Pallenberg, and Michelle Breton.

The film was not without its psychic fallout. Fox was so affected by the film that he did not work again for ten years, becoming deeply involved in Christianity, whilst over the years Pallenberg was beset by a series of problems including drugs and accusations of witchcraft. Recently scriptwriter Donald Cammell committed suicide and Michelle Breton died destitute and drug-addled in Berlin. Cammell summed the film up well when he said that the Turner/Jagger character was a figure on the edge of lunacy, "trying to grab at poetic ideas of being possessed by someone else's demonic energy".

Sympathy for the Devil was conceived and incubated at roughly the same time as *Performance*, and all the while the Altamont festival loomed on the horizon. If Woodstock was the exclamation mark to the hippy generation's wild outdoor bacchanalia then Altamont was the full stop, following but months after.

** The album lay in the vaults for many years, although the best tracks like *Cabinessence, Our Prayer* and *Surf's Up* were cherry picked for various Beach Boys albums like *20/20* over the next few years, and the rump of the album was released as the mildly disappointing *Smiley Smile* in 1967. Several large chunks including bits of the full 8+ minute version of *Heroes and Villains* appeared on a box set in 1993, but in 2004 the unbelievable happened. Together with a band called *The Wondermints* who were apparently enormous *Beach Boys* fans, Brian Wilson went into the studio and re-recorded "an approximation" of *Smile*. It may not have been as magickal as the original, but it would have to do...

With the Hell's Angels as Jagger's Praetorian Guard, the blasted heath locale was a fitting crucible in which the dark forces, made manifest through a heady mix of music, drugs and violence, could bend minds and break bodies.

Watching the film of the event now it's plain to see that although Jagger may have been able to evoke the forces of darkness to visible form, he had no idea what the hell to do with them once he had! His vain struttings as the Prince of Darkness on stage paled into insignificance compared to the real hell being played out in the audience where the luckless Murray Hunter was being slaughtered by the Angels. Rock lore has it that the horror took place during *Sympathy for the Devil*. In fact it was during *Under My Thumb*. Either way, the devil went down to California that night.

When Cammell heard about the disaster at Altamont he commented, "I remember saying 'I told you so... you see what rock and roll can do'. I felt a little bit prophetic." This rock'n'roll prophecy may have had its genesis in the fact that Cammell drew strong influences from Aleister Crowley, his father having been author of the first Crowley biography. Cammell junior simply "dug Magick and wanted to find out more". *Performance* was that 'more', his final statement on the subject neatly squaring the circle: "This movie was finished before Altamont, and Altamont actualised it."

OH MISTER CROWLEY

Crowley's influence on rock musicians down the years has been pervasive. After all, he did say "every man and woman is a star!" One early acolyte was Graham Bond. A stalwart of the '60s R&B scene, his early bands featured such soon-to-be's as Jack Bruce and Ginger Baker before they went on to stardom in *Cream*. Bond fell so far under Crowley's spell that he came to believe he was Aleister's illegitmate son. His burgeoning obsession meshed with the wild London underground scene and he soon began naming his bands *Initiation* and *Holy Magick* and could be seen striding through London in flowing robes, carrying magical regalia. His record label, Mercury, even allowed him to use part of one of their buildings as an occult temple. **

Unfortunately one of the prices Bond had to pay for this occult infatuation was a growing addiction to heroin and all the problems the White Lady brings. Shortly after being discharged from a mental hospital in 1974 he threw himself under a tube train The official reason was that his mind was disturbed, but legend tells that he was seen struggling with some unseen force immediately prior to his fatal accident. I recently met an old friend of Bond's, who shared his occult preoccupations, and who believed that his death may have been averted had he only returned a book on the Quabbalah to Graham in time.

This tragedy raises the age old problem of exactly what is a mental illness and what is occult possession - are they just different names for the same thing? And as for possession by spirits, isn't heroin one of the most powerful agents of possession known to man, another form of the pact with the devil? Always promising mastery of self but inevitably leading to subjugation of the soul, and death. Deal done. Game over.

STAIRWAY TO HELL?

Zeppelin's Jimmy Page was also fascinated by the Crowley myth, and his involvement with the magus has reached legendary proportions in rock lore. For instance, whether or not it is true that Page had read Crowley's *Magick in Theory and Practice* at the age of 11, as he claimed, is immaterial. It's the sort of

---

** Bond's cat also disappeared under mysterious circumstances and was later (according to whom you believe) found having been killed in a ritualistic manner. To this day, occultist David Farrant denies having had anything to do with this, and refuses to discuss it further.

thing he should have been doing as a nascent rock god. As his fame and fortune grew, Page was able to indulge himself by acquiring one of the largest collections of Crowley artefacts in existence.

One of his American friends, 'Miss Pamela'[**] recalled to Zeppelin biographer Stephen Davies, "I believe that Jimmy was very into that stuff... and probably did a lot of rituals, candles, bat's blood, the whole thing." Miss Pamela also recounted a persistent rumour about the band, claiming that "they all made this pact with the Devil, Satan, the Black Powers, whatever, so that Zeppelin would be such a huge success."

In 1970 Page bought the ultimate piece of Crowley collectanea, the magician's former home of Boleskine House on the shores of monster haunted Loch Ness. This was where Page's section of the Zeppelin film, *The Song Remains the Same,* was shot. Another occult sideline of Page's was ownership of the Equinox occult bookstore in London. In short, he was no dilettante, despite press attempts to trivialise his beliefs, and the unobtrusive engraving of Crowley's 'Do What Thou Wilt' dictum on his belt buckle only served to underscore this. Page's response to journalists eager for a sex/devil/drugs soundbite was the sincere "I don't worship the devil, but magic does intrigue me. Magic of all kinds."

Musically, this occult fascination was bound to out and it did on *Led Zeppelin III* where again the 'Do What Thou Wilt' message appeared,[****] this time scratched on the run off to the record. Zeppelin's fourth album is also riddled with occult influences.

Each of the band chose a symbol which was to represent them on the cover. Page is the only member to refuse to reveal what his represents, but it looks like a magical sigil, a figurative distillation of desire intended to be lost to the conscious mind; all the better to work out its destiny on the astral plane. The album's gatefold sleeve opens to reveal a dramatic painting of a hermit. Not just any old hermit but one representing the Hermit of the tarot pack. Page summed it up thus: "He's on top of the mountain and there's this person who is aspiring towards him, but it's a long ascent. A general philosophy, I suppose, of ever onward."

Zeppelin IV, as every occultist and Rolf Harris fan knows, culminates in the awesome *Stairway to Heaven,* which states "there are two paths you can go by, but in the long run there's still time to change the road you're on." Which path had Page chosen, I wonder?

Christian fundamentalists were, as ever, certain. It was the left hand path. Proof? Well, according to the fundies, if you play *Stairway to Heaven* backwards you can clearly hear a voice intoning "Here's to my sweet Satan", "There's power in Satan" and "He will give you 666". The claim is made that Zeppelin intentionally back masked these words onto the record to have a subliminal effect on its listeners. Don't try this with your CDs kids!

Page made his occult ambitions clear after a gig at LA's Forum in 1977. Queried as to what he wanted out of life he replied, "Power, mystery and the hammer of the gods." You really only have to listen to his riffing on any of the live tapes of that period (or the triple CD *How the West was Won* to know that he got all three. During the '70s Page became involved with cult filmmaker Kenneth Anger, with both men sharing the Crowley obsession. Anger invited Page to contribute a soundtrack to a satanically oriented

---

[**] Miss Pamela aka Pamela des Barres is a very colourful character. She was wife of singer/actor Michael des Barres between 1976 and 1991, and author of the notorious book *Groupie* as well as singer with Zappa produced band *The GTOs* whose one album is magnificently peculiar.

[****] There were etchings on both sides of *Led Zeppelin III*. Side one proclaimed 'Do what thou wilt', and side two 'so mote it be'. Bizarrely the b-side etching disappeared on some later pressing.

film called *Lucifer Rising*.

Despite various disputes between the two. Page eventually submitted around 28 minutes of mind-blowing, eerie, occult music. The guitarist also appeared subliminally in the film, a flash frame showing him gazing at a photo of Crowley whilst holding the *Stele of Revealing*, an occult text.

When Zeppelin drummer John Bonham died, the press seized the chance they had been waiting for. The *London Evening News* ran the headline 'Zeppelin Black Magic Mystery', with the usual "unnamed source close to the band" hauled out to claim that "Robert Plant and everyone around the band is convinced that Jimmy's dabbling in black magic is responsible in some ways for Bonzo's death". [**] The myth continues to the present day. During Plant and Page's 1995 world tour a fan, probably possessed by nothing more than stupidity and a surfeit of rock legend, rushed the stage clutching a knife. After being restrained by police, he claimed he had heard Plant and Page playing 'satanic' music.

REPETITIVE BEATS

Time and the heat go on. The 1980s saw another slew of bands taking up an interest in the occult This time, post-punk, it was the chaotic aspects of magic which appealed. Bands such as *Psychic TV* tuned into a more chaotic magic. Weaving a multimedia sorcery and using such instruments as Tibetan human thigh bones, Genesis P Orridge (Neil Megson to his mum) and friends formed their own religion, *The Temple Ov. Psychic Youth*, and ventured where other magical musos had feared to tread.

More recently even the title of *Orbital*'s synapse-crunching single 'Satan' was enough to send the tabloids and culture nannies into frenzy, fearful that the dreaded demon spawn could be conjured up simply by a contentious word and a driven beat. Maybe they're catching on. Remember that 'repetitive beats' are enshrined as part of the Criminal Justice Bill. The powers that be don't want scantily clad people dancing outside in large numbers to the devil's rhythm, and they don't want it to such a ludicrous extent that they are prepared to legislate. Think about it. But it's too late, there's a bad moon risin' and techno, ambient, and trance-dance have all taken up the baton (or should that be wand) of music as magick, whilst the upsurge of interest in green issues in the 1990s has seen both pagan- and earth-mysteries oriented rock develop. Music, like magic, has the power to change consciousness in accordance with will. When both are combined it seems that on occasion they can let some power through into our otherwise mundane universe. But as The Dead's Micky Hart muses, "What door, what power?"

Hard evidence for either is slim, that's the problem; but the mystery and thrill of the beat and its uses bedevil you still, bringing musicians and audiences back time and time again to try their luck, knock, knock, knocking, on Satan's door.

** These stories first surfaced three years before, when in 1977 Plant's son Karac died of a mysterious infection, two years after Plant and his then wife Maureen were seriously injured in a car crash in Rhodes, Greece. Both incidents were blamed by an increasingly credulous tabloid press upon Page's Crowley obsession. In 1989 when I met and interviewed John Paul Jones, he told me at the beginning of the interview that he would talk about anything except for "Pagey and that black magic bullshit." Make of that what thou wilt. **Jon Downes**

UFO: what the nurse saw

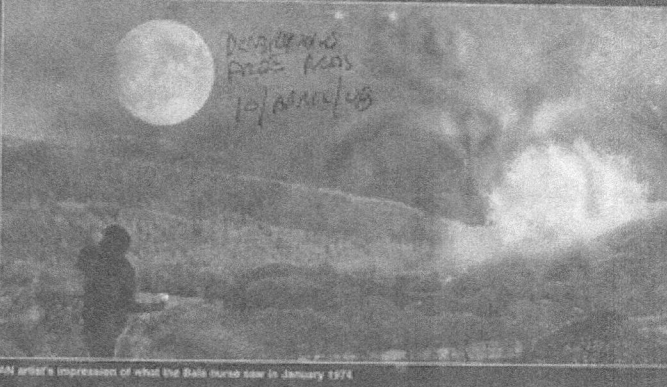

AN artist's impression of what the Bala nurse saw in January 1974

EXCLUSIVE
by NATALIE JONES
natalie.jones@nwn.co.uk

THE nurse who witnessed the UFO 'crash' near Bala 34 years ago has spoken exclusively about her experience.

Last week the *Free Press* revealed that confidential Ministry of Defence files on Unidentified Flying Objects are set to be made public in the coming weeks.

Among these declassified papers is expected to be evidence of the suspected UFO crash on Cader Berwyn on January 23, 1974. Dozens of witnesses across Lancashire and Cheshire phoned the police, earlier that evening, after seeing a strange formation of green lights flying erratically over the skies.

At 8.38pm something registered onto the Berwyn mountains and the resulting tremor - which measured 4.5 on the Richter Scale - was felt in Wrexham, Chester, Liverpool and some areas of Manchester.

Reports at the time said a nurse who lived near the scene of the impact saw a flying saucer the size of the Albert Hall had smashed into a mountain, throwing debris and bodies for over a mile.

The reports also said she walked up to a body, and realised it wasn't human, but before she could describe what she had seen, two MoD officials ordered her to remain silent.

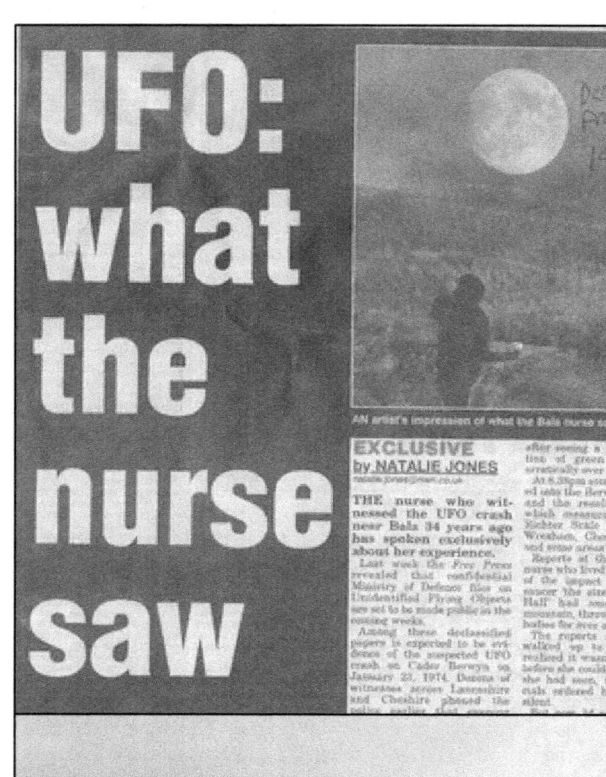

... nurse puts the record straight in an exclusive interview with the *Free Press*.

"All these reports are a load of rubbish. I did not see any bodies and no-one stopped me," said the nurse.

"We heard this almighty tremor, the house shook, we thought an aircraft had crashed, and being a nurse thought we could help."

Along with her two teenage daughters, who were St John Ambulance members, in the darkness of a winter night, the three set off in their car.

They were not prepared for what they were about to witness.

"I saw a huge pulsating mountain, with a few little lights almost like fairy lights flashing about. It was much much bigger than the moon, and we got to line, then one mile away from it.

"I regret we didn't stay to see what happened or see it take off again.

"There was not another soul in sight while we were up there, no military, no MoD, no one.

"We drove as far as a layby and turned round and came back home, the girls were a bit nervous. We were not needed, our errand was first aid," she added.

"I was not approached by anyone after the event and what was written in many newspapers afterwards about me was a load of rubbish," she ...

The view from where Nurse Pat Evans stood when she saw the 'UFO'

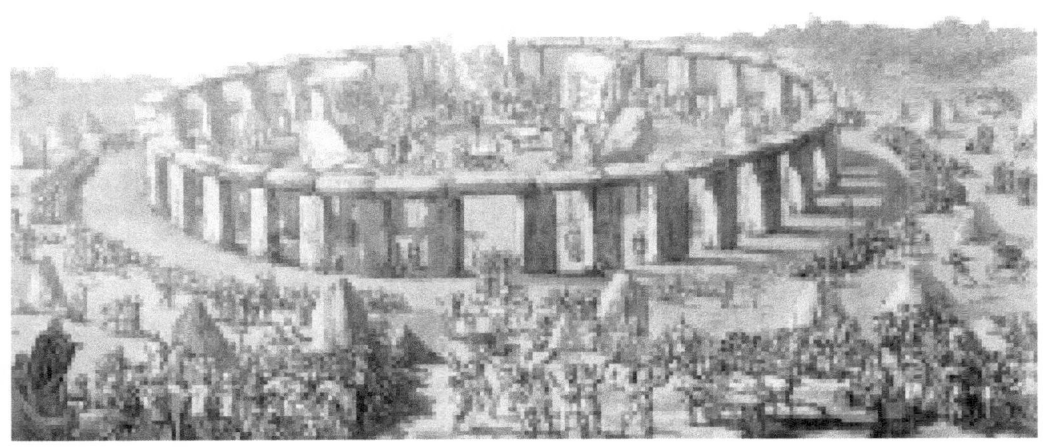

THE BERWYN MOUNTAIN UFO CRASH - A
BRITISH ROSWELL?

In 1958 Gavin Gibbons wrote *By Space Ship to the Moon*, which featured a UFO landing on the Berwyn Mountains. Sixteen years later those same mountains would again be the focus for a story involving a downed UFO. But this time, some said, the story was for real.

The Berwyn Mountains divide central North Wales, separating Shropshire from Snowdonia. Prehistoric man lived and worshipped here, leaving a dramatic ritual landscape to which many beliefs have become attached. Folklore records these peaks have been haunted by a multitude of aerial phenomena over the centuries and contemporary paranormal puzzles abound, including 'phantom bombers', ghosts, lake monsters and that most modern of mysteries the 'alien big cat'. Although ever popular with tourists the Berwyns can be dangerous and rescue teams are frequently called out. Cader Berwyn, the highest peak, rises to 827 metres and several aeroplanes, both military and civilian, have crashed on its slopes over the past fifty years. In winter the area is remote, an ideal spot if ever there was one, for UFO activity.

It's against this backdrop that an incident took place on 23 January 1974 which first perplexed locals and later the UFO community. The events spawned a cascade of rumours, leading many to conclude that an extraterrestrial craft had landed or crashed on Cader Berwyn. It's further claimed that the alien crew was whisked off to a secret military installation, the whole fantastic business being hushed up by the UK government.

The Berwyn Mountain Incident has been described as '...the best example of a UFO retrieval in Britain', and likened to the Roswell and Rendlesham events. A preposterous claim? Certainly. But even the most bizarre story must have its genesis in truth, no matter how mundane or exotic that truth may be. Imagine for a moment the consequences if aliens had fallen to earth that night in January 1974? If this were proven we would finally know we were not alone in the universe. Such proof would also demonstrate that the government had been keeping The Greatest Story Never Told hidden from us and would blow the lid on the alleged global UFO cover-up.

But if it can be argued that there was no alien craft, then what does lie behind these claims? Could it have been the crash of a secret military craft such as one of the 'flying triangles'? Or perhaps a failed missile test from the rocketry ranges at nearby Aberporth? A hoax even? Or something far more sinister. And if it is any of these then why have the claims of UFOs, alien cadavers and military cover-ups persisted for over three decades?

Comparisons with Roswell and other UFO crash retrieval events show the Berwyn Incident to have many of the same motifs and therefore worthy of study. Yet whilst rumours of this crash have been in existence for thirty years it has only recently drawn any serious attention from the UFO community. The Berwyn Incident, far from proven, is a kaleidoscope of rumour and fact concerning crashed UFOs, alien bodies, military retrieval teams, earth tremors, meteorites, weapons testing, disinformation agents, Men In Black and geologically created lights.

The story is complex and I have pieced together a composite account from the witnesses, informants, ufologists and newspapers, of what allegedly happened on and around January 23rd 1974. This is 'the story', the generally accepted account, variations on which have become enshrined in the ufolore and which is seeping out into the public's consciousness. Prior to the Berwyn Incident the north of England, had been plagued by the 'phantom helicopter'. Over a hundred sightings were made of this anomaly, seen flying at night over dangerous terrain and in appalling weather. These sightings took place between spring 1973 and spring 1974 and ceased immediately after the Berwyn Incident. Despite the numerous sightings and keen police interest no one explanation was ever found. But something, was flying around the northern skies and many of the witnesses concurred; 'it seemed to be looking for something'.

Wednesday the 23rd of January 1974 was just another winter's day in Bala and the nearby villages of Llandrillo and Llanderfel and UFOs were the last thing on the villagers' minds. But as night closed in an event took place which was to change all that. Just after 8.30pm locals were jolted from their musings by a large explosion, followed immediately by a terrible rumbling lasting four or five seconds. Furniture moved, buildings shook and animals voiced their terror. Terrified people shot to their windows, and flooded into the streets in an attempt to discover the cause of the disturbance. Many recall seeing huge lights streaking across the heavens and, looking toward the mountains, saw fingers of light projected into the night sky.

Hundreds of people telephoned the emergency services, believing a disaster had taken place and one nurse was convinced an aircraft had crashed and drove towards the mountains. Once she was on the high mountain road she halted, astonished at what she saw. There, high on the barren mountain before her, was a glowing sphere. It was too far from the road to be reached on foot and she could only watch in silence as the sphere pulsated, changing from red to yellow to white, while other white lights could be seen moving round it on the hillside.

As the nurse drove back to her village she was stopped by a group of police and soldiers who forcefully ordered her off the mountain, saying the road was being cordoned off. Official reaction was quick to the initial explosion, suspiciously quick some said, with the police and military arriving within minutes, turning other curious villagers away from the mountain roads. In the following few days a large military presence appeared in the area. Roads remained closed and the farmers complained they were forbidden from tending their stock. Clearly something was being sought, or why would military helicopters be criss-crossing the area and strangers combing the mountainsides? Even more suspicious were the dark-suited officials who arrived in the area, asking questions the events on the mountain. The incident at-tracted serious TV and radio coverage and *The Guardian*, *The Times* and the Welsh regional and local press carried detailed reports.

Speculation was rife; an aircraft crash would have accounted for the noise, lights, and for the official involvement and one newspaper was certain that the event involved a crash of some kind, noting:

'There is a report that an Army vehicle was seen coming down the mountain near Bala Lake with a large square box on the back of it and accompanied by outriders'.

But the authorities refused to acknowledge that anything had taken place. Meteorites and earth tremors were also suggested as being the cause, and indeed would have explained some of the mystery.

But what could possibly explain the sphere and beams of light seen on the mountain? They were swiftly dismissed as the villagers' imaginations, shooting stars, or more ludicrously as people out poaching hares. Such natural phenomenon was also unlikely to lead to roads or large areas of mountain being closed by the army.

The media soon forgot about the incident and the locals too let the matter fade deep into their memories. But UFO researchers realised that something had occurred which had not been satisfactorily explained. Lights in the sky, and mysterious explosions, coupled with unusual military activity are avidly noted by the UFO community as indicators of a UFO crash, yet in 1974 the subject of UFO crash retrievals was barely mentioned in the UFO literature, especially in the UK. Various UFO journals reported the events but no investigation was undertaken and no real conclusions were offered.

But shadowy forces were at work and within months UK UFO investigators began to receive official looking documents from a group called Aerial Phenomena Enquiry Network (APEN). These documents claimed that an extraterrestrial craft had come down on the Berwyns and was retrieved for study by an APEN crash retrieval team!

APEN also claimed there had been a key witness to the UFO crash who they were recommending for hypnotic regression. In 1974 hypnotic regression was unknown in the UK UFO community and besides being used in the 1961 Betty and Barney Hill 'abduction', hypnosis virtually unknown with n the subject. Some researchers have speculated that APEN may have been a government psy-op, spreading disinformation via UFO mythology to divert attention from secret weapons testing. APEN issued similar enigmatic communications in conjunction with major other UFO events, notably the Rendlesham Forest case.

The Berwyn Incident lay dormant throughout most of the 1970s and 80s, being little more than a footnote in the literature. But intriguing pieces of information surfaced over time, later becoming part of the lore surrounding the case. Jenny Randles was a frequent visitor to the region in the late 1970s and recalls the locals discussing military activity on the mountains in the wake of some crash-like event. Jenny was very interested in the case and initially put it down to a possible 'earthlight', transient lights caused by geophysical stresses.

By the late 1990s the Berwyn Incident had featured heavily in UFO books and magazines along with national newspapers and TV documentaries. Most significantly in 1997 it was the focus of a chapter in Nick Redfern's best-selling book, *A Covert Agenda*. From its humble beginnings the Berwyn Incident had evolved into a 'British Roswell', firmly enshrined in ufo-lore as one of the UK's few UFO crash retrieval cases. This publicity caused new witnesses to come forward, their testimony adding dramatic dimensions to the case.

In *UFO Magazine*, ufologist Tony Dodd recounted an anonymous informant who claimed to have been in a military unit put on stand-by several days before the date of the Berwyn Incident. This unit was sent to Llanderfel to collect 'two large, oblong boxes' and ordered to take these to Porton Down in Wiltshire, a UK government research establishment. There the boxes were opened, Dodd's informant recalling

'We were shocked to see two creatures which had been placed inside contamination suits. When the suits were fully opened it was obvious the creatures were clearly not of this world and when examined were found to be dead. What I saw in the boxes that day changed my whole concept of life. The bodies were about five to six feet tall, humanoid in shape but so thin they looked almost skeletal with covered skin.'

These and other extraordinary claims made by ufologists Nick Redfern, Tony Dodd and Margaret Fry led me to a re-investigation of the Berwyn Incident in 1998. I was sure that somewhere, between the witness accounts and the claims of the ufologists, lay the key to what really happened on that January night in 1974.

Ufologists stress the importance of the 'paper trail', official documentation which any event, however secret must generate. It seemed eminently reasonable that the Berwyn Incident would have left some trace in official records. Ufologists who pursued the case prior to 1998 had failed to follow this line of enquiry, even claiming the documentation no longer existed. They hadn't looked hard enough, because I discovered a plethora of official documentation which I balanced against the witness statements, to piece together the true events of January 23rd 1974.

What follows is the results of that re-investigation.

In *A Covert Agenda* Nick Redfern suggested that the 'phantom helicopters', seen in the months prior to the Berwyn Incident, were flown by military UFO crash retrieval teams and were on permanent stand-by having received advance knowledge of a UFO landing. But the 'phantom helicopters' are a red-herring. Although the phenomenon had been called a 'helicopter' most of the witnesses were in fact describing an unknown light of many shapes and colours. The 'phantom helicopter' was more Unidentified Aerial Phenomenon than Unidentified Flying Object. Commercial helicopters were found to be responsible for some sightings; others remain a mystery to this day. But no 'phantom helicopter' was seen in the Balam area, and there is no substantive connection between the 'phantom helicopters' and the Berwyn Incident other than the circumstantial link made by Nick Redfern.

The night of January 23rd 1974 was strange by anyone's standards, a display of *son et lumiere* on a scale rarely seen. Villagers near the Berwyn Mountains reported a great deal of aerial phenomena throughout the evening and besides the strange lights on the mountain reports describe at least four incandescent balls of light which streaked across the skies between 7.30pm and 10.00pm. Ufologists have implied that these were UFOs, one of which came down on Cader Berwyn. Farmer Williams said, 'I saw this object coming along the mountain, about the size of a bus really, white in the middle, it came across the mountain and dipped. I thought it was going to crash.' A dramatic description, but one for which there is a rational explanation, just as there is for all the other aerial phenomena seen that evening.

Records kept by the Astronomy Department at Leicester University show that a number of outstanding bolide meteors were seen that night over the UK, coinciding with the times given by witnesses in Wales. The first was at 7.25pm, others at 8.15pm, 8.30pm and 9.55pm. Bolide meteors are considerably brighter and longer lived than ordinary 'shooting stars'. They can appear to be very low, and often trail 'sparks' of blue and green across the sky. Bolides are responsible for many misperceptions of UFOs and often fool the emergency services who are called out to 'plane crashes', only to discover that witnesses had seen a bright bolide meteor.

At exactly 8.38pm the Bala area was rocked by a huge explosion, closely followed by a deep rumbling. One witness recalled it as being 'like a lorry running into a house'. Crockery rattled, furniture moved and

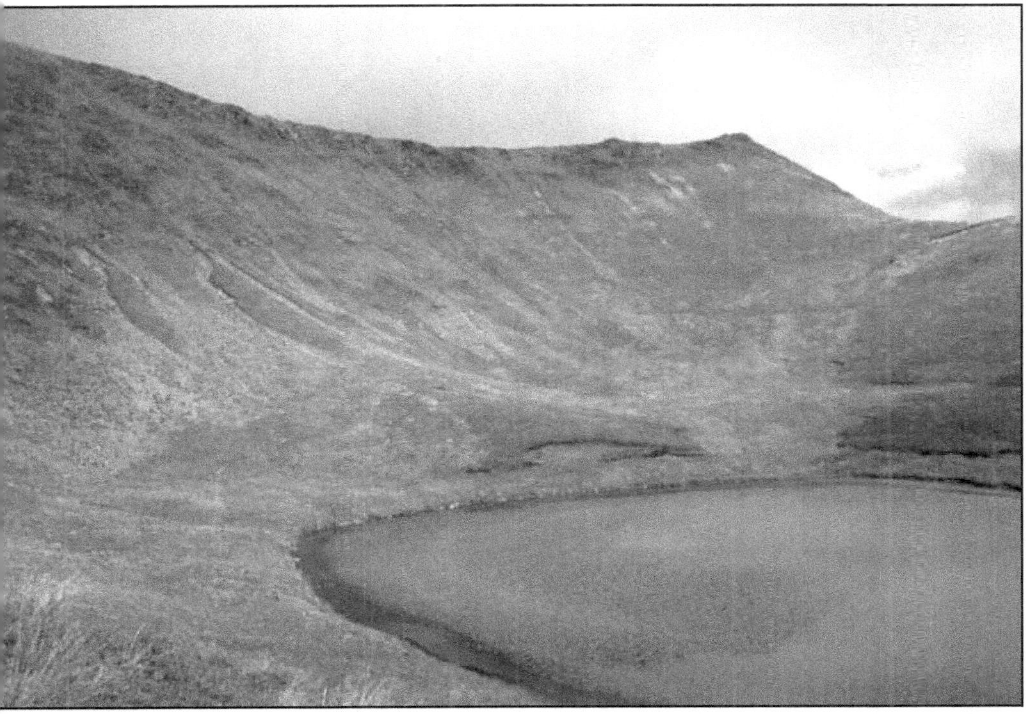

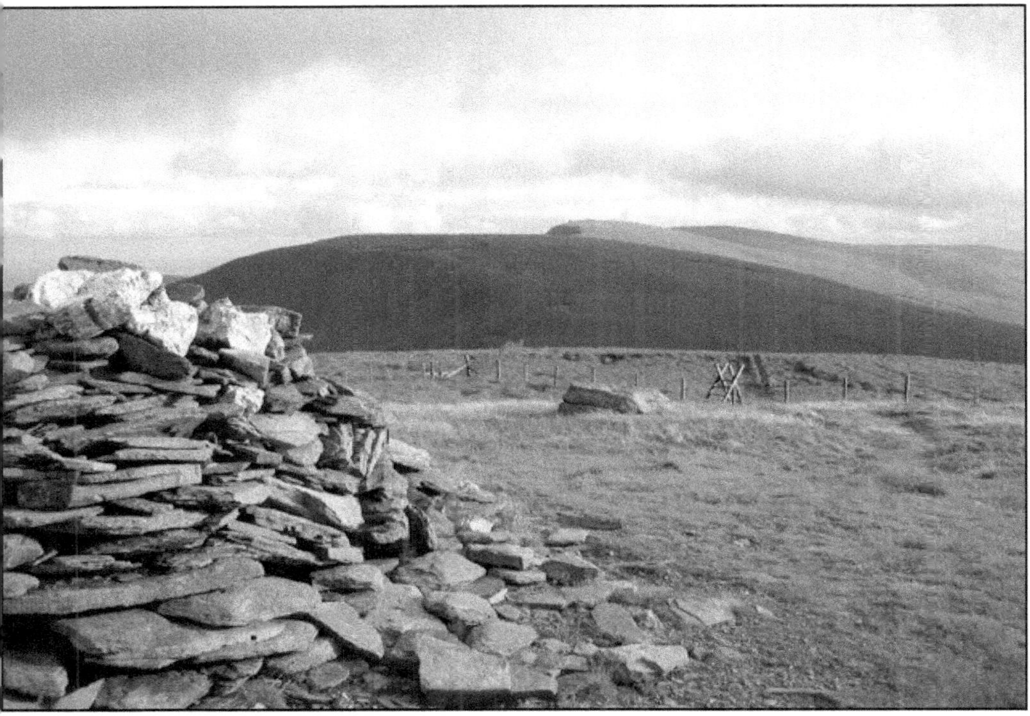

Views of the Berwyn Mountains

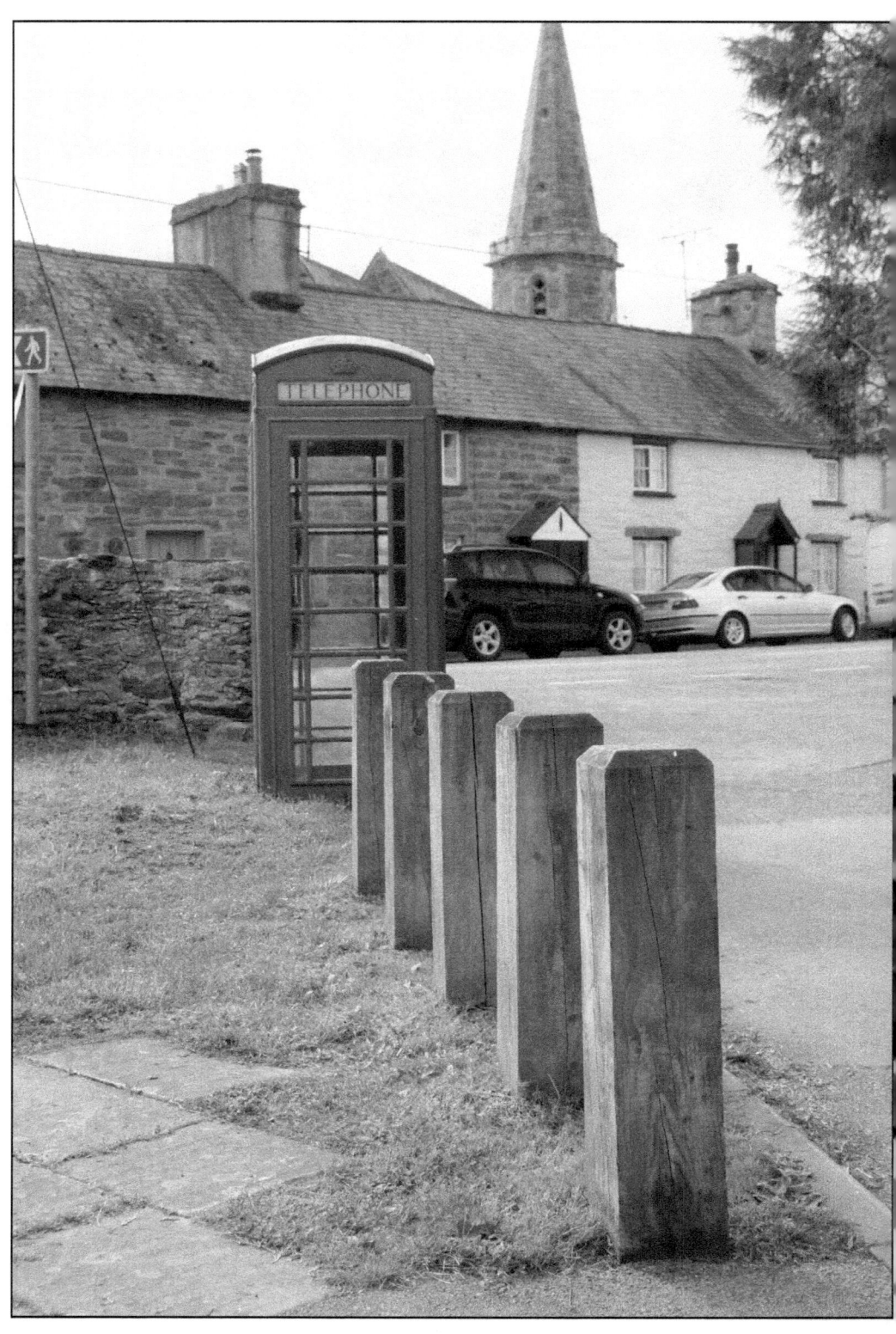

The phone box in the centre of Llandrillo, where villagers gathered during the event and which was used to help jam the switchboard of North Wales Police

walls rippled slightly. Some were certain it was a plane crash on the mountains. Others remembered earth tremors from the past and assumed it was the latest tremor along the geological rift called the Bala Fault.

This is the primary series of events which subsequently caused a number of UFO researchers and their followers to believe that a UFO crashed. In effect they are claiming that the explosion and rumblings was a UFO impacting on Cader Berwyn. Yet the crashed UFO story only came out years after the event. At the time confusion reigned as to what had caused the disturbances. Reports of lights in the sky on that evening fuelled the idea that something crashed on the Berwyns. Witnesses across North Wales claimed to have seen a bright object in the sky 'trailing sparks' immediately prior to the 'crash'. But this was actually seen at 8.30pm, eight minutes before the explosion, astronomical records indicating that it was a bright fireball meteor. Nonetheless, in the minds of many, it has become conflated with the 'explosion' to create evidence of a crash.

The explosion was heard only in the Bala area but the tremor was felt as far away as Liverpool and within hours seismologists had determined the explosion and tremor were caused by an earthquake of 4-5 on the Richter scale. Its epicentre was the Bala area, at a depth of eight kilometres. To cause a reading of that magnitude, a solid object - meteorite or UFO - would have weighed several hundred tons and left a massive crater. Therefore, unless a UFO had crashed at the exact moment of an earth tremor, it can be safely assumed that the disturbing sounds were the result of natural processes.

Following the explosion Llandrillo district nurse Pat Evans ran into the street. She saw no lights but the explosion and talk among villagers convinced her that something had crashed on the mountains. The 'phone lines were jammed with 999 calls, but eventually she spoke to Colwyn Bay police HQ. They suggested it could have been a 'plane crash so she drove up the mountain road, intending to offer help until the emergency services arrived.

As Mrs Evans reached the point where the B4391 road levels out she was puzzled by what appeared to be an illuminated ball of light on the mountainside. A light drizzle was falling, but apart from that the night was clear and she remembered, 'There were no flames shooting or anything like that. It was very uniform, round in shape...it was a flat round...'. As she watched the light changed colour between red, yellow and white. Smaller lights, 'fairy lights' in her words could be seen nearby. It was too far away to reach on foot so she returned home.

Many who have written about the Berwyn Incident have claimed that Evans was turned back from the mountain by soldiers. This canard arose from a misunderstanding when she was first interviewed by ufologists. Evans is furious that she has been misrepresented in this way and has stated unequivocally that she saw 'not a living soul' on the mountain that night. More importantly a letter from her exists, predating any interview, noting that she saw no-one. This is significant because the mal-investigation of her experience has become fundamental to claims that a crash retrieval team was on the mountain shortly after the explosion.

Nonetheless what she saw on the mountain slopes was crucial to the case and I sought evidence untainted by time or ufologists, turning to records held by the British Geological Survey (BGS), in Edinburgh. These records, untouched for twenty four years, revealed that a team of investigators was dispatched to the area within days of the event. This is almost certainly the source of rumours of 'officials' who stayed in local hotels, questioning villagers. Six BGS interviewers conducted detailed door to door enquiries working to a set questionnaire, asking 'odd' questions such as 'Were you alarmed or frightened?' and 'Did you hear any creaking noises?' Over two hundred people were interviewed. Nurse Pat Evans was one of them. The BGS field notes were enlightening. Most ufologists have assumed that Pat Evans was on the mountain immediately after the explosion, arguing that the lights that she saw surrounding the anomalous 'glow' must have been from a pre-alerted crash retrieval team, as no-one else could have got on the mountain so quickly after the 'crash'.

But the BGS records from her 1974 interview are specific about time and note Evans, 'left house during 'Till Death'....'. This appeared to be a reference to the TV sit-com *'Til Death Us Do Part* and the TV schedules revealed that *'Til Death Us Do Part* started at 9.30pm on that night. Knowing that the Evans' left the house sometime after 9.30pm means she would have observed the anomalous ball of light sometime after 9.40pm, an hour later than was previously thought. That hour's difference is crucial. Fourteen-year-old Huw Thomas was also watching television that night. At about 9.20pm he answered the door to several policemen who wanted to commandeer the farm Land Rover, because a 'plane had crashed on the mountain.

Huw's parents were out, so - with a neighbour driving - they set off up a mountain track, with police following by car. As they neared the open mountainside they stopped to move a car blocking the track, Thomas recognising it as belonging to local poachers. Once through the gate several policemen spread out on foot with torches, whilst the Land Rover and police car drove up the narrow track. The time it took Thomas to drive up the mountain and move a car from the road places the police search team on the lower slopes of Cader Berwyn from 9.40pm onwards. The BGS also interviewed one of the poachers, whose car Thomas had moved, confirming their time and position and stating they 'carried on work for 45 minutes (after the explosion) and were almost back at the car when met party (police etc) coming up.'

Huw Thomas confirmed these details in a 1998 interview.

The BGS records also contained a map on which witness locations and sightings of lights were plotted. This was a revelation, showing the 'sphere' seen by the nurse, the location of the poachers and the police search party to be all in the same small area of hillside. Even more remarkably the times given to the BGS by all three parties place them there at the same time. Suddenly, witness testimony and official records gelled.

The conclusion is inescapable. Neither Huw Thomas nor the police saw the glowing sphere seen by the nurse. Conversely the nurse did see the police, albeit unknowingly. Her BGS interview clearly describes 'vehicles' and 'torch lights'. This was the search party. Between them, close to both, is the 'sphere'. Therefore whatever she saw must have been visible to the search team and the poachers. So it seems that either Thomas and the police lied to the BGS in 1974 and myself in 1998, or it wasn't noteworthy at the time.

But what was it the 'sphere', which has been claimed as the downed UFO? There is one possibility which could account for it. The BGS notes record the poachers used powerful lamps made from car headlights. Pat Evans recalls the weather was clear but drizzling. Lights seen in those conditions can appear to change colour and to 'glow'. As for the size, which she described as larger than vehicle lights, this may be a misperception as Evans was looking across two miles of dark mountainside and expecting to see a 'plane crash or similar scene of devastation. On the evidence available it is certain that the nurse saw the poachers with their lamping lights at the point they met and talked to the police.

Some ufologists claim that although bolide meteors were seen throughout the evening, the lights seen on the mountain immediately after the explosion were connected to the UFO crash and BGS notes do refer to villagers seeing beams 'on the brow' of the hill. These accounts were puzzling until I examined the locations of the witnesses.

All who witnessed 'light beams' were located in Llandrillo, from where the land rises sharply to the south. From the village the 'brow of the hill' is just a few hundred metres from where the poachers with lamps were. The BGS note the poachers, 'continued work for half an hour to forty five minutes' after the 8.38pm earth tremor, and it was within this time frame the beams were seen. One witness told the BGS he had seen the poacher's lights on previous occasions and they were exactly the same as the beams seen that night.

Claims that a military presence was on the scene immediately following the 8.38pm explosion and in subsequent days also crumbles under examination. As we've seen nurse Pat Evans was not stopped by soldiers or police and saw no-one on the mountain roads. She left for work at 7 00 a.m. the following day and saw nothing unusual in the village or on the roads. So how did stories of a military presence arise?

To understand, we need to return to the paper trail.

Following the 8.38pm earth tremor the police opened a Major Incident Log which records they initially thought a 'plane had crashed, Fire and Ambulance services being put on stand-by. At 9.09pm the police contacted RAF Valley Mountain Rescue Team (VMRT) and a three man unit arrived in Llandrillo at 00.10am. Their log records the incident as 'Unidentified lights and noise on hillside' and comments, 'VMRT requested to investigate lights and noise on hillside. Advance party covered relevant area with negative results. Incident produced much local excitement.' At 7.00am on 24th January VMRT, together with local police, combed the mountains, abandoning the search at 2.15pm. Huw Thomas was also out on the Berwyns that day, acting as guide for Dr. Ron Madison, a scientist working on the theory that a meteorite may have impacted. Madison and Thomas recall seeing no-one on the mountain other than the police and VMRT.

But this low level of official activity wouldn't account for reports of closed roads, the military presence, or the aircraft and helicopters seen overhead. But none of the original police, VMRT or BGS documents from 1974 mention this alleged military activity and the only contemporary record of a military presence comes from the Border Counties Advertiser, the source of unsubstantiated rumours of boxes being brought off the mountain. In looking for an explanation to this particular component of the story there are two crucial factors.

Firstly, none of the Berwyn Mountain Incident witnesses were interviewed by ufologists until after two decades had past, and secondly at least two other events took place in the area which contained similar elements.

On 12th February 1982 an RAF Harrier carrying top-secret equipment crashed on Cader Berwyn. The RAF descended on the area in force, using Gazelle and Wessex helicopters, together with Harrier and Hercules planes, in the search. Llandrillo was the epicentre of the search and was alive with military vehicles and personnel for several days, with the crash site being sealed off until the wreckage could be removed.

A similar crash also took place on the same mountain in the winter of 1972, two years before the alleged UFO crash and once again the area was sealed off by a large military presence. It is very likely that these incidents, which occurred at the same time of year on the same mountain, were conflated with the 1974 events in witness's minds when recalled years later.

But, say believers the UFO crash theory, what about the claims made by the 'military informants'? After all, when military personnel are prepared to speak out surely there must be something in their story? Perhaps, but the informants who contacted researchers Nick Redfern, Tony Dodd and Margaret Fry did so only *after* the story had been in a 1996 issue of *UFO Magazine*, which fuelled the controversy with speculation but offering no pertinent facts. Nick Redfern has since told me that his informant's telephone number is 'dead', whilst Dodd refuses to expand on the identity of his contact. Notwithstanding this, Dodd's informant generates more questions than answers. If the military had discovered alien cadavers would they really move them by truck rather than the more efficient and secret helicopter? Nor, surely, would Porton Down compromise security or contamination by opening the boxes in the presence of what were essentially the 'delivery boys'.

These 'revelations' surfaced at a time when several prominent UK ufologists were being contacted by alleged military sources offering UFO-related information, none of which amounted to anything tangible. Researcher Kevin McClure suggested that this was a well organised hoax, and based his suppositions on the number of contacts made within a short time-span and the absence of any useful information. APEN, the organisation which circulated official-looking documents following the Berwyn Incident are also regarded by serious ufologists to have been one of many hoaxes perpetrated by ufologists on ufologists. This sort of document hoax is not new to the UFO community, the most famous being the MJ-12 papers which fooled ufologists for over a decade.

That's basically where the Berwyn case stands today, more than thirty years after the incident occurred. There are still some inconsistencies; the symmetry of any UFO case is rarely perfect, especially when abandoned to rumour for decades. But the account I have given is, I suggest, probably the most plausible explanation for the disparate events which coalesced into the Berwyn Mountain UFO Crash. Of course,

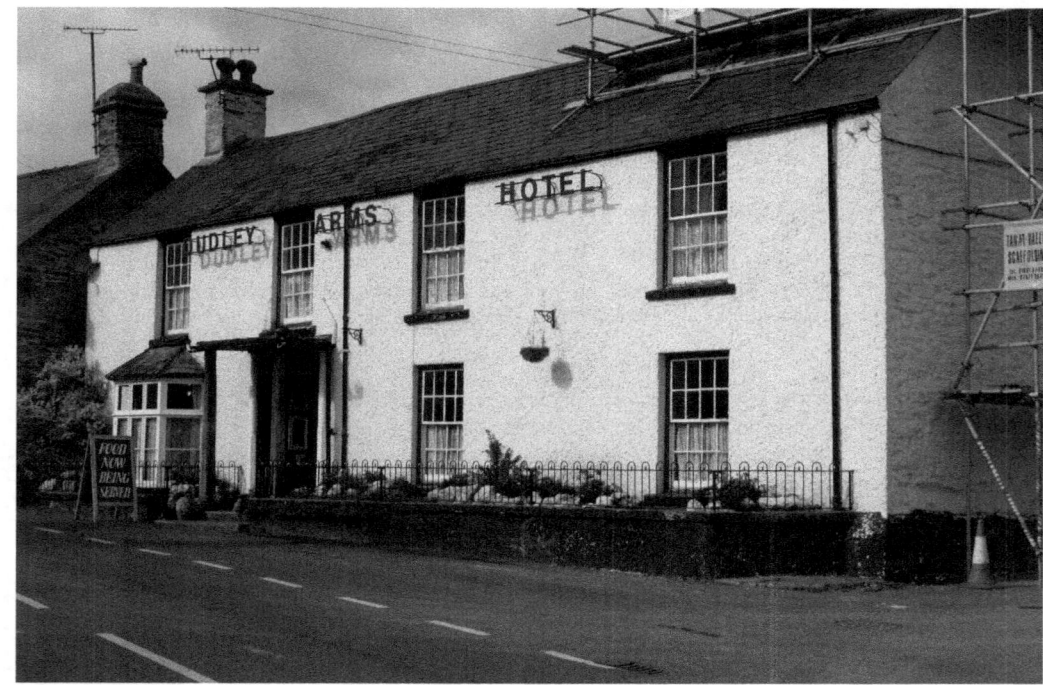

The Dudley Arms Hotel in Llandrillo

there are those who continue to believe a UFO crashed and who insist that official documents have been destroyed or falsified, that witnesses have been misquoted and so on. That's their prerogative and is quite understandable in view of the complexities of this case and the power of belief in the extraterrestrial hypothesis. My conclusions, however, are based not on belief but on the 'paper trail' left by police, RAF, VMRT and the BGS, and the pattern which has emerged from those sources is largely consistent with, and clarifies, witness reports. So until more solid evidence is produced I am afraid that I think the notion that an alien spacecraft crashed in the Berwyn Mountains is redundant.

It's hard to believe that a concatenation of prolific meteor activity, an earth tremor and poachers could lead to the conclusion that a UFO had crashed. Yet it did, proving once again that the truth about a UFO case is invariably far stranger than any fiction. Although I've been investigating Fortean mysteries for thirty years now, each case teaches a lesson. The Berwyn Mountain Incident taught me never to trust material originated by ufologists, but to always go back to source documents and witnesses, and try to reconcile the two. It also taught me more about the flaws of perception and of the care that is needed in unravelling witness observations from their interpretations. However certain a witness may seem of what happened, memory frequently conflates fact and fiction to create a powerful and convincing reality which seems to admit the 'other' into the affairs of mankind.

Charles Fort, had much to say about the connections between earth tremors and meteorites, and it may be that there are deeper factors at work in the Berwyn Incident. Perhaps earth tremors and bolide meteors are in some way connected by mechanisms which are at present outside our understanding. Or maybe extraterrestrials have covertly learned how to enter Earth's atmosphere under cover of meteor showers, even disguised as meteors!

In lieu of hard facts the speculative possibilities are as endless as they are futile. On the other hand it could all be just a gigantic cosmic coincidence, a tangle of belief and wishful thinking from which ufologists have spun yet another saga in the continuing extraterrestrial mythos.

You decide!

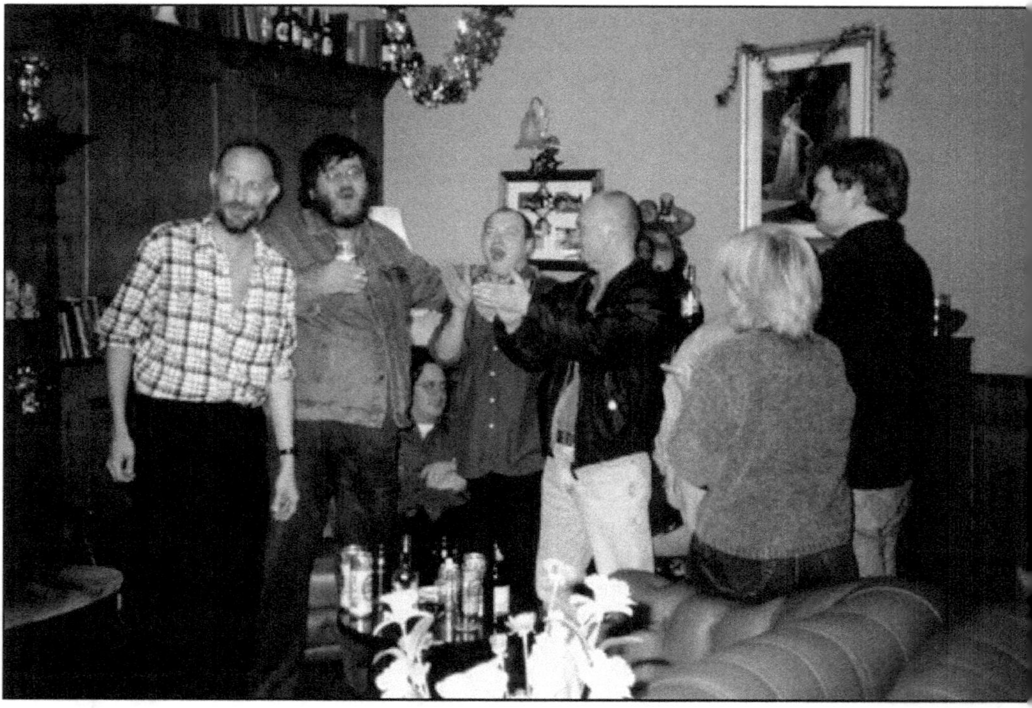

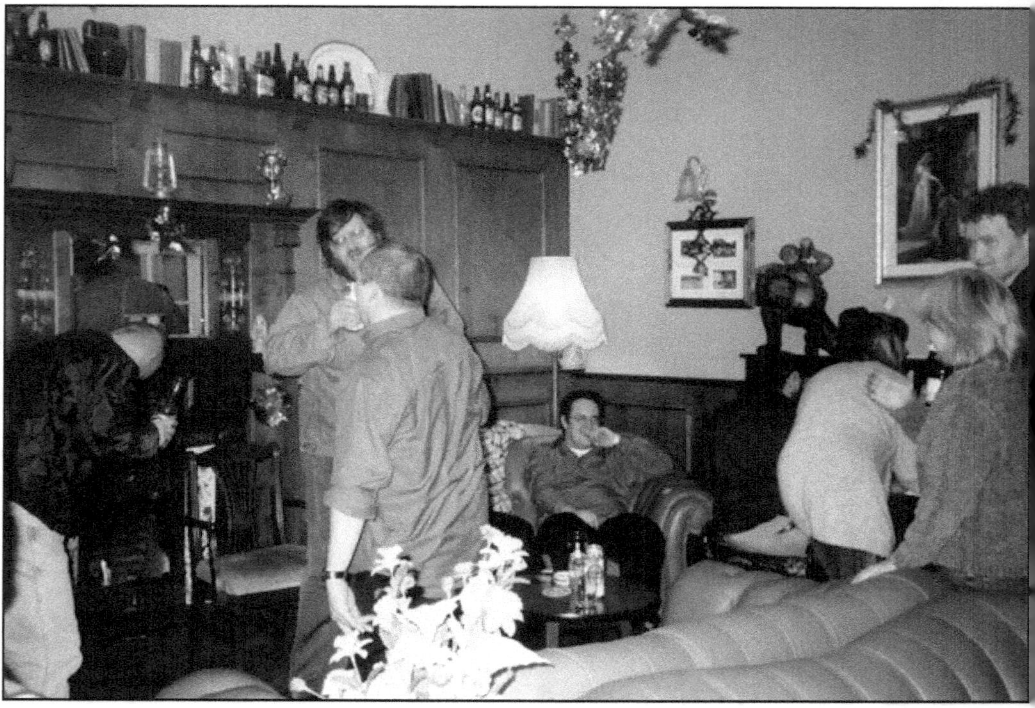

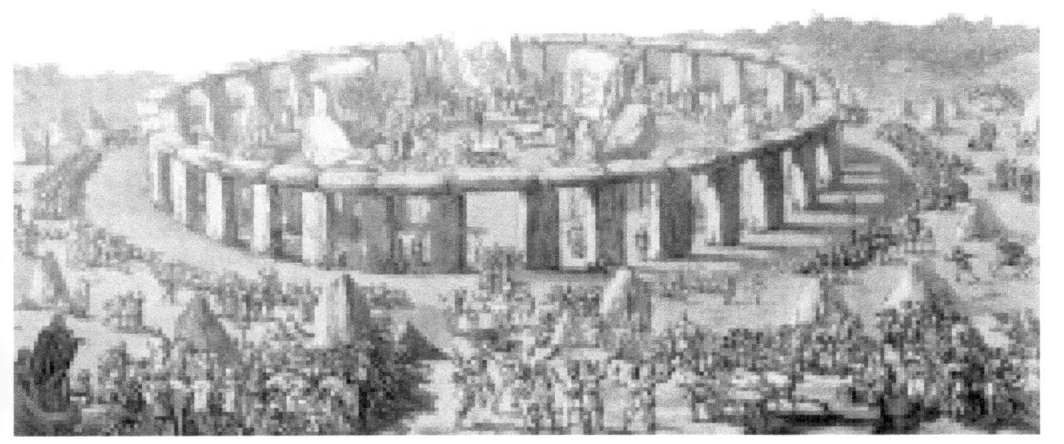

TAKING LA PIS

This piece of scurrilous Fortean journalism first appeared in issue four of The Armchair Ufologist

First sight I saw was Jon Downes trying to flog his pathetic wares[**] from behind a desk which was clearly out of proportion to his size. He regaled me with tales of the goings on at the hotel on the previous night......clearly I had missed something as observing ufologists in their social interactions is far more interesting than any stupid stories that they hawk round the conference circuit.

Jon gives a new meaning to the phrase 'largeing it' and is clearly ufology's answer to Blackadder's Bishop of Bath & Wells. But who has the drawings? All say in a breathy voice "Dear boy, I don't give a flying fuck what you think of me" and rightly so Jon. Great guy, and the only other person in ufology besides Neil Nixon who you can have a cracking conversation about music with. He knows his stuff. Surely by now there should be some form of test whereby if you don't know whom, say, *Mighty Baby* are, you aren't allowed to be a ufologist?

Straight into Jon and Nigel Wright's lecture. This was loosely based on their book *Rising of the Moon*, a Keelesque romp through various 'paranormal' and ufological events in the south west a couple of years ago. Fascinating I'm sure, but it seemed to me like they'd just stitched any old cobblers together and made an adventure story out of it. What's more the only visual aid present was the arrival on stage of a four pack of Stella Artois. Apparently, Jon had been asked if he needed any visual aids and he (in jest) requested said four pack. The audience gasped at the sheer audacity of the man. Jon just drank up his breakfast and rambled on.

Down somewhere on the front row you could see a hunched figure in a parka cringing. A thought bubble appeared above his head saying "preposterous, that would never happen at a YUFOS conference and the fat bastard would have to wear a suit anyway", yes it was Graham Birdsall, well out of his natural habitat at someone else's UFO event. Bet he didn't pay for the ticket!" "But what's this? Lurking at the end of the

---

[**] My current selection of 'pathetic wares' includes this very book, dear boy. JD

---

foyer, looking ever so slightly nervous, was Tim Matthews. Tim had to make an appearance because well, because, that's what he does, just so people don't forget him. All that you need to know is he was handing out leaflets for some rally or other and acting furtive with Downes - who would have to be in very deep cover indeed for anyone not to spot him. Luckily I caught them flagrantly giving Nazi salutes and I sincerely hope someone uses this as proof that they were there and I had a camera.

After dinner we all decanted into the piano room for a few hours of the most bizarre ufological post gig 'fun' I have been present at, and I've been at a few. Simple Beatles songs soon gave way to rock standards belted out by a man who I spoke to much but know only as Dave from Geordieland, aided and abetted by a free flowing permutation of Jon Downes, Nigel Wright, Sir Malcolm of Robinson, and many others including Miss Bott on backing vocals. *Louie Louie, Stand By Me,* all the old ufological classics were trotted out and then it was into the Irish rebel songs such as the touching version of *The Armagh Sniper* delivered by Jon (bar bill for the night £65.00) Downes, now doing a passable imitation of Citizen Caned while the most responsible of us such as Posh ufologist, Nick Redfern, merely looked on in disbelief. Matthew Williams skulked in an earnest fashion and then went off to ring his mummy.......we were joined again by the Hull people one of whom was well oiled and confided to all and sundry that he was a bouncer, and kept showing parts of his anatomy whilst questioning the availability of leeches for it.

Clearly I was missing the ufological context he was getting at here and his friends eventually took him away. It is perhaps best to ignore Jon Downes' frequent and desperate pleas to Irene Bott for something called 'executive relief'. Thankfully Irene is far too expensive for Jon to merit even a look of disdain. Just because he's a media whore and arts editor of the *Planet on Sunday* (didn't Clark Kent work for them?) it doesn't mean to say he can get away with this sort of behaviour.

So, that was LAPIS 1999, it was good and you should have been there. LAPIS also hold the distinction of holding the last UFO conference this millennium (depending, of course on when you believe the next millennium starts).

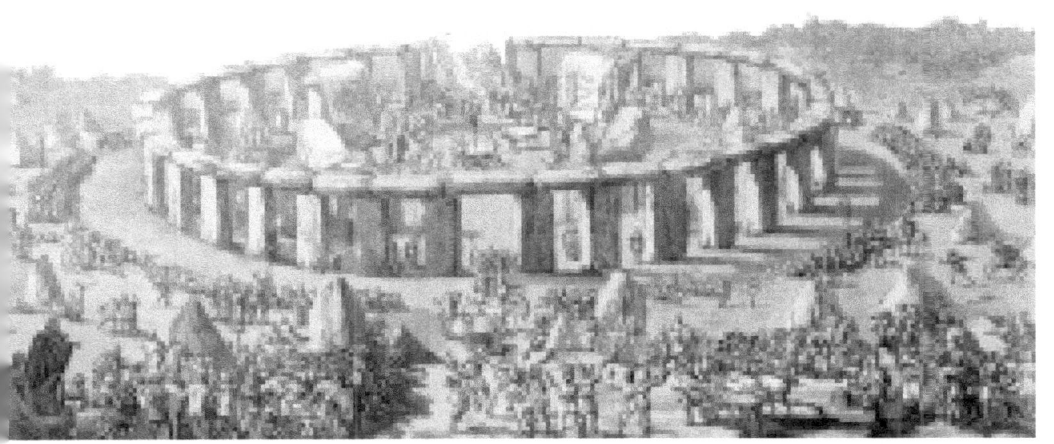

THE JOHN KEEL INTERVIEW

Published in *UFO Brigantia, issue 53/54 1992*

Ever since I was about 11 years old and read Keel's first book, *Jadoo,* I was obsessed by him. Others felt like that too apparently, as I later came to find out. He's one of the few people to have revolutionised how we think about ufology and strange phenomena general y and I'd long wanted him to speak at a UK UFO conference. It took three years to get him here but as many of you know Keel spoke at the annual IUN conference in August this year. Although debilitated by jet-lag, the effects of diabetes and the unwanted attentions of the Men in Black from BUFORA Keel still managed to give a stirring speech to the troops which left many people leaving the hall shaking their heads and muttering "that's wiped the floor with Bill Moore's explanation for Roswell". This was the first time he had ever publicly spoken in the UK and he may not come this way again. If you missed it, it just serves you right. I spoke to Keel at length over the three days he spent in Sheffield and learned many things, some of which I agreed with, some I didn't. But what really struck me overall was Keel's grasp of ufology, the perspective he has and his sense of humour. When the conference was oven I managed to get a 'formal' interview with John - here it is.

AR: John, would you like to tell me how you first became interested in Fortean subjects, and in UFOs in particular?

JK: It was so long ago. You know, I read Charles Fort when I was very young, when I was about 14 or 15 years old. So, I was reading *Amazing Stories*, in those days, and they were getting letters to *Amazing Stories* about things people had seen in the sky - this is before 1947. I was writing a newspaper column at that time for my home town newspaper and I did a couple of columns on that kind of thing, lights in the sky and people would see contrails high over head and they would think that that was some kind of spaceship or something and they'd write to *Amazing Stories* about it. In those days, in the '40s contrails were very rare; an airplane usually has to be high altitude to leave a contrail. Anyway, I was around when the whole UFO thing broke and I remember I was standing in a carnival in my home town and I was standing in the middle of the Midway in the carnival and a friend of mine came up and said 'Hey Keel, have you seen this newspaper story about this guy out West who saw some strange things over the mountains", and it was like a shock to me I thought "Oh my God, it's starting". I remember thinking that, that it's starting now and of course that was the beginning, that was the Arnold story but I hadn't yet seen it in the papers. The Kenneth Arnold report did not get much play in the papers in the northeast; it was mostly in the West. It took a while for it to reach the East in the magazines and so on.

AR: Do you think that the Arnold sighting and the subsequent UFO hysteria was a bit of a reaction to

WWII? The world had been used to Earth-threatening excitement for several years and then peace broke out. Do you think we were waiting for 'something' perhaps and that the Arnold sighting triggered that 'something'?

JK: Yeah, but it was also what we called the silly season. In the newspaper business in those days the summer months were very slow news-wise, there wasn't much news. So they would seize on something like that. One year it would be Loch Ness Monster sightings, the next year it would be UFOs. We don't really have a silly season any more we have a silly season the year round now.

AR: What did you believe UFOs were at that time?

JK: I assumed, after reading Fort, that they must be spaceships. Fort didn't really come right out and advocate the ET thesis but he said there was something there and that it had been around for a long time because he'd traced reports all the way back and Fort was very persuasive if you could get through his style. He had an odd style of writing, a humorous style which a lot of people to this day don't quite comprehend.

AR: Do you think you've copied your style in any way from Fort's? You have also got a very distinctive writing style which I think 'tricks' people intentionally into believing....

JK: I sort of sometimes satirise on Fort. Fort used to use certain phrases like 'I have a theory, that the stars are hanging from strings and the sky is only 800 feet up' and that would be a joke and people would seriously quote that and say "well Charles Fort thinks the stars are hanging on strings". But I think my own style sort of evolved over the years. I was writing a humorous column as a kid.

The way I got into the writing business was I wrote a letter to the editor of my hometown newspaper, I was about 12 years old, he thought it was a very funny letter and he called me into his office and he asked me to write a column and we called the column 'Scraping the Keel'. And so it was a column of alleged humour and I would make little kind of childish jokes and it was quite popular so in my little hometown was about 5000 people so in a very short time I was the most famous person in the town. Then I started the high school newspaper there and I called it *The Jester* because I was making fun of the school, let's face it. Then when I turned 16 I got so bored with school because in this town there was no course for me to take in this school.

I took all the science courses in one year, courses that were considered the toughest courses, chemistry and physics and so on. I passed them like that and the only courses left were, they had an agricultural course but I wasn't about to become a farmer. They had a business course but I wasn't really interested in business and so I left school when I was sixteen and I started writing full time, or as much as I could, I was working on the farm too. I started sending stories to the magazines in New York City and sooner or later people started sending me cheques! My first cheque was for two dollars! And I was really thrilled by that and by the time I was 17 I had sold quite a few short pieces for a very small amount of money and I decided that I was going to go to New York and make my fortune. So I left my family - they didn't believe I was going to go to New York they thought "Well, he'll be back tomorrow". I arrived in New York with 75 cents, didn't know a soul except editors that I'd corresponded with but I didn't know them well enough to socialise with them.

I was just a country bumpkin in the big city, but there was one magazine editor that owed me some money and I went to see him and I thought I'd be able to live on this money for a while because they owed me quite a lot of money. Quite a lot was like 30 dollars.

But they were going broke and they paid me off 50 cents at a time and so I would go up there every day and get my 50 cents and I slept on park benches, I did all the homeless things but in those days you were safe, today you'd get murdered the second day. Can you imagine a 17 year old boy in a big dangerous city like New York?

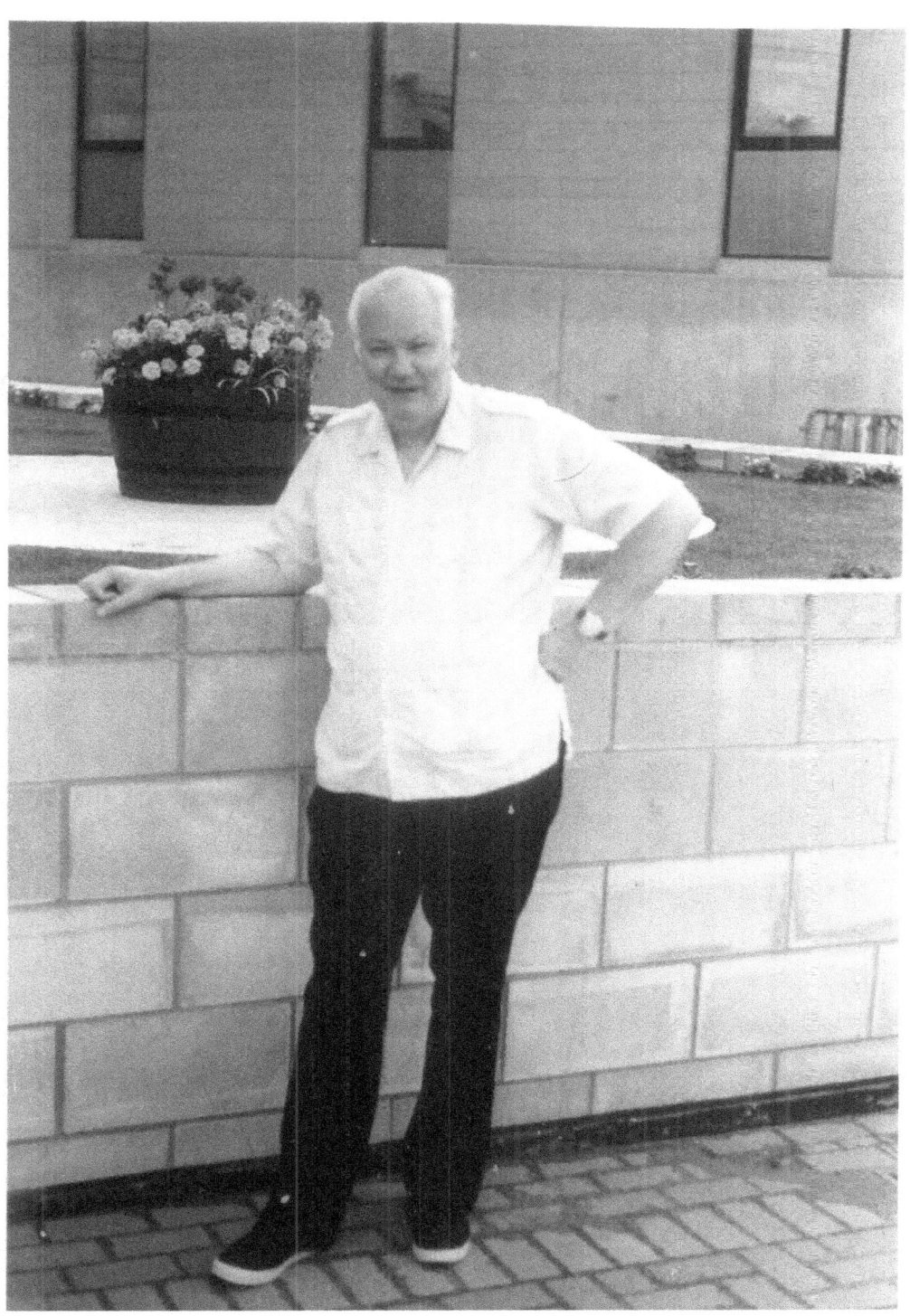

John Keel. IUN International UFO Conference, Sheffield 1992

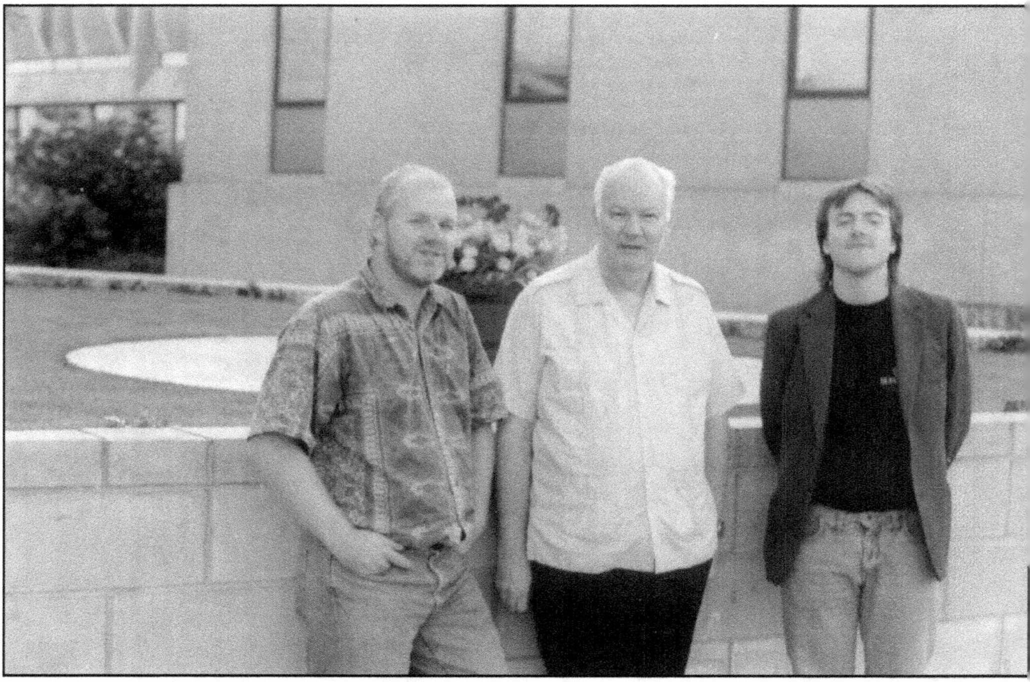

Andy Roberts, John Keel and a rather smug looking David Clarke
at the IUN Conference

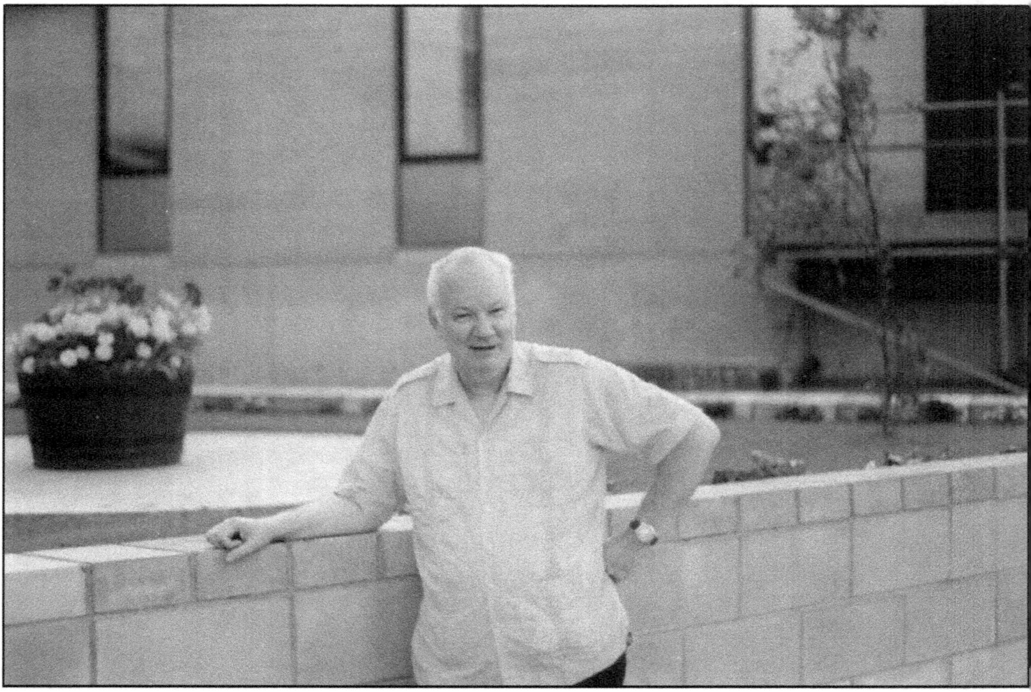

I quickly settled in Greenwich Village where all artists and writers and within two weeks I everybody and I became editor of a poetry magazine, had a little office there in Greenwich Village, and that's how all started.

AR: When did you start travelling?

JK: That was years later when I was drafted into army in the Korean War. Instead of shipping me to Korea they shipped me Germany which was a very good move on their part, 'cos they were shooting people in Korea! They assigned me to a radio station in Germany, I done some work in radio New York and TV was just beginning in New York and I'd done a little TV and the army, believe it or not, they saw my record there and they assigned to a radio station – in fact the biggest radio station in the world at that time, American Forces Network. I started writing radio programmes for them and within one year I was promoted to the chief of productions for the whole network, at 20-21 years and I'm practically running the whole network!

Then when my two years in the army were up they offered me a civilian job and I had a choice – return to New York or stay with the army, and I stayed another year as a civilian in Frankfurt and they gave me a nice apartment and a very good salary and so on. But I used to dream up my own assignments. I sent myself off to Egypt to do a broadcast from the Great Pyramid! We had a soldiers' singing contest where I had to go around to all the army camps in Europe and pick out the best singer in each army camp and so I took a tour of France! I had a chauffeured limousine that took me around France and I judged this singing contest, but that was just one of the many, many scams that I had going.

AR: Sounds like Sergeant Bilko!

JK: I also did a radio broadcast from the Castle of Frankenstein, there really is a Castle Frankenstein, I did a Halloween broadcast from there, which was a very big success, the newspapers and magazines like *Time* compared me to Orson Welles because Orson Welles had pulled off this famous Halloween radio programme of 1938. So by now *Stars and Stripes* was always writing about me and running pictures of me and I was suddenly the most famous soldier in Germany! But after being there as a civilian for a year I'd saved almost all of my salary during that year they offered me a better contract to stay on and then I had a big decision. Whether to stay there, forever - I could still be over there! But I decided that I would take a wild chance and take the money I had saved and go around the world, which I had always wanted to do. I especially wanted to visit India. So I took my savings and I left Germany and I went first back to Egypt where I'd done the broadcast from the Great Pyramid.

AR: Any particular reason why you went back to Egypt?

JK: Because I felt a strong relationship to Egypt, a lot of people feel that, it's rather mysterious, you almost feel like your ancestors are from Egypt and I wasn't the only one to feel that. I've heard other people talk about it too, although I felt no kinship at all to the modern Arabs, the modern Egyptians, but I felt something about the land of Egypt. I really felt a strong relationship to it. So I lived there for almost a year.

AR: Was it during this time that you saw the UFO at the Aswan Dam?

JK: I saw a UFO at the old Aswan Dam, they later built a new one, but there was an old Aswan Dam and I was down there and there were a lot of people around there must have been a scattering of like a hundred people all visiting the dam and so on and we saw this circular thing that was spinning. It appeared in a clear blue sky and this was in 1954. Later I found out there were sightings all over the Middle East at that time in 1954 and of course 1954 was a very big year in France and think Britain was also included. That was a major year. This thing that I saw was like the Saturn-shaped objects you've seen drawings of. In other words it appeared the centre of it was not moving but the outside was spinning. A very odd thing and various people were looking at it with me and I asked some of them what they thought it was and what the altitude was.... and everyone had a different answer. You had 200 witnesses and you had 200 different answers! I thought it was about 200-300 feet in the air, but some people thought it was 1000 feet, 5000 feet and because you don't know the size of the thing you can't judge the altitude of it. Right there, in two seconds I was convinced that flying saucers existed! There was no way anybody could ever tell me after that that there's no such thing as flying saucers.

AR: Where did you go from Egypt?

JK: I lived in Egypt for a while, and then I moved on across the desert. I went to Baghdad and I arrived broke in Baghdad which had become my normal condition because I had an agent in New York who would send me money and sometimes the money would be delayed or some SNAFU. I was broke in Baghdad and I quickly learned, whenever I was broke, to check into the most expensive hotel and then because I was an American and had that famous green passport they never questioned me and just though "Hey, he's an American, he must be filthy rich!" So I would check into the best hotel and eat in their restaurants until the money came through and I never got questioned once! From Baghdad I took the long trip down through the Persian Gulf on some kind of funny boat and ended up in India and then I spent a great deal of time in India because it's a fascinating country.

AR: Yeah. In *Jadoo* you travelled through India, sort of debunking the so called paranormal events such as life burials, snake charmers, and the rope-trick and so on, could you tell us a little about that?

JK: I always had a childhood interest in magic and I continue to this day to have an interest in magic, and I wanted to find the famous street magicians of India and when I did find street magicians they were all doing card tricks! Which they had bought by mail from London! It was very hard to find anyone doing the famous Indian tricks. I searched for the Indian Rope Trick and I found various forms of it being performed but they were not the authentic Indian Rope Trick. They were all little faked tricks for the tourists.

AR: What was so special about out snake-charming?

JK: Snake charming had always fascinated me as a kid on the farm. I started studying herpetology and reading books on the subject and I had a neighbour who used to go out and catch rattle snakes and sell them to some company that needed rattlesnakes. I used to go out with him and so at a very early age I learned quite a lot about snakes and reptiles so I actually studied snake charming with some of these snake charmers except there's not much to study because the charmer is owing a pipe and moving his hands back and forth and the snake is trying to strike at his hands.

The snake can't hear so it's all showmanship, the people watching think the snake is dancing to the tune of the pipe but the snake is just trying to kill the piper!

AR: Did anything unusual happen to you whilst in India?

JK: I had many Fortean type experiences in India.; One strange thing that happened more than once was strange people would come up to me and say they'd been waiting for me to appear - this was probably baloney and they'd say, "There's an American tourist, let's take him for big bucks".

I got very sophisticated very fast and I went into the Himalayan Mountains because at that time in the '50s there was a lot of publicity about the Abominable Snowman. There were a number of expeditions into the mountains looking for the Snowman, I think the *Daily Mail* in London sent a big expedition, and I figured I might be able to get a photograph of the Abominable Snowman and sell it to *Life* magazine or something. So I went into the mountains and to the little country of Sikkim and I crossed the border into Tibet, not very far though 'cos I'm six feet tall and Tibetans are four feet tall and the Chinese were in there and they would see this six foot tall guy and say "That is not a real Tibetan". At least I could say I'd been to Tibet.

AR: Whilst in *Jadoo* you debunk the common or garden yogic tricks, when you get into the Himalayas you seem to become less sceptical and have some experiences of the 'remote viewing' which the monks do. Any comment on that?

JK: I was very impressed with what some of these monks, lamas, were doing. They seemed to know every move that I was making. It was like I was being watched through the whole trip and so I would arrive at a monastery and they were expecting me and they had dinner ready! I was quite impressed with a lot of that.

AR: How do you think they did it - was it because of the time they spent training their minds?

JK: Yeah - what else is there to do there!? I had the experience of running into a lama on a snow covered mountain and he was almost stark naked and he didn't mind the cold at all. They weren't surprised to see me and in some of these areas, this is in the '50s, they had never seen a white man before. I think in Sikkim at that time there had only been 400 white men 'throughout their history in that little country. Nepal was practically inaccessible and Bhutan was inaccessible. You could cross into Bhutan and never come out again.

AR: Did you actually see the Yeti?

JK: I was with some natives, I hate to use the word natives, I was with some of the people who lived there, and I was the stranger. And across the lake we saw a brown figure; a large brown figure moving around in the brush across the lake and the natives with me said that was a Yeti. Now it could have been a bear, or it could have been anything but they told me it was a Yeti because they knew it would make me happy and so that was my Yeti! I saw the Yeti footprints a couple of times, the famous Yeti footprints which are huge. If you see the footprints you say "Well maybe I don't wanna meet this guy".

AR: Do you Yeti exists in the physical realm?

JK: Then I did, yes. Although all of the stories about the Yeti which I heard from different people seemed very demonic. They believed it was bad luck to see one of them. Everybody had a story to tell about the Yeti in those days, everybody who lived in those areas. But now I'm not so sure the Yeti is a real animal. At that time I was absolutely convinced.

AR: I know you don't want to talk about the Mothman but I'll just ask one question. I'm still puzzled by one bit of *The Mothman Prophecies* – the chapter entitled Beelzebub Visits West Virginia where you relate the story of how you called at a house to make a 'phone call and because you were not from the area people misidentified you as the Devil?! Is this part of your tricking device which continues through the book - to make people see that everything isn't as it seems?

JK: As you know the was written several years after the events and it was very difficult to get a New York publisher interested in it and I needed a strong opening and this was a true story. My car had run off the highway on a very rainy night and I was dressed in a neck tie and a full suit. You didn't see that very often back road in West Virginia, a black suit, and I went around pounding on doors to get somebody to call a truck for me. It turned that the people finally made the call people that were on the bridge that later collapsed. Next day told everybody they knew that a strange man in a black suit, and a beard, which were rare in those days, called and he must have been the devil so that made me part of folklore and I found years later that people were still telling that story that the devil had come around to these houses on this back road.

AR: I think that says a lot about human beings. The majority of your Virginia sightings seem nave been just odd blobs light into which people have read something else- are you saying then that we live in an environment which still has many hidden, but natural mysteries with which we interact and interpret?

JK: Yeah, we seem to be surrounded by almost invisible world that can manipulate us in any way. In fact I just had a letter before I left New York. I had a letter from a man named Henry Belk. His family are very rich, they own a chain of 400 stores in the south and Henry for many years has investigated psychic surgery, that's his thing and I was astonished to get this letter the other day, he said that after these years investigating psychic surgery he had decided that the psychic surgery was being done by invisible force. The surgeon was just an instrument for it and Henry is evolving now a whole theory about invisible entities and so on and for him, he's very scientifically oriented, it's a surprising thing for him to come out with.

AR: Do you think that this phenomenon, the one behind the lights, helping psychic surgeons and so on, do you think it is conscious or merely reactive?

JK: When I was investigating UFOs I realised that somebody was playing games with us in fact there's a chapter in *Operation Trojan Horse* about the cosmic Jokers, a phrase which caught on by the way and people all over the world are using that phrase 'cosmic jokers' now, You get involved in a situation which seems very real at the time and then as it progresses, if you're smart enough, you realise it's really a joke and somebody's playing a joke on you and it has no meaning at all. Now some people are too dumb to realise that and then it just keeps growing and developing because this phenomena sort of feeds on it.

AR: Can you give us an example of how that manifested itself to you?

JK: Yeah, 'They' had me running around New York looking for a mysterious gold cross (AR: shades of psychic questing!) that if I could only find this gold cross I would save the world! And for a while I was playing these games. A very well known American ufologist named Ted Bloecher, well Ted spent 30 years of his life, he's in the theatre, he's a song and dance man but he spent 30 years of his life spending all his spare time researching UFOs and he would be with a dance troupe in a small town he'd go to the newspaper and go through their files and get all their UFO reports. Well he finally got involved in some contactee stories in New York state where there were landings and UFOs supposedly contacting people and so on and he got deeper and deeper into these and then it finally occurred to him that 'somebody' was playing with him, that it wasn't real, that it was a joke that they were playing on him and that whatever his interpretation was the phenomenon would then mould itself to it. So he quit ufology and he's made statements to people that he's very sorry that he spent 30 years on it, he regrets now that he wasted 30 years when he could have been out chasing women or whatever.

AR: Do you think there was any connection between the collapse of the Silver Bridge in *The Mothman Prophecies* and what was going on.

JK: Well some of the people who died on the bridge were people who'd seen the Mothman and it was all very strange, there were millions of coincidences and strange, interrelated events for example there was a family in West Virginia with the rather unusual name of Walmsley. Now the Walmsley family was an integral part of the Mothman mystery because several people in this family had seen the Mothman and as you know in small towns in America one family will have three hundred different units in the area, cousins and grandparents and so on. Well in Budd Hopkins' first book he talks about the first UFO sighting in New Jersey that he got interested in and it's the Walmsley family in New Jersey! And a couple of the Walmsley people in West Virginia went down with the bridge. There does seem to be a lot of things interacting with us on this planet that we don't ...

AR: Why that particular area, why West Virginia for so many strange occurrences?

JK: We're not smart enough to figure it out! Some of these things of course have no meaning at all and some of them there may be real meaning like these two men who materialised on a street to a women, dressed in clothing that was way out of fashion, clothes from the 1940s and these men seemed very odd and sinister to her - they may have been on a special mission of some sort. Their mission was to go to a store and buy all the Keel books and take 'em back to the next dimension!

AR: In several of your books you mention that you've been contacted by witches and magicians who've had similar experiences to you. Do you think that's perhaps because witches and magicians can manipulate, 'call up' if you like, these energies by the power of emotion?

JK: They have studied the same thing but they haven't studied it from a ufological point of view. They've studied in from almost a religious point of view and incidentally in Point Pleasant where the Mothman was appearing, after all the, publicity that Mothman received, the town was inundated with witchcraft cults and things and the power plant where the Mothman was first seen, the walls inside the power plant are now covered with graffiti from witches and magicians, pentacles and that kind of thing.

AR: Do you think that as a result of an interaction with an invisible environment that we the humans are actually meant to understand the universe and its mysteries or are we fighting a losing battle doomed to play, as you say in one of your books, "It's the only game in town"?

JK: I think the human race is going very slowly, step by step, towards some goal that we don't understand and I think you can see in the last forty ears how we have evolved with our new age movements and things, now this doesn't mean the whole human race. It means a fragment of the human race has gotten an understanding they didn't have before and it really started in 1848 with the Fox sisters and spiritualism. That was the first real new age movement. A lot of other things happened in 1848 but it was like that one was the beginning and whatever the phenomenon is it's outside of us so each generation is carried a step further but our generation doesn't matter. As you know many of our ufologists are now dead and they died without knowing anything about all of this.

Some of them carried it a little step forward. It may take another hundred years or another five hundred years before we know what this ultimate goal is.

AR: Have you any ideas what Mans' 'ultimate goal' may be?

JK: Well, a very smart fellow, an Englishman by the way, named Arthur C. Clarke, wrote a book called *Childhood's End* which is about this very thing, about the evolution of the human race until the logical end of evolution is a spiritual state and no longer a physical state and that's in his book. I have come to think that that's true too, that our physical bodies are very limited and very fragile and not worth very much, but our spiritual existence, whatever it is - we don't understand it, is the key and if there's such a thing as evolution and reincarnation and so on it's the endurance of this fragment of energy that we each carry around with us.

AR: Do you think it's connected to the Earth in any way. In your talk last night the first slide you showed was of the Earth from space and that's the first time I've ever heard a spontaneous round of applause during the lecture at a UK UFO conference.

JK: Yeah I think it's the Earth. The American Indians you know believed that they were part of the Earth, that the Earth owned them, and that they didn't own the Earth and I think that's probably true. I think the Indians and a lot of these so-called primitive people had a great understanding of all this and it was unfortunately lost when the white man came over. Look what happened to the Indians in South America, we destroyed their written records in the name of religion. On Easter Island they had written records and the first thing that the Spanish priests did when they arrived there was destroy the written records as being the 'work of the devil'.

AR: A long time ago, I don't know if you can remember it, you once said in the pages of *Fortean Times* that "We are the source of the phenomenon". Have you anything to say on that subject, for instance about contactees, are we contacting ourselves?

JK: It's like do you hear the sound of a tree falling in a forest? If we weren't here would there be UFOs here? I think the UFOs are definitely connected directly to us and we're only seeing what they want us to see, what we think we're seeing.

AR: Who are the 'they' then?

JK: It's a force. I tried to define it in very simple terms in my book *The Cosmic Question*. I also went into the problem of mystical illumination which has always fascinated me because it happened to me when I was eighteen. When I was living in New York as an eighteen year old I was living in a furnished room and I woke up one night and the whole room was bathed in this very peculiar light. I thought the building was on fire! Then I started having, you can't call them hallucinations, a flood of Material was coming into my mind and suddenly I understood everything. I swear I understood the meaning of every-thing, how the world was created, how it was going to end. I knew it all! And I said "This is terrific, boy I'll write this all down tomorrow when I wake up", and the next day of course when I woke up I couldn't remember anything!

I remember the experience and I remember the room being bathed in this light but I couldn't remember any of this material, it must have entered into my unconscious mind. And for thirty years I thought I was the only person in the world that had had this experience, I never mentioned it to anybody and then I started reading some of this stuff about cosmic illumination and then I started meeting other people who'd had the same experience and I realised that many people in each generation has this experience and many of them don't necessarily do anything with it and other: it changes their whole life.

AR: In what way?

JK: They become teachers, scientists, politicians. I think John F. Kennedy had probably had that experi-ence and I think also that if someone like JFK has the experience it dooms them - he got into his position of president too soon. He would have changed the world. If he had lived in 1963, there would have been no Vietnam, there would have been a major space programme because he would have devoted all of move, for warfare into the space programme which was his plan, and we would be of Mars now

AR: Do you think this is why contactees often "self destruct", because they have 'the secret' and want to do something with it, they try to do it too fast and they burn out.

JK: No, contactees only get part of the experience. For contactees it's like false illumination. They only get part of it and they get crazy, they misinterpret it. There are a lot of people in religion who have this experience and put it to good use. There are a lot of priests and nuns and holy people who've, that's why they get into religion, they have this experience and they spend their lives helping other people. Mystical illumination is a very important key to this and there are books on it, books written by people who've had the experience, books by people who've studied the experience. A Dr. Bucke wrote the first book on it in the early 1900s and after he wrote the book he slipped on the ice, hit his head and killed himself. There are many people who have the experience and don't necessarily remember seeing a light or seeing anything, it just happens to them and they change overnight and they don't know why.

AR: What do you think about the current fascination in the USA for the extraterrestrial hypothesis?

JK: Well, it's been a propaganda campaign, it's been a very small group of people propagandising this, proselytising a new religion and the new religion is this notion that there are extraterrestrials out there. Now science on the other hand has backed away from the whole extraterrestrial thing. In the 60s many scientists thought that there was a very good chance that there were extraterrestrials.

Carl Sagan for example founded exobiology and now these scientists, including Arthur C. Clarke by the way, who has made a number of statements in the past few years saying that he no longer believes there is any chance for extraterrestrials to exist. The ET premise has been promoted by the movies and by the UFO buffs and the average person in the street now sort of accepts it, because they haven't given much thought to it and they've seen the movies or they've heard UFO buffs on the radio or TV and they say, 'well that makes sense, we're being visited by extraterrestrials' - they just simply accept it.

AR: Do you think the US government has the faintest idea about UFOs or is the only cover up one of ignorance?

JK: I think they're pretty dumb about this. I've spent a lot of time trying to find files that would really have significant material and I've known a lot of people in the government and in the military and there are a lot of people who are interested in the subject but there's never been no unified effort to study it or discover anything, and how do you study it without actually making contact with the UFOs? So the UFO buffs have kind of dreamed up a whole fantasy world where they think the government has made deals with the UFOs. That's just the UFO buff's way out, of protecting himself, otherwise, if he didn't think that then he would be in a very vulnerable position as a UFO buff, so he says that the reason that we don't know anything about UFOs is because the government is keeping it quiet. And the alternative to that is the reason we don't know anything about UFOs is they don't exist.

AR: In *Operation Trojan Horse* you issue a warning to people wishing to become ufologists, basically warning them off the whole idea. What brought this on and do you still advocate that caveat?

JK: Yeah, in a lot of my speeches I usually end up with a statement like that. I usually point out that individuals and civilian organisations don't have the expertise or the money to do anything and that it's a waste of time to try to investigate these things. The best they can do is go and sit on a hill and watch the lights in the sky, and say 'hey, there goes one!' In order to really investigate this you might need twenty million dollars, to build the right instruments. This is a big project and I don't think even the government has ever undertaken that.

I don't think any government has ever undertaken that. The governments around the world all assumed the American government was gonna do it. You may remember in the 1970s Idi Amin - remember good old Idi Amin? Well in Uganda they were seeing UFOs all the time and Idi Amin had his ambassador to the UN stand up in the UN and say 'hey do something about this', and it was a famous speech at the UN, and of course the UN officials said 'what are we going to use for money?' and 'where are we going to find the experts'. When you think about it there isn't a single real expert on UFOs in the world because nobody has had that kind of experience to be an expert.

You can be an expert on submarines, because it's tangible, you can study the structure of submarines and you can ride in a submarine and all that but nobody can really do that with a UFO. So if a UFO landed tomorrow in Trafalgar Square, who would the British government call in to study it? It would be a big problem.

As I said they would probably have to call in first of all aeronautical designers- you wouldn't call in physicists and astronomers, and if there were beings on board you would call in your very best medical people, forensic pathologists, and biologists. The last person you would call in would be a ufologist, 'cos he'd be useless, he'd stand there and stare and say 'my god, it's real!'

AR: Are they real then?

JK: I'm talking about the lights and things. People do see something because I've seen them myself, but I don't think they are machines.

AR: One final question John, which I'm sure an awful lot of British ufologists have wanted to ask you for a long time. Just why didn't the moon come up on the night of April 3rd 1967? (note to baffled readers consult your copy of *The Mothman Prophecies*).

JK: (laughs) Yeah, I got the information from the local newspaper; I put that in almost as a joke because it was a humorous incident. I'd seen the moon the night before and then that night there was no moon – and also one night I saw the moon come up and I thought it was a flying saucer. A lot of people have done just that I'm sure.

AR: Thanks John, a most interesting interview.

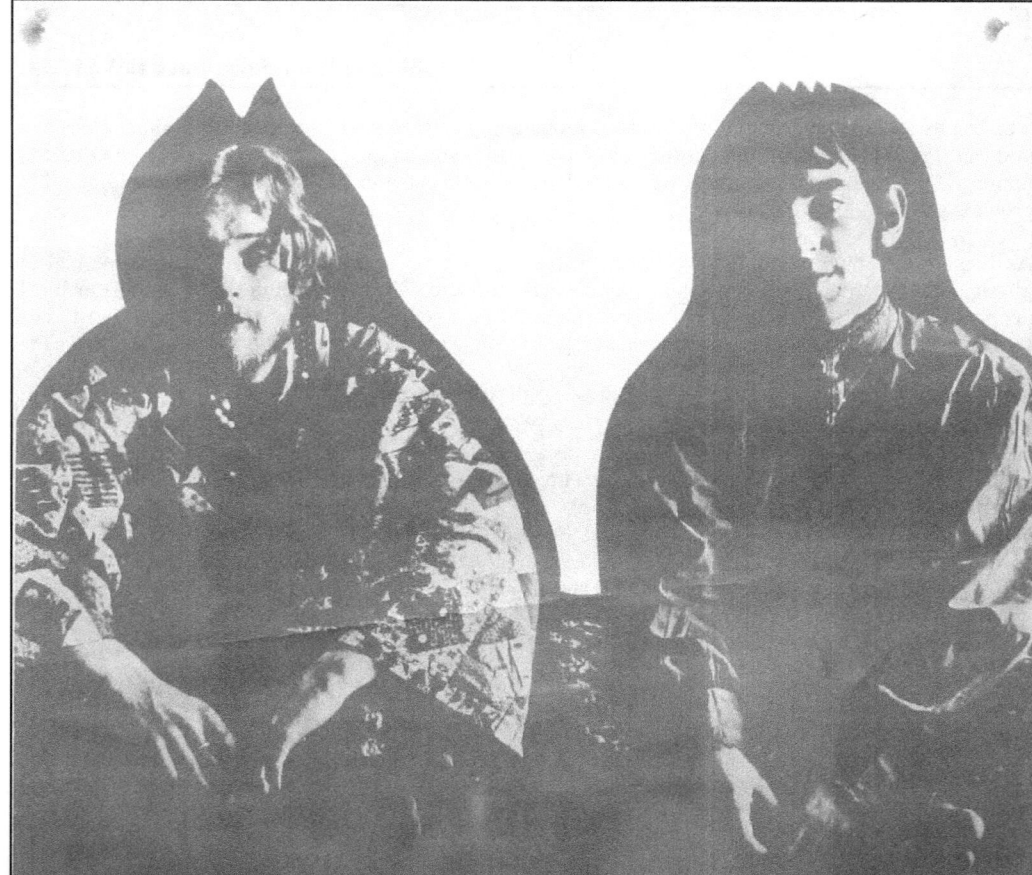

THE
INCREDIBLE
STRING BAND
A MYSTICAL PANTOMIME
GLASGOW CONCERT HALL
OCT. 13 8P.M.
5s. and 7s.6d. at Cuthbertson's

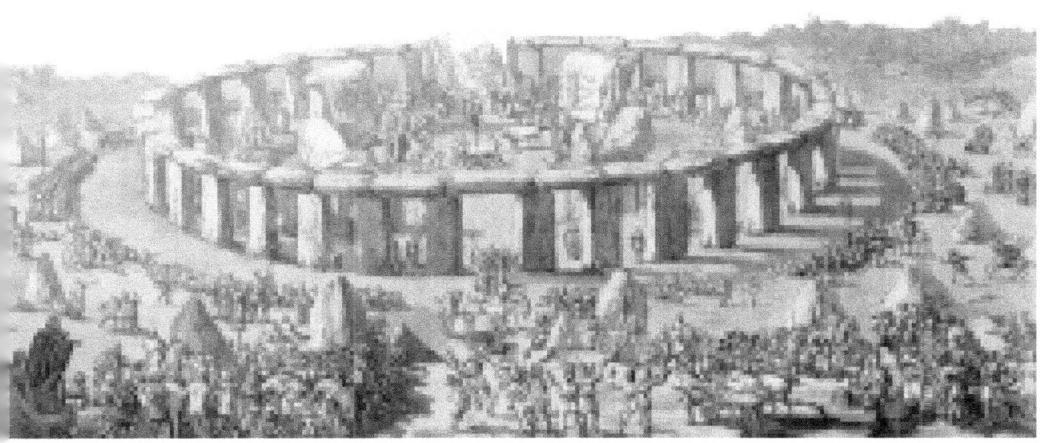

THE LORD OF WEIR—A FAIRY STORY?

A brief look at a very Fortean song from a very Fortean band
First published in *Be Glad For The Song has No Ending*

The Dancing Of The Lord Of Weir is probably the strangest song that Robin Williamson of the *Incredible String Band*, ever wrote, both lyrically and musically. Its first public exposure came in October 1971; Robin introduced it at a gig with the following words:

> 'Some people hold that fairies are the life or consciousness from anything, like a plant or a small forest, a wind or a sea - the consciousness of natural things. And some people say that fairies are, in fact, legendary memory of a different and non-human race that lived probably in Britain and Europe and possibly survived in remote places until as late as the 15th-17th Centuries.'

At another gig, Weir was prefaced by:

> 'This song is another quite new one. I got the idea from hearing this story that a long time ago in Britain there was different races living here apart from human races. There was this race of people who lived in the outlands and in the moors and in the very high places and they were accredited with supernatural abilities and they lived life in a very crude way, herding deer etc. And they were very wild, and they're supposed to have given rise to legends of fairies, and I wrote this song taking that as a viewpoint'

And from an interview:

> 'It's a fantasy story about a remote, imaginary past. It's based on the idea that there were actually fairies that were a race of people who lived in wild parts of Britain and were slightly different from ordinary mortals They lived there for a long time until they eventually got wiped out by persecution.'

An interesting idea and one widely held by many scholars in one form or another, the idea being that rather than the fairies being a 'different and non-human race', they were Neolithic peoples who retreated before the advent of metal users and fled to remote places where they lived simply, often underground in the 'hollow hills', revering the spirits of nature. The country inhabitants knew of their existence but were wary of their ways and magics and left them to themselves.

This legend may be the origin of many a medieval 'wild man' story, and several counties have tales of 'Brownies' and the like who came from the hills to help at harvest time, without whose help the harvest would fail and the milk curdle. Further explorations of this idea can be found in the works of Margaret Murray. The William Golding book *The Inheritors* takes a similar angle too; as does John Buchan's story *The Watcher on The Threshold*. The same theme is covered in a poem from early last century which begins:

> 'Up the airy mountains, down the rushy glen / We daren't go a-hunting for fear of little men / Wee folk, good folk / Trooping all together / Green jacket, red cap /And white owl's feather.'

Suffice to say that folklore was obviously the source of the song and it demonstrates Robin's deep knowledge of and influences drawn from the period where ancient history and folklore overlap; mythic times when deeds became legends and magic was definitely afoot. Weir was certainly an intimation of what was to come with Robin's later focus on Celtic myths and legends.

The song tells the story of how the local lord ('Weir' is an adaptation of an old Scottish word for 'war') gets above his station and steals one of the fairy tribe's women, 'she of the wild eyes, she of the wild hair'. Using their 'small magics' the tribe enter Weir's hall disguised as minstrels and play the fairy dance, compelling the mortals to dance against their will out into the world to be saved only when they think 'one kind thought'. Their kinswoman is rescued and they return to their home beneath the ground.

Weir is, like its subject matter, otherworldly. The instrumentation actually sounds like it's being played by people who have a different concept of music to the rest of us, while Robin's voice wails and skirls the story over the top. The version on *Myrrh* is an outstanding track; it resonates with an incantatory force which reinforces Robin's reputation as a modern bard.

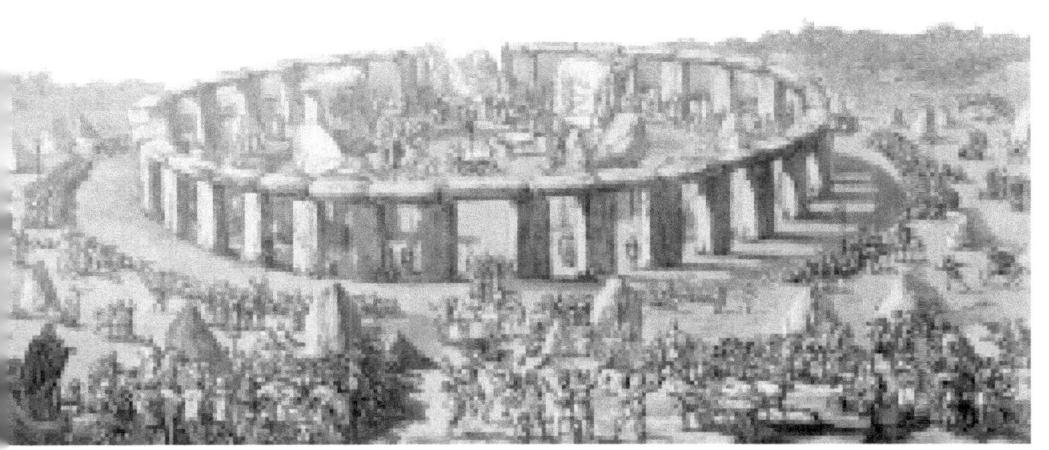

THE OLD STRAIGHT TRACK
TO THE NEW AGE
Saucers, psychics and free thinkers

The term 'New Age' is a familiar one, but to what does it refers? The new age movement has no creation myth, no overarching creed, and is in a state of constant flux, which varies with the mystic fashions of the day. Thus, we take the term to indicate that nexus of belief that includes everything from crystal healing to speaking with dolphins, by way of shamanic drumming groups and extreme dietary practices. Most new age beliefs can be defined as being based on opinion and aspiration rather than possessing, or requiring, any basis in fact. In the past fifty years, the new age movement has grown exponentially by accreting a steady stream of fringe belief that has been co-opted under its banner. It should come as no surprise to learn that flying saucers are one of those beliefs.

Mainstream ufological belief in the fifties and sixties, of the kind most often proclaimed in the media, reasoned that the nature of flying saucers was straightforward. They were physical, structured 'nuts and bolts' objects of unknown origin, almost certainly from outer space or beyond. World governments knew all about them and it was only a matter of time before 'the truth about flying saucers' would be revealed. Opinion as to their purpose was less clear and it is at this point where new age ideas began to seep into the subject, through the ideas of the contactees, organisations such as the Aetherius Society or those who believed that saucers were demonic in origin. We will meet these and other groups with similar outré agendas in later chapters. But any discussion of how rapidly ufological belief has broadened to take in aspects of other belief systems must include a discussion of how new age ideas influenced and interacted with the subject.

For those people interested in flying saucers, but who rejected as too simplistic the belief they were purely physical creations of other civilisations, new age ideas offered an alternate way of thinking. As with most other areas of UFO interest the new age elements within it are not discrete units, and many of the key figures in ufology moved effortlessly between the different aspects of the subject, their lives a constant pick'n'mix of belief. The new age vision of flying saucers was more often than not one of the acceptance of telepathic contact, salvation and validity of experience over absolute scientific proof.

The new age movement's involvement with flying saucers did not suddenly appear in the 1950s. Its roots lie deeply embedded in Theosophy and Spiritualism, both of which held that there were other layers to reality, worlds of experience other than those of everyday existence. Spiritualist and Theosophical beliefs whilst being self contained have embedded within them all the elements which formed the basis of new age thought in the mid to late 20th Century. Theosophy contended that the divine or the 'other' could be experienced directly without mediation from priest or dogma, whilst Spiritualism predicated on the premise that the soul survives after death and can interact with the living. The concept of spiritual and mental salvation was a core belief in both movements, as was the notion of other intelligences operating independently of humankind. These ideas recur time after time in re-worked ways throughout the history of ufology and it is easy to see why so many with a broad spiritualist or theosophist background were attracted to the study of flying saucers, or sought to try and integrate saucers and their potential into their pantheon of beliefs.

The Spiritualist movement in the UK was somewhat perplexed when flying saucers began to be reported in the late 1940s and early 1950s. Some psychics and spiritualists dismissed them immediately. Others were intrigued, believing the saucers and their occupants to be another aspect of the spirit world. Several spiritualists also believed that the flying saucers represented both a means to contact other intelligences and the possibility of salvation from further human conflict.

A number of spiritualist mediums believed they had made contact with flying saucers and an example of this occurs in a 1954 *Psychic News* article, which reported, 'Speaking through the well known medium Ralph Watson, his control Tabiti answered questions by experts about Flying Saucers during a trance sitting in Hastings…For two hours the sceptics bombarded the medium with questions, but his control was ready with the answers. He replied in technical language to questions about the makers of Flying Saucers'.

This low-level interest from the spiritualist community bubbled under throughout the 1950s. However, although individuals with spiritualist beliefs toyed with the idea of contact with saucers the spiritualist establishment was too clearly defined and dogmatic to accept the multiplicity of possibilities was came attached to the subject. Whilst ufologists in the UK wrote several books on the flying saucers during the 1950s, spiritualists could only come up with one. This one was called *Venus Speaks: Direct Revelation Regarding Flying Saucers and Life on Venus* (1954). The booklet consisted of communications received whilst the sitter, 'M.T.', was in trance, and purported to be from 'The Chief Scientists of Venus'.

The cover illustrations were obviously based on the UFOs allegedly seen and photographed by George Adamski, whilst the text was a barely intelligible stew of pseudo-technical information. Most of it was about the propulsion systems that powered the saucers, mixed with the usual contactee message about how humans were causing ecological disaster, and topped off with a healthy dose of paranoia about diet and healthy living.

Although unable to provide tangible evidence to support their own beliefs the spiritualist establishment, through their main publication *Psychic News* mostly frowned upon the upstart belief system of flying saucers. By the time saucer contactee George King, was encroaching on their territory spiritualism had lost patience completely with the saucer movement. Flying Saucers featured rarely in the spiritualist press after 1960.

Yet there were many people, some linked to the spiritualist movement who believed that mental contact with extraterrestrials was possible. This notion also fed into the flying saucer contactee movement, and was a direct result of the groundwork laid by Spiritualism. The combination of saucers and spiritualism led to some bizarre, if not unintentionally hilarious, scenarios being played out among small groups of UFO buffs throughout the UK.

One such faction, which straddled the line between spiritualism and saucer belief, was a disparate group of individuals known as the Attingham Group. They were so called because they had met or they had connections with the new age centre based at Attingham Park in Shropshire From the 1950s onwards, under the auspices of Sir George Trevelyan, Attingham Park became a focus for all things new age. By the mid 1960s, Attingham had become a melting pot of new age ideas. During the week, Attingham played host to adult education courses, but each weekend saw a new age invasion with courses offered on topics such as The Dark and the Light taking place. Many new agers who attended these Attingham courses were also interested in flying saucers. And so in the warm seclusion of the Georgian mansion like-minded souls were able to discuss the deeper meanings of flying saucers in isolation away from the strictures of mainstream ufology and its emphasis on nuts'n'bolts craft. Trevelyan himself was only mildly interested in saucers but there was small pressure group of Attingham regulars who were working to persuade him to set a UFO study group. This would essentially be a saucer study group for the New Age and had the Attingham Group been successfully formed and publicised it would have provided a viable opposition to the idea that saucers were merely physical craft. That the group barely got past the discussion stage was largely due to the naïve new age reasoning which lay behind it.

This potential study group included some very interesting and well-placed society establishment and establishment names. Air Marshal Sir Victor Goddard was the key player. In 1967, he wrote to several distinguished pillars of the scientific establishment in an attempt to get them involved in flying saucer research by way of the Attingham Group. One of his targets was astronomer Sir Bernard Lovell who ran the Jodrell Bank radio telescope in Cheshire. Goddard should have known better than to approach Lovell who was well known for being an objective and sceptical scientist. His brusque response to Goddard's entreaties was to the point, 'I ought to say then straight away that I find the whole of this business most alarming'. He continued in the same tone with, 'I have repeatedly gone on record in the past to the effect that there is not the slightest piece of real scientific evidence to support a belief in the UFO phenomena.'

Undaunted, Goddard pursued his attempts to set up a new age saucer study group and tried to involve the well known Buddhist judge Christmas Humphries and spiritualist and property developer Instone Bloomfield. Other new age aficionados who hovered on the fringes of Goddard's would be Attingham Group included Michael Parker, a member of Prince Philip's staff, the former MoD scientist Frank Houghton-Bentley and Lord Clancarty, a.k.a. Brinsley le Poer Trench. Johann Quanjer was also heavily involved. It was one of Quanjer's friends, Lady Cynthia Sandys, who exemplified the often-ludicrous results of mixing new age beliefs.

During the course of his correspondence with Sir Bernard Lovell back in 1967 Victor Goddard tried to impress the pragmatic astronomer. He did so, not by demonstrating his scientific knowledge, but by claiming him that Lady Sandys was in psychic communication with dead American contactee George Adamski. Lady Sandys believed herself to be psychic. Johann Quanjer persuaded Sandys to attempt contact with the spirit of the recently deceased Adamski. Adamski was something of a hero to the new age saucerers and Lady Sandys claimed that she had made contact with his spirit on several occasions. 'I was told that he was working all over the Solar system, sometimes in Venus, Saturn and so on', being a typical example of her communications. Adamski, speaking through Lady Sandys also stated 'Oh, I like that fellow at Jodrell Bank, we think alongside each other, but he must go further', and, 'Science talk is interplanetary, so to your group who are waiting to meet the saucers, I would say collect your scientists first. Lovell I should like to name, but he must be given proof first.'

It was these vapid psychic messages from the dead Adamski that eventually prompted Goddard to write to Sir Bernard Lovell, suggesting he help the putative Attingham Group. Goddard was so confident that Lovell would be keen to support his cause that he had booked a roof table at the Royal Garden Hotel for 18 July 1967 so they could meet to discuss matters further. Goddard had drastically misjudged Lovell.

Besides his letter displaying a scepticism in the subject of UFOs generally Lovell had a few sharp worlds about Adamski, 'As for Adamski, I have never met that gentleman but I did attempt to read his book, and I must say that judging by any standard which you and I would normally apply to such works it really was the most unutterable rubbish'. If that weren't enough to get the message across to Goddard, Lovell hammered his feelings home, writing, 'I am sure there is no need for me to say more to make you realise my personal attitude to these so-called phenomena, and to the people who believe in them.'

It was hardly surprising that, given tactics such as those employed by Sir Victor Goddard, the Attingham Group never made an impact on the UFO scene. The Attingham Group disintegrated before it had really formed. In any case, Trevelyan's new age interests were much too eclectic for him to be mired in a new age UFO group. Although the Attingham Group foundered and whilst Trevelyan himself would never go public with his interest in UFOs, Attingham Park had played its role in the new age saucer interest, as it was acting as an introduction point for those people whose beliefs were too outré for the mainstream. One of those who used Attingham as a touchstone was Peter Caddy, who gate crashed a conference of New Age leaders held at Attingham Park in the summer of 1965. Caddy's place in the new age saucer nexus is crucial. His name may sound unfamiliar but the location from which he made his name almost certainly won't be.

Ask anyone with an interest in the new age about Scotland's Findhorn Community and you'll receive a nod of recognition. Ask what they know, it and you'll be told a half-remarkable story of a spiritual centre where people live in harmony, communicating with the spirits of nature. The Community has been dubbed, 'The Vatican of the New Age', and includes among its patrons such diverse personalities as Prince Philip, Shirley Maclaine and Mike Scott from the *Waterboys*. Findhorn is worth over £5 million pounds a year to the area, yet still strongly polarises opinion. Some believe that the community attracts vitally needed employment and tourism to the area. Others are more cynical, one neighbour commenting, 'If they were any good to anyone they wouldn't be at the Findhorn Foundation', another noting that members of the community are often seen hugging when they meet, 'It's just not our way'.

Yet whatever its detractors may say the Community is embedded in the spiritual psyche of the UK and one of its founders, Eileen Caddy, was awarded the MBE for 'service to spiritual enquiry'. According to the Community's newsletter, 'Eileen chose to hand the medal to God'. What God thought of the award was not recorded, but it may have been more pertinent to ask, 'What did the aliens think?'.

Yes, aliens. The official Findhorn website states, 'The Findhorn Community was begun in 1962 by Peter and Eileen Caddy and Dorothy Maclean. All three had followed disciplined spiritual paths for many years and had been specifically trained to follow God's will.' However, 1962 was merely when the trio moved to Findhorn. The Community's true origins lie in the 1950s, in the maelstrom of post-war fringe ideas and philosophies that eventually coalesced into what we now call the New Age.

Central to Findhorn's origins is a secret that the current leaders of the community would very much like to play down, flying saucers. One of the core beliefs held by Findhorn's founders was that flying saucers existed, and that their occupants were in psychic contact with them. It was also an article of faith that physical contact with the saucers was not only possible, it was certain.

Findhorn's principle mover and shaker was Peter Caddy, together with a close-knit circle of partners and spiritual travellers such as Eileen Caddy and Dorothy MacLean. All were heavily involved in the flying saucer contactee belief system, but it is Caddy's story that binds them together. As with many spiritual leaders, Caddy evolved through a series of religious, philosophical and occult beliefs of which flying saucers were just one aspect. Caddy married Nora Medling in 1941 and after a 'good war' Caddy's life became a whirlwind of meetings with remarkable men and women. He soon realised the limitations of his marriage to Nora, when he met another spiritual seeker, Sheena Gowan. Their spiritually intense meetings soon turned into a physical relationship, Sheena receiving 'guidance', by way of what we now call channelling, from God, which led to Caddy being instructed to end his marriage to Nora.

It's easy to suggest that the post war 'spiritual' milieu in which they existed was merely a justification for extramarital relationships. Indeed, reading Caddy's autobiography it is hard not to see the post war spiritual scene as a hot bed of partner swapping, a sort of *Confessions of a New Age Disciple*. By his death in 1994, Caddy had been married five times and had numerous 'special friends' during his voyage through the spiritual, but fecund, waters of the New Age.

In the 1940s a chance meeting in the Philippines with Anne Edwards, a.k.a. Naomi, spun Caddy off on a new series of adventures. Naomi was a channeller and the first sensitive Caddy met who claimed contact with aliens, 'Naomi had received many messages from beings in space, concerning their space ships, their purpose and mission'. Naomi remained in the Philippines whilst Caddy, Sheena and Eileen settled in Scotland.

By 1954, Caddy, via Naomi, had amassed numerous telepathically channelled messages from what he termed the 'space brothers'. In line with others who were receiving channelled communications during the 1950s, such as George King of the Aetherius Society, the message coming through Naomi was that extraterrestrials were fearful about the state of Planet Earth, and warned of impending ecological disaster if humanity didn't change its ways. Caddy received an 'inner prompting' to compile a detailed report on the nature of these messages, called An Introduction to the Nature and Purpose of Unidentified Flying Objects, which would clearly define who and what lay behind the increasing numbers of UFO sightings.

Once the 8,000-word report was completed, the problem was how to distribute it to the twenty-six people Eileen's guidance had decreed. Former Prime Minister Clement Atlee was handed his copy by his aunt! Lord Dowding, already an outspoken proponent of flying saucers and spiritualism, received his copy at his London club. After reading it Dowding wrote to Caddy saying, 'I am personally convinced of the existence of spaceships, and I think it highly probable that they are manned by extraterrestrial crews…I think that the government ought to take the subject of spaceships very seriously, and to let some senior and responsible official take on the task of collecting evidence as a preliminary step to formulating an opinion, and perhaps a course of action.'

Caddy's main target for the report was Prince Philip, known to have a keen interest in flying saucers and to subscribe to *Flying Saucer Review*. Prince Philip had tasked his Equerry, Squadron Leader Peter Horsley, to investigate flying saucers on his behalf. Horsley relished the role, often using his master's influence to interview key UFO witnesses at Buckingham Palace. Horsley was an old friend of Caddy's, and together they hatched a plan for getting the saucer report to the Prince during a North African stop-over the royal pair made whilst returning from Australia. Through Horsley Caddy's contact in the Royal entourage was Commander Mike Parker, who was the Prince's Naval Equerry and another flying saucer aficionado. Parker immediately leapt at the chance to get the report into Prince Philip's hands, saying, 'Oh good! Anything to have a crack at the dome-headed boys', meaning the scientific establishment, most of whom had no time for fanciful notions concerning UFOs and alien visitors.

In March 1957, the Caddys took over the Cluny Hill hotel in Forres, overlooking Findhorn Bay. Eileen had channelled guidance from God that they were to establish a 'Centre of Light' there. As the Cod War hotted up in the late 1950s so did Caddy's interest in flying saucers and how their occupants could save the earth the expected nuclear conflagration. Eileen Caddy had received the channelled message, LU-KANO, which appeared in her inner eye written in letters of fire. The Caddys could find no meaning for this word and were prompted to ask their most powerful sensitive Naomi, who, Caddy claimed, '.. could be in instant telepathic contact with any name given to her...'. Naomi tuned in and discovered that LU-KANO was the captain of a Venusian 'mother ship' who wanted to make contact with the Caddys.

Caddy wrote, '...we were told the time had come to make that contact'.

From then on there was almost daily-channelled contact between Dorothy, Lena, Eileen and Naomi, Caddy's sensitives, and the Venusians. Expectations were high that physical contact was imminent and Caddy's circle believed that the saucer folk would evacuate specially chosen earthlings. Caddy and his coterie of female followers saw themselves as the chosen ones and Caddy and Lena would often go to a possible flying saucer landing site on the beach near Findhorn to await the sky-saviours. As a measure of how serious this belief in physical contact with the saucers was, the otherwise ecologically minded Caddy noted, 'I had the trees cleared from the mound behind the hotel in preparation for the landing.'

The much longed for landing never came. But the media found out about Caddy's activities and they ran articles about the goings on at Cluny Hill Hotel. The front-page headline in the *Sunday Pictorial* for 20 September 1960 screamed, **THE MARTIANS ARE COMING, HE SAYS**. The exposé trumpeted that Caddy believed 'great numbers' of flying saucers from Mars and Venus would be landing on earth within the next few months to warn earthlings that they were on the brink of disaster. 'The main thing is to be nice to them', he said, 'They have to be met with friendship. They are trying to help us.' Caddy explained he had created the landing strip on Cluny Hill at the aliens' behest claiming, 'I was instructed to do so by a kind of telepathy from them', and then went on to outline to his readers exactly what his belief in flying saucers meant,

> 'I believe they will offer people on Earth a chance to leave this planet with them before the catastrophe. They are like us in many ways, but the chief difference is that they have no understanding of such emotions as hatred, greed, jealousy or spite. Their only emotions are love and friendship.'

The adverse publicity these media revelations caused the Cluny Hill Hotel almost got Caddy the sack.

The summer of 1961 saw political relations between Russia and the West deteriorate to the point that there was widespread belief that nuclear war was imminent. Caddy's team of sensitives and channellers were reassured that an extraterrestrial rescue plan to save the Earth was under way, and they were among the chosen ones to be saved. Eventually a message came through that seemed unambiguous, 'Each one of you should be in readiness, you will be given very little warning'.

The extraterrestrials telepathically informed Caddy that they had tried twice to land on the Cluny Hill landing strip, once on Christmas Eve 1960 and again on New Year's Day 1961, but were foiled by a combination of climatic conditions and atomic bomb testing. Caddy and Lena mounted watch for several hours a night in the hope that the third attempt at a landing would be successful, but sadly, the aliens stayed away. In November 1962, the Caddys left Cluny Hill and parked their caravan at the Findhorn Bay Caravan Park and the beginnings of the Findhorn Community as we know it today were formed.

Caddy decided they would become self-sufficient and they planted a huge variety of fruit and vegetables in the poor soil of the Moray coastline. Against all reasonable expectations the garden thrived, a fact that the Findhornians attributed to their daily meditations and contact with the nature spirits, or Devas.

Although the Community was now working closely with nature spirits, Caddy's flying saucer fascination continued unabated. He forged links with many saucerians who shared his vision, including American contactee Dan Fry. During this period, Caddy also met with New Age maven Sir George Trevelyan who was making tentative enquiries among the flying saucer elite about the possibility of forming a national UFO authority within the UK. Through Trevelyan Caddy also met the writer Brinsley le Poer Trench (Lord Clancarty), Air Marshall Sir Victor Goddard and Johann Quanjer, and many other dedicated flying saucer fanatics.

Johann Quanjer, an enigmatic ufologist who has been written out of the subject's histories, came to know the UK flying saucer scene very well, and he wasn't impressed with much of it. Through his connection with Caddy, Quanjer became aware of the flying saucer contacts and near-landings reported at Finchorn. Quanjer's belief in flying saucers was strong, '...there is no doubt in my own mind that these extra-terrestrials and their saucers *do* exist and that they are seriously intending one day to make their presence known to people on earth.'

By the mid 1960s, Caddy had set up a telephone contact system to alert a select group of people when the saucers were due to appear. Quanjer recalls, 'One morning, in May 1966, an urgent phone message came through to me from Edinburgh, Scotland: 'The bells are ringing'. These four words, breathlessly sounded out for me on the trunk line, were apparently a 'code' for something like, 'Flying saucers might be landing on a previously indicated spot somewhere on the North Coast'.

Although he had not as yet visited Findhorn, Quanjer was somewhat sceptical about their detailed claims of extraterrestrial contact, writing, 'These saucers had thoughtfully planned to burst upon an astonished world during the Whit week-end of 27-30 June, so that everyone with a job (as I had) could attend without great inconvenience.' On arrival at Findhorn Quanjer's reservations were proved correct, 'What I had been led to believe would be a bucolic paradise of new age initiates, was really a huddled mass of mild eccentrics...'. Quanjer's view of Caddy was dim, '...here was their leader, a healthy middle-aged man who preferred to accept unemployment money and family benefits rather than a job to support himself and his family'.

The Findhornian's attempts at self-sufficiency didn't impress Quanjer either and he referred to their, '...small but luxuriant vegetable garden...' as being, '...perhaps their only visible hold on reality.'

After introductions to Peter Caddy, Robert Ogilvy Crombie (Roc), and the other invited guests Quanjer was informed a channelled contact had sent instructions that a flying saucer was going to come in from the north east, flying low over the North Sea to avoid being captured on radar at nearby RAF Lossiemouth.

This was it! The landings had begun.

As darkness fell, the excited group of new agers drove to the beach where they waited eagerly for the saucer. For a while nothing happened and then, 'Suddenly, the actor (Roc) with arms aloft, exclaimed that it had arrived. 'Yes, it was here.' No one else saw anything though it was concluded that our space guest must still be in another dimension.' Quanjer had, by now, had enough of the naïve pretensions of the Findhorn set and sent his own thoughts out, '...much further and higher in silent prayer that they please not land here among this inauspicious human welcoming party.'

After the failed landing Eileen Caddy received a channelled message confirming contact had been almost made. 'Let none of you have any feeling of disappointment regarding last night (the landing of our space brothers). All was in preparation for something far, far greater than any of you have ever contemplated.'

The message went onto advise that what Caddy and his friends believed would be a flying saucer sent as part of the extraterrestrial plan to evacuate their supporters, was in fact merely delivering a message that

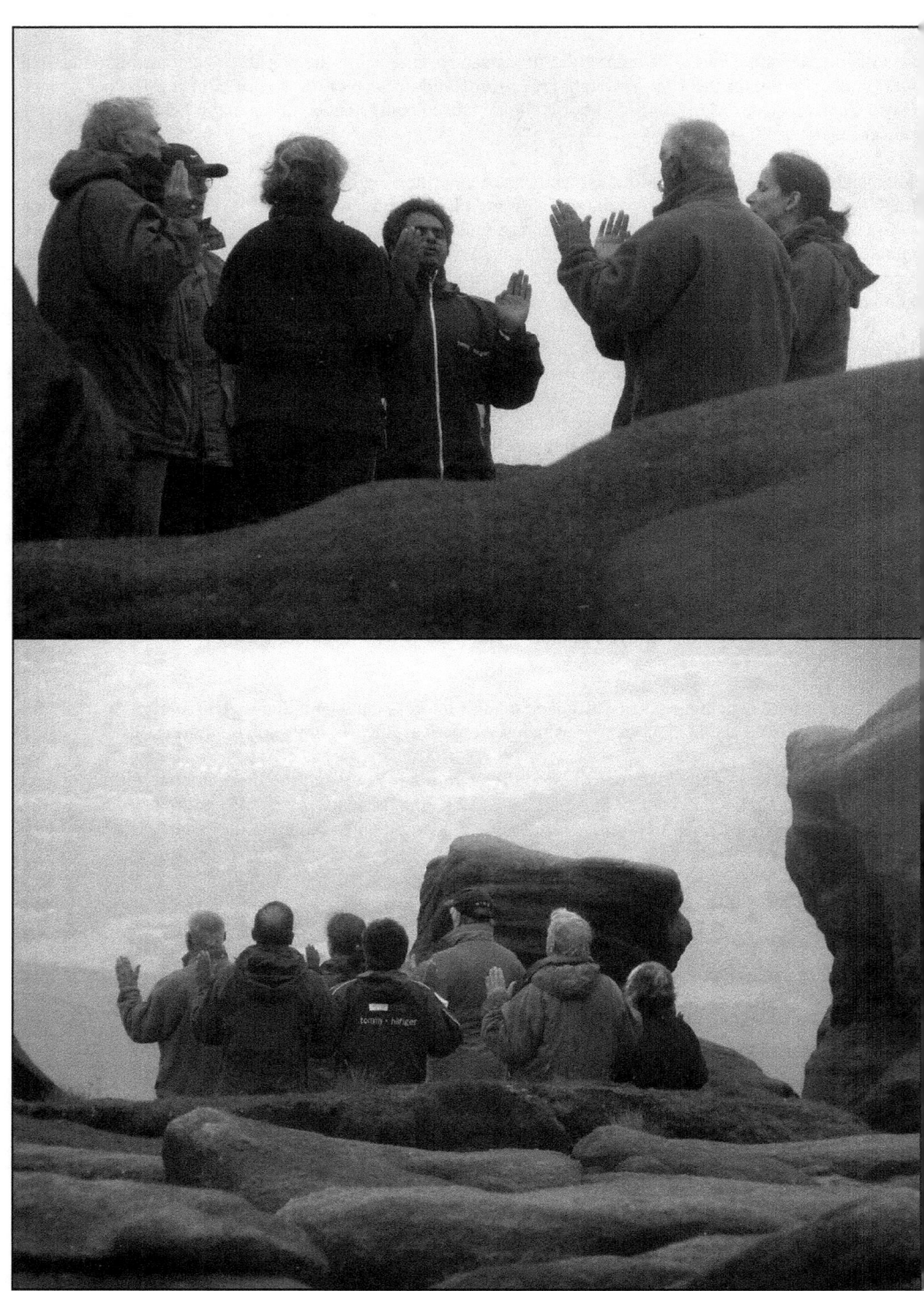

The Aetherius Society on a pilgrimage to their Holy Mountain of Kinder Scout in 2006

everything would be okay. Findhorn's reputation as a New Age community was now spreading rapidly, and not just within New Age circles. A growing number of hippies, inspired by the idea of living simply and communally, in harmony with God and nature, became aware of Findhorn. One such seeker was Neil Oram, a flamboyant character on the hippy scene who was deeply interested in the metaphysical aspects of flying saucers.

Oram and his family arrived at Findhorn in 1968 and were immediately disappointed, 'It felt like Noddy land. Utterly UNREAL. Like ceramic pixies and gnomes cavorting in the garden. Phoney. 'Croquet on the lawn' type of atmosphere. There was an instant culture clash between the two tribes, and the distrust was mutual. For all Caddy's protestations of unconditional love for the human race his first impressions of meeting Oram and family were, '...to my dismay they were dirty, dishevelled hippies....They had to learn that dirty, torn and slovenly clothes were not acceptable at Findhorn, particularly in the Sanctuary.'

During this initial meeting, Oram recalls Caddy saying, 'You see the trouble is a lot of you hippies have been taken over by the sex drive and that's why you can't channel God, the angels, or our advanced space brothers.' The irony of this, considering Caddy's interwoven personal relationships as well as Oram's later claim that Caddy had been, '...screwing the hippy chicks who started arriving. As usual all being done behind Eileen's back', was decidedly rich!

Oram's hippie sensibilities grated with Caddy's ascetic leanings and tensions grew between the two men. This came to a head one evening when Caddy barged into a caravan ordering him, 'You're wanted in the Sanctuary!!!'. Oram ignored Caddy, who repeated, 'I said you're wanted in the Sanctuary now!!!' Once again, he shouted, 'This is your last chance! Are you coming with me now or not?'. Oram declined but was later berated by one of Caddy's sycophantic followers, 'What were you doing man? What were you doing refusing to come to the Sanctuary? You were meant to be a CHANNEL, man! A CHANNEL for our space brothers! The mother ship was HERE!!! Right above the Sanctuary man! Right ABOVE...and it was calling for YOU!!! And you let us ALL DOWN MAN!!! You threw away the opportunity for HUMANITY to EVOLVE onto a HIGHER LEVEL!!! You've let us ALL DOWN, MAN! You're a BETRAYER of our movement. A JUDAS!!!' The following day Oram and family left Findhorn.

When Peter Caddy left Findhorn in the 1970s, the focus of the Community slowly changed Channelled messages from the space brothers and belief in flying saucers were replaced by deeper work with the nature spirits and more direction from God itself. Alfresco flying saucer welcome parties were out, and spiritually earnest seminars and conferences were in. Prophecy turned to profit and Findhorn became a commercial venture, setting itself on the ideological course that has brought it to financial fruition today. Their response now to questions about the part flying saucers paid in their development is simple but evasive, 'There's no 'official' community line regarding UFOs and we have no policy on publicising the subject or otherwise.'

To the vast majority who visit Findhorn this obfuscation will not matter, but the story of Findhorn and flying saucers is a piece of the jigsaw of the UFO subject in the UK. It could be said that Findhorn is nothing more than an apocalyptic 1950s flying saucer cult that got savvy and moved with the times, dropping one of its original tenets and replacing it with others more in keeping with the mores of the New Age market place. Others may believe, especially when they are considering Oram and Quanjer's comments, that Peter Caddy was a hypocrite; a con-man using cod-spirituality for financial and physical gain, utilising and manipulating whatever elements of the supernatural currently fashionable to attract adherents and money. However, it is much more likely that Caddy and his followers were a group of sincere but flawed human beings who were desperately seeking *something*. That something, like the goal of all spiritual seeking, was a desire for certainty, guidance and purpose in a chaotic universe. During the period between 1954 and 1970, flying saucers, or rather the *idea* of flying saucers provided them with that something. Their shared belief in the impending apocalypse and the possibility of salvation from the skies enabled them to form strong relationships and to build a thriving community which was based on their communal philosophy and hopes. By their own accounts they were happy, and if their belief in extraterrestrials provided them with that happiness, then that cannot have been a bad thing.

Fringe, new age beliefs about flying saucers didn't always revolve around psychic contact with the craft or their occupants. Other strands of new age saucer belief drew on other ideas from the early 20th Century and made just as much, if not more of an impact on ufology.

One early free thinker whose ideas provide a direct route from the early 20th Century to the nascent new age saucer beliefs of the 1950s and beyond was Alfred Watkins. In June, 1921 Watkins, a down to earth mill owner from Hereford had a mystic hilltop vision that revealed to him that specific locations in the landscape were connected by straight lines. These lines, he believed, were real and consisted of ancient track ways. Watkins' 1925 book *The Old Straight Track* expounded this theory and introduced a potent new phrase into the new age vocabulary when he called these lines of connectivity ley lines. Watkins chose the term 'ley' to apply to the lines because of the frequency with which the word appeared as part of names along the tracks. Many of the leys appeared to go through ancient sites such as stone circles, holy wells and churches.

In the latter half of the 20th Century, Watkins' basic ideas were appropriated by the new age and hippie movements, becoming attached to many of the beliefs we deal with later in later chapters. However, the poet W. H. Auden summed up the essence of Watkins' vision in his 1956 poem, *The Old Man's Road*, one stanza of which reads:

> 'By stiles, gates, hedgegaps it goes
> Over ploughlands, woodlands, cow meadows
> Past shrines to a cosmological myth
> No heretic today would be caught dead with

After the first flush of interest in ley lines diminished, the idea fell largely dormant until the late 1940s, when ex-RAF pilot Tony Wedd re-vivified the subject. His 1941 sighting of an unidentified flying object and the surge of flying saucer sightings during the 1950s made him think deeply about the subject and to begin to formulate theories about the mysterious sky craft. He had read Watkins' book in 1949 and had started to interpret the landscape, and noted that certain clumps of pine trees appeared to be in direct alignment with each other. Why, he didn't know, but he believed he was onto something of significance.

During the 1950s, Wedd attended meetings of the Tunbridge Wells Flying Saucer Club. This was one of the earliest flying saucer clubs and was patronised by Air Chief Marshall Lord Dowding. At a meeting in 1955, Wedd saw Desmond Leslie give a talk about the contactee George Adamski. After that, Wedd was hooked and he read everything he could about flying saucers. He was keenly interested in the contactees and the messages given to them by the space people, and especially in the information on energy and technology. This led him to make a variety of unusual devices, many of them based on the idea of free energy.

The French ufologist Aime Michel also intrigued Wedd. His 1958 book, *Flying Saucers and the Straight Line Mystery*, argued that many of the UFO sightings in France's huge UFO flap of 1954 were along straight lines. Later research has proved that Michel's theory was deeply flawed, but the idea sparked Wedd's imagination into thinking about the connection between flying saucers and the landscape. He looked for straight lines connecting certain landscape features and read significance into place names which included variations on the words 'mark' and 'ley'. Through his interest in Leslie and Adamski,

Wedd must also have come across Desmond Leslie's speculation that saucers may have travelled by, '... following certain definite magnetic paths now known to surround and interpenetrate the planet'.

Through his friendship with contactee Philip Rodgers, Wedd met Mary Long. Long claimed to be in frequent telepathic communication with the space people who were feeding her with pseudo-scientific information from their spaceship that remained in more or less permanent geostationary orbit above the Pacific Ocean. Ideas of ley lines, earth energies, contact with extraterrestrials whirled like a kaleidoscope in Wedd's mind and he eventually drew these unrelated new age strands together, forming a synthesis.

In August 1960, Wedd learned of two separate UFO sightings, one along a ley that he believed existed running from a pinewood on Lyewood Common, and others seen at Keston Mark. Wedd connected the two events, noting, 'The conjunction of the two place names was too big a hint to miss – and I began to suppose from that date that the saucers' crews knew about the leys'. It should be noted that whilst this join the dots reasoning sounds utterly specious now, Wedd and many others took it to be gospel truth. It is an excellent example, were one really needed, of how ufologists often reach to conclusions, using one unproven speculation (in this case, leys) to justify a theory about another unproven speculation (flying saucers).

Wedd detailed his theories in 1961s Skyways and Landmarks. This publication was significant because it was the first time flying saucers and leys were linked in print. Wedd's somewhat woolly assumptions outlined in the pamphlet became the basis for many of the beliefs in flying saucers held by the hippie counterculture and the new subject of Earth Mysteries.

The mainstream ufological establishment at that time, which comprised of a number of local and regional groups, which was soon to come under the umbrella of the British UFO Research Association, was somewhat intrigued by Wedd's ideas. However, they were regarded as essentially too new age in nature although in 1970, BUFORA organised a symposium on the subject, which concluded that there wasn't enough evidence to connect UFOs to leys. Wedd was unsurprised, like many free thinkers his ideas had already moved on from their origins, noting, 'A contactee informs me that navigation by the old leys is difficult nowadays for a flying saucer, because the leys are in poor shape.'

Although the new age connection with flying saucers is tenuous it's obvious how much the new age belief system has seeped into other areas of ufology. For instance George King's Aetherius Society drew heavily on new age ideas, as did the hippie counterculture. Whilst the mainstream ufologists tried to keep the subject focused on physical, nuts and bolts craft and government cover-ups, those who comprised the new age saucer study groups were quite different. They were accepting of any and all ideas about the saucers and hopeful for the future of humanity. Above all the various different beliefs upon the flying saucer spectrum of the new age stressed the idea of interaction. It was possible to meet and speak directly with space people; it was possible to use the latent powers of the mind to send and receive messages across the vast gulfs of space. For the new agers the saucers weren't here to study or harm us, they were here to contact us, to teach us and to help assist in humanity's often painful struggle to rise above itself.

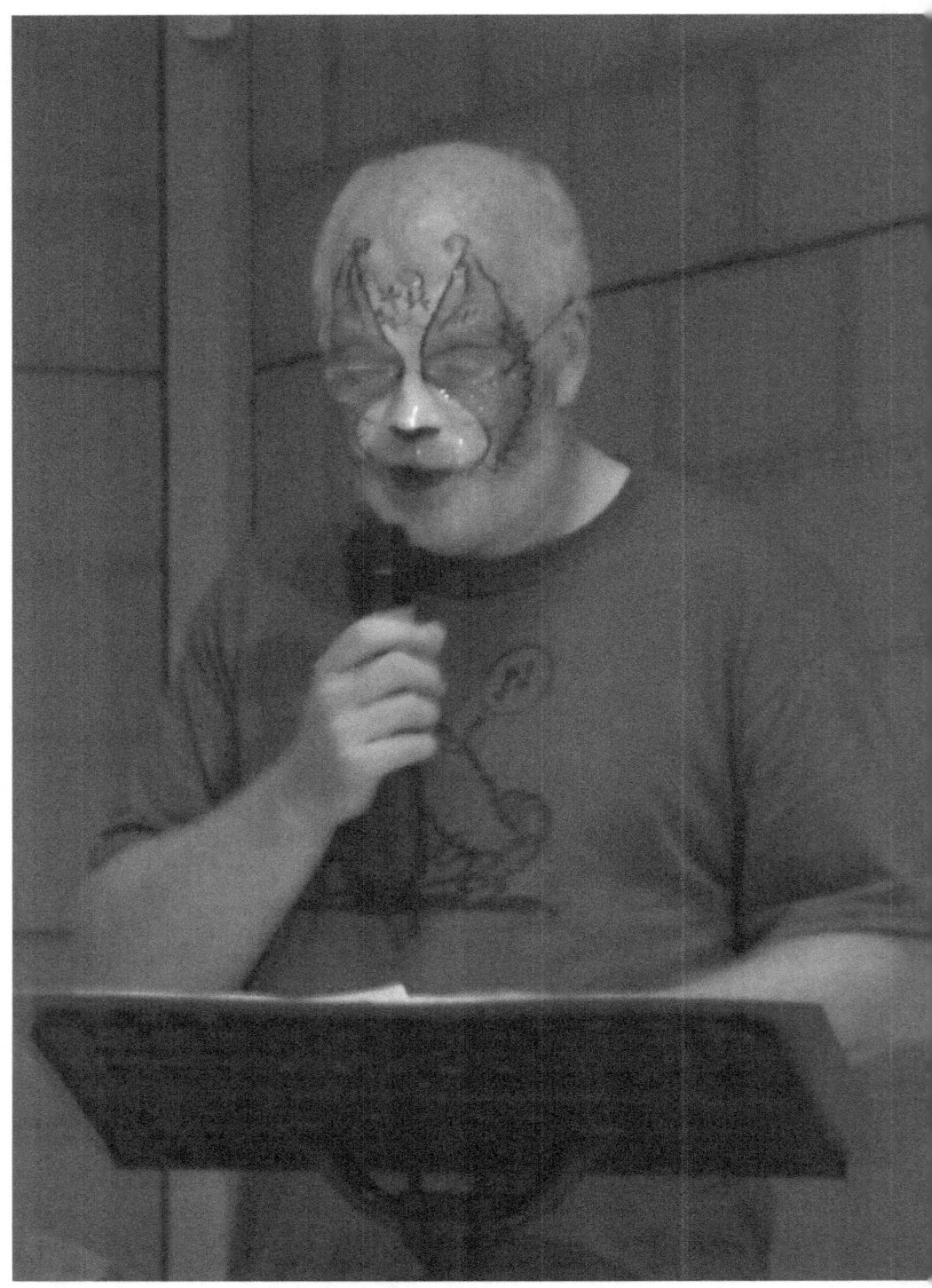

Portrait of the artist as a middle-aged hippie: On stage at the 2009 *Weird Weekend*

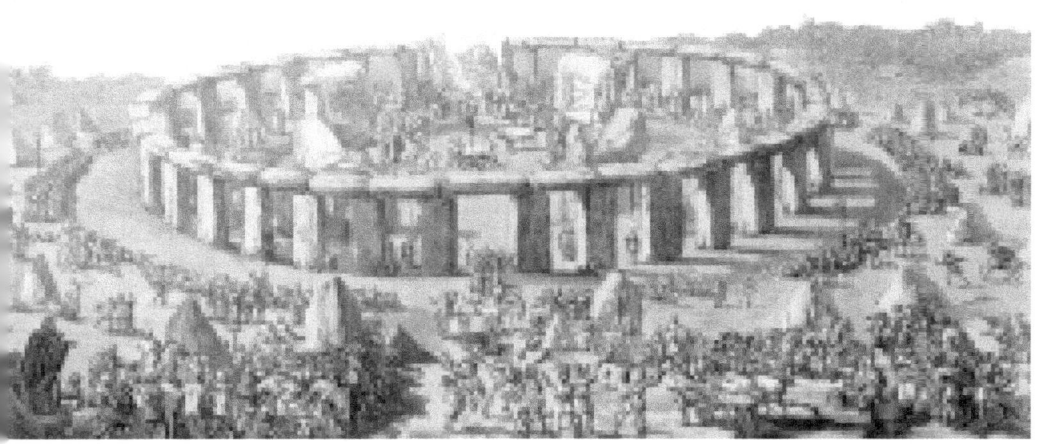

THE BAD BOY OF BRITISH UFOLOGY SPEAKS OUT

Talk to the Devil: An Interview with Andy Roberts
Dateline: Monday, August 8, 2005 By: STUART MILLER
Phenomena News Editor

For the few of you reading this who may have no idea who Andy is, well, within ufology he isn't the most popular guy around. Andy is a sceptic, but then quite a few people are. What marks Andy out as a bit different is that he's generally not nice with it. He sneers, scoffs, scorns and generally talks to people in a combative and aggressive manner. It would be easy to read into his tone that he regards most ufologists as stupid, unable to see the reality of what they believe in and are extremely reluctant to change their views once more detail is revealed about a case. He and I have "fought" many times on message boards and I'm not the only one who has had run ins with him by a long way.

Andy though is a lot of other things besides the above. On his own and also with his writing partner Dr. David Clarke, he is probably the most prolific published writer within the ufological and Fortean field in the UK. I would imagine within the world stage he'd not be far off the top of that too. His books and articles stand out for the obvious depth of research and sheer hard work that has gone into them. You may not like what he has to say, but you've got to admire the way it's been put together. Love him or hate him (there seems to be no middle way). British ufology in particular would be much the worse without him. Unquestionably.

He has always interested me simply because it was obvious that the bluff, aggressive exterior was almost certainly a cover for a personality of probably the opposite countenance. It's difficult to put your finger on it but amid the mocking and sneering, there appeared to be a vulnerability. I'd recognise that yet I was still dumb enough to get trapped in the web and frequently picked up the verbal cudgel to fight back on behalf of all ufologists everywhere. Between the two of us, there was enough arrogance to go round the entire north west of England.

It was during our last verbal altercation quite recently that an idea that had been bubbling away for a while came to the surface. Would he do an interview with me? It is entirely typical of the two of us that while publicly we were calling each other virtually every name we could think of, privately we were corresponding and arranging this dialogue. What a couple of sad bastards.

In his usual modest manner, he pointed out to me that he rarely did interviews and that this would be a bit of a scoop. He was right. I could not remember ever reading one before and if they have taken place in the past, then it would be the distant past. Yes, he's been on the telly and the radio and spoken, and I think I've seen the odd bit here and there where he's been quoted in an article or two, but that was about it.

I didn't want this to be just an interview about his professional career. I wanted to get to know the man a little better too. Dare I say it but I wanted to try and find out what made him tick as well. He was great! He was prepared to answer any question I could throw at him and he answered with an enthusiasm and eagerness. Nothing was off limits. There were even suggestions about topics. If you've followed his career and his public pronouncements, then this might just change the way you see him.

SM: What drew your interest to the subject for the first time? How old were you? And how did you get involved?

AR: As a child I'd always been interested in 'fantasy' type stories, myths, ghosts, legends and the like, which resulted, when I was about 10, in me devouring all Dennis Wheatley's occult fiction and starting a lifelong interest in all things strange. UFOs must have been on my mental radar throughout that time but the first time I *consciously* remember them was a summer's day in 1967. I was in Scarborough, on holiday with my parents. I recall seeing a one-off publication called *UFO* on a newsstand and persuaded my Dad to buy it for me. It was fantastic! Full of pictures of UFOs. I was lucky enough to find a copy second hand a few years ago and now realise it was complete rubbish!

But after that I devoured everything in the local library's adult occult section (using my mother's card) and then found Keel's *Jadoo*, Vallee's *Passport To Magonia* and all the Shuttlewood books, which were coming out in the late 60s and early 70s, along with stuff by Crowley and the occultists. I then became completely obsessed with UFOs, ghosts, and any other kind of strange phenomena, which has probably not done me any good at all!

SM: What made you want to write and where were you published for the first time?

AR: I always had a talent for writing at school and always wanted to be an author. However, the various vicissitudes of adolescence and generally growing up put this on the back burner. Then, just after my first wife and I had our child, she decided to work and I stayed at home to become a house husband (pretty radical in the early 80s, I can tell you). Whilst this was a fantastic experience I was quite isolated and needed something to stop me going completely mad. Initially I took to writing text based computer adventures for the ZX Spectrum using a programme called *The Quill*, which I sold through the computer magazines.

So I suppose that was my first publication, if you call computer games a publication. Then I revived my interest in ufology and, via the West Yorkshire UFO Society, took up being an active ufologist at the end of 1983. Because I wasn't working, I began to devote all my time to it (whilst doing house-work, child rearing etc.) and wrote a number of articles for their magazine, *UFO Brigantia*. By 1985 I had taken over editorship of *Brigantia* which - over the next six or seven years – became the best UFO magazine the UK has ever seen. I wrote a lot for that, as well as other UFO magazines, and *The Ley Hunter* and various other small circulation publications like *Earth Mystery* magazine.

I was also published in a few newsstand magazines of the period. One was *The Supernatural* and another was *Exploring the Supernatural*. During the mid 1980s I was one of the first people in the UK to take a serious interest in what are now know as 'Alien Big Cats'. I wrote and published an A5 booklet (recently updated and re-published by CFZ Press) called *CATFLAPS! - Mystery Cats In The North*, which was a round up of ABC's from folklore to the present day. I approached the subject with the same rigour with which I approach UFO study and it sold extremely well and became a classic.

Throughout the late 1980s I had various chapters in books of UFO essays (*Phenomenon, UFOs 1947-87*) and besides editing *Brigantia*, wrote lots for local and regional newspapers, as well as contributing research material to other authors, such as Janet & Colin Bord for their book on Holy Wells.

One day, whilst driving down to Paul Devereux's in Brecon with that young whippersnapper Dave Clarke, we were discussing UFO books and just thought, let's write one. So we drew up a synopsis, whacked off a couple of sample chapters and within a couple of months we had a contract with Robert Hale Ltd to write *Phantoms of the Sky - UFOs A Modern Myth?* Since then I've written or co-authored in some way seven or eight more books, plus zillions of magazine and newspaper articles and researched and/or contributed to over 20 radio and TV programmes, the most recent of which was the BBC TV *Timewatch* UFO program.

Between 1994-96 I had a bit of a break from ufology and was co-owner of a record label and did quite a bit of road managing for various bands (mainly versions or variations on people who had been in the 1960s psychedelic folk band *The Incredible String Band* - who were highly praised by the *Beatles*, *Stones* etc and were the only Scottish band at Woodstock!) I also ran their high quality fanzine for a few years, organised some huge fan conventions and did various bits of music journalism. Also, between 1988- 1993 I was one of the people who founded the now legendary Sheffield UFO conferences, which were the forerunner of *UFO Magazine*'s conferences. I was extremely proud of these because we brought people like Keel, Vallee, Hopkins, Bill Moore and the like to the UK.

I was also a founder member of the IUN, BUFORA Council member (until I realised BUFORA was full of twats and liars) and co-edited their magazine *UFO Times*. For a while, I amused myself with writing and publishing *The Armchair Ufologist*, which was a *very* cynical look at ufologists and those who inhabit ufology. It's on the net somewhere if you can be bothered to look. More recently, besides the above, I've spoken at a lot of *Fortean Times* UnConventions and written a monthly UFO column for FT, as well as being a frequent contributor of articles. There are many, many other instances of where I've been published but I can't remember them all off hand.

SM: What did you "believe" initially about the subject and how did your thinking change if indeed it has at all. If it did, what caused that change and development?

AR: Because I came to ufology from reading about ghosts, witchcraft and other strange phenomena, I was never one of those sad people who came into it via sci-fi and were ETH believers. I loathe most scifi with a vengeance and the ETH seemed, and seems, ridiculous - why would a civilisation obviously so advanced as to be able to travel across the universe want to visit a planet where people have no respect for each other or the planet they live on?

Because of my background reading, and after coming into contact with people like Keel and Vallee, I initially believed that UFOs occupied the same 'reality status' as ghosts, or perhaps were indigenous inhabitants of our planet or atmosphere, all that kind of thinking. That lasted through my teens and my experiments with the occult and psychedelic drugs. Within a year or two of becoming an 'in the field' Ufologist and researcher, I was disabused of those beliefs and realised that there is no evidence of alien visitors and that UFO experiences are just another aspect of human belief in 'the other', in the same way people believe in the literal reality of ghosts, Bigfoot, elves, fairies etc. That's not to say these things don't have *a* reality, just that they are not literal and physical. As I get older and more experienced in ufology I become more and more sceptical about the literal reality of UFOs, aliens etc, but more and more amazed at the human capacity for misperception and belief.

SM: How did you team up with Dave?

AR: I knew of Dave from reading articles of his in the mid 1980s, but had never met or communicated with him. In, I think, the summer of 1986 I was getting involved in Earthlights research and organised a meeting at my house to which Dave came (with Nigel Watson). For some reason we appeared to hit it off and have been good friends and colleagues ever since and have shared many ufological adventures. If you think I've done a lot of research, investigation and writing, you should take a look at Dave's output. Phenomenal, the man never rests whereas I do - often!

SM: How did you get involved in the Fortean and mythology side of things? Did that come first before ufology?

AR: I think the answer to this is implicit in the above answers. Despite the fact that I'm known for my work in ufology I've done huge amounts of research in many other areas of Forteana. I've done - and published - research projects on Screaming Skull legends, The Search For The Death Ray and Mountain Panics, among several other areas of Fortean interest. Ufology is only a tiny area of interest to me really and I'm always amused when ufologists rant and rave because *very* few have actually done a tenth of the research and investigation I've done in ufology, never mind any other area of research.

Besides my ufological activities I have several Fortean things on the go at any one time - sometimes these will see the light of day, often they are just for my own interest and entertainment. Fundamentally I'm interested in why humans believe in strange things, how this is demonstrated, what they admit as 'proof' and why they just can't accept the world as the amazing place it is. I'm just a nature mystic at heart and don't see the need for complicated mythologies or belief systems. Life's too short to be serious about believing in aliens, ghosts or whatever.

SM: If there has been a highlight to your career so far, what would you say it was?

AR: Well, the fact that I've done what I've done is a highlight to me. But I suppose the 'biggies' have been solving big cases such as Cracoe or Berwyn. Solving any case is a huge adrenalin rush because they are like multi-dimensional puzzles, which many people have worked on and failed. Therefore to be able to put the clues together and to come up with an answer is a highlight. I also like to see the reaction in those people who invested strange beliefs in a case, when it's taken apart into its component parts!

Of all the many ufologists I've met, the ones who impressed me the most were Bill Moore - because he didn't take it too seriously. Meeting John Keel was a big disappointment I'm afraid. Jacques Vallee was just enigmatic!

SM: Do you get nervous about media appearances?

AR: A bit. I think anyone who says they don't is a liar. However, once you've done a few and realise that the media know fuck all about ufology and also realise that you will be standing about for hours and/or having to repeat the same sentences numerous times, you soon lose nervousness. Some media people are the most intelligent and amusing people I've come across, but I'm afraid that more often than not they are stupid, shallow individuals who are more interested in style over content. I won't do anything for the media without being paid - for the simple reason I'm not that arsed and I've put a lot of time and money into my research.

If they want some of it they can pay for it or they can go talk to one of the many morons who will give them rubbish information for free!

SM: You mentioned being married once before. Presumably you got divorced. Has there been much pain in your private life?

AR: I was married between 1977 and 2003, although separated from my first wife on and off since 1997. Lived with someone else on and off between '97 and '01, eventually re-married in March 2004 to Gaynor

Wootten (nee Sunderland, subject of Jenny Randles' book *Alien Contact* and one of the founders of the Psychic Questing movement). As for 'pain' - well it's much better to experience intensity of emotions than none at all, and I can assure anyone who is bored enough to be reading this nonsense that the series of emotional upheavals often codified as the 'mid life crisis', is a far more powerful and potent event than adolescence which, for me, was a breeze. Can't wait for my dotage!

SM: The impression given of your writing career, even from quite early on, is that you were always quite positive and progressive. Were you "pushy" and good at self-promotion in terms of getting work and projects or were you constantly approached because you had the time and skill?

AR: A bit of all of the above. The simple fact is that, although many people want to write and believe they can, most are hampered by the fact that they either can't string a coherent article or book together, or they haven't got the ideas and material to do so even if they can write. Luck came into it, as well as the fact that Dave is far more pro-active in these areas than I and I've been lucky enough that I've written many things with him that he's done a lot of the initial leg work for in terms of contracts etc. He will go to heaven, although I doubt if I'll see him there.

SM: Your views about BUFORA are now very well known. What caused the initial change? Are you idealistic or maybe argumentative?

AR: I'm not idealistic, more pragmatic. Am I argumentative? You bet your sweet bippy! BUFORA is a disgusting, parasitic organisation, which charges a great deal of money for a very small service. Anyone thinking of joining BUFORA should realise that they can get a trillion times more information free on the Internet. Anyone in BUFORA should leave immediately. The cream of UK ufology has been through BUFORA in the last thirty years and without exception, have left with a bitter taste in their mouths. It pretends to be a democratic organisation yet it is run entirely by a council, of which a small minority actually decide what happens. I am speaking as an ex-BUFORA Council member who has had extensive experience of the organisation over the years, so I know what I talk about. Ask any real UK ufologist and they will tell you the same. Even Jenny, who is a model of restraint, has had hideous experiences at their hands and little good to say about them.

They are a total anachronism and should be destroyed by any means possible - and believe me, I've tried! I refuse to waste any more words on the stupid little enthusiasts club it has become, other than to say if enough people leave and no more people join, it will wither and die.

SM: How do you cope with failure if an article or book is not well received? When you decided to stop doing something like *Brigantia* or *The Armchair Ufologist* (I have seen it), if the reason was a lack of interest or reader apathy, how did that feel?

AR: If something's not well received, quite frankly, I don't care. By the time something is written and out there, the research and creative process is long gone and I'm well into something else. I write and research first and foremost for my own satisfaction - having it read by others and being paid for it is a bonus. I could quite easily have continued doing *Brigantia* forever, and often wish I had because I enjoyed it so much, but I stopped doing it when I went into previously described musical projects between '93-'95. Unfortunately *Brigantia* stopped completely because Stuart Smith, who had taken it over from me, died. *The Armchair Ufologist* was again something which would have continued but my personal life was 'difficult' in the mid 90s so it just slipped away.

The interesting thing about the *Armchair Ufologist* was that although it seriously took the piss out of people, many of those people actually *begged* to be in it and couldn't wait for the next issue! But times change and things change with them, sometimes you've got to let things go and move on.

SM: The reasons you gave for not accepting the ETH seem a bit pessimistic. Are you disappointed by people and "the way we are"?

AR: I'm constantly disappointed by people because I think most people are wasting their lives and there is a lot of ignorance and stupidity out there. People, by and large, seem easily satisfied by superficial trappings. I blame the decline of the Grammar School system and the fact that advertising is the very

Devil's Work. I think modern life is basically rubbish, although I enjoy the products of wealth such as CDs and cars etc. If I had the money I would be living in a very remote place indeed and few people would ever see me again - which would make a lot of people very happy! It would make me ecstatic!

SM: You mention that within a relatively short time of being in the field as a ufologist, you realised there was no evidence of alien visitation etc. Did you reach that point so quickly because there was no hard evidence that satisfied you or was it because of the people you were meeting and interviewing?

AR: Entirely because of the lack of evidence and nothing to do with the people. Most of the UFO witnesses I've interviewed (and witnesses to any other Fortean phenomena) have been perfectly ordinary people who genuinely believe in whatever it is they have told me.

I too believe they have had that particular experience. But I don't believe that the experience has been a literal one. I think the next question expands on this one somewhat. I do, however, think many ufologists are dangerous, barely literate nutters, who should be taken into secure units for their, and society's good.

SM: Why do you regard "belief" in ET as flawed? Is your natural inherent nature to accept something purely on the basis of solid fact?

AR: Sort of. I believe many things that other people would laugh at - but I don't expect them to believe it, because I know these are subjective beliefs. The problem with the ETH'ers is they appear to be on a religious mission to make us believe something, for which there isn't even the tiniest scrap of physical evidence. It's far too much like evangelism or fundamentalism for me.

I don't know - or care - whether life exists anywhere else in the multiverse, but if someone is telling me something exists in physical form then I want proof, not waffle. So for me, the ETH can only be proven by the scientific analysis of some material which several laboratories, under blind test conditions, all believe to be some form of life or fabricated material, which didn't originate on Earth. It's not too much to ask, yet despite all the bluster, it's never happened.

And I don't believe it will, because in the history of Fortean phenomena *nothing* which is claimed to be alien or supernatural (ghosts, cryptoids, elves, fairies, Loch Ness Monsters etc) has *ever* been proven to be physical in nature and is invariably found to be misperceptions based on the current cultural fashion in whatever country it takes place in. Who sees fairies now? Who saw UFOs when fairies were being seen? Why does southern Ireland have a long tradition of apparitions of the Blessed Virgin Mary but no real abduction tradition? Why was it that Arnold didn't see 'flying saucers' but they were termed that, and then people started 'seeing' flying saucers? True believers can't - or won't address themselves to these questions, the questions which are only the start of obtaining meaningful and relevant answers to the question of Fortean phenomena.

SM: After the above question, and this is not meant to be a trick question, but are you religious or do you regard yourself as particularly spiritual?

AR: Religious? - nah, kill 'em all and let their Deity of choice sort 'em out is what I say. There have been more deaths in the name of religion than in any other cause. I hate, detest, loathe and laugh at organised religion and the poor saps who fall for it. Spiritual? Well, I believe the multiverse is itself God; I'm a Zen pantheist with Taoist undertones and a lay preacher in the First Church of the Last Laugh. Hail Eris! I almost died in a near drowning accident whilst on holiday this summer - your life doesn't flash before your eyes and nor are any last minute religious truths revealed. I was rescued and I emerged from the water laughing my head off in a combination of shock and joy at being alive. As I walked, soaking wet, through the three miles of forest back to the car I was, yet again, struck with the realisation of just how fantastic the natural world is; it's perfect in every sense at all times, doesn't aspire to any particular state other than that it is in at any given time and doesn't intentionally cause harm or suffering to anyone/thing else.

Now, *that's* spirituality. Like I said, I'm an old nature mystic at heart.

SM: Is it possible to explain the link for you personally, if indeed there is one, between psychedelic drugs and understanding or appreciating the occult/ufology etc.?

AR: That's a very big question! My *personal* view, which I never seek to impose on anyone is that I think that everyone on the planet should have at least one psychedelic experience in their Lves, in an appropriate setting, with a guide who knows what's what.

Despite the government making LSD illegal there are many psychedelics which are still entirely legal in this country and elsewhere. Psychedelics taught me about the nature of belief and how easy it is to get snared by any one belief. They also taught me not be scared of mental and spiritual bogeymen, or indeed of anything else. They taught me to take responsibility for myself and to be utterly aware of the world around me at all times and they taught me that most things people take for granted, or get caught up in materially, are a distraction from the main event.

I've had experiences and times on psychedelics which have been revelatory beyond words. I've also had times which have been the exact opposite. They are both utterly dangerous, dangerously fabulous and all points between and beyond. Often both at the same time. I both believe what they have taught me, and I disbelieve what they have taught me. But I have never regretted using them. Talking about psychedelics is like talking about war. If you weren't there you have *no* idea what it is like because, like the war experience, you *cannot* describe the psychedelic experience in words, any more than you can, say, dance about writing. I could go on, but you get the picture, they taught me things.

SM: You mention Dave Clarke's output but you don't come over as a slouch either. How do you keep it going? What sparks the interest and ideas?

AR: Because I have so many interests and new ones all the time, there isn't enough time to even scratch the surface of what I'd like to. The advent of the Internet made research much easier and obscure books and papers easier to acquire, and all my spare time is taken up researching or thinking about research. I'm not very sociable, hardly drink, rarely enter a pub unless it's to see a band, or otherwise mix with humans if I can possibly avoid it outside of work, and I use my time wisely. I would hate to get old and have spent my life just going to work, going to the pub and watching TV.

SM: You seem very frustrated by people and their belief systems and almost appear to be on a mission to wake them up and shake them out of their stupidity. Do you think you make a difference - do people "hear" you or do you feel you're banging your head against a brick wall?

AR: I think the answers above sort of answer this question. Yeah, I think that most people, through no fault of their own, and usually because of circumstances or cultural conditioning are 'asleep' in many ways. And in ufology, many certainly are - that's why so few people stay in the field for any length of time; because they are looking for some answer, some explanation of a literally supernatural kind. When they don't find it, they either leave and hunt for it in some other, even more woolly Fortean phenomena or they go the opposite way and denounce it all as being 'of the devil', or become hard core debunkers.

Like heroin addicts, they are just belief addicts and lurch from one to another. Didn't one of Keel's entities say 'wake up down there'!

SM: As I understand it, you work with, or run a hostel for young people with drug problems. What's involved and how did you get drawn into this?

AR: I've worked with young people (i.e. under 25s) since March of 1989 when a friend of mine who managed a hostel needed some relief cover. I said, 'yeah, I can do that' and a few days later was in sole charge of eleven male ex-offenders overnight in a hostel in Halifax. The learning curve was, err. steep. Believe it or not, until I started working with young people I was shy and retiring and wouldn't say boo to the proverbial goose. However, you are soon eaten alive in the hostel world if you are like that so I willed myself to change. I soon realised I had an aptitude for dealing with 'difficult' people and worked my way up to Project Worker and eventually ended up as a Hostel Manager. During the intervening years I've been threatened by seriously baaad people more times than I care to recall, had death threats made against me and my family, been held hostage by a knife wielding maniac for several hours and generally seen some serious weirdness.

I've also met some very interesting young people and had lots of laughs. That's why the bunch of pussies who inhabit ufology just amuse me, because they have no idea what the real world of the underclasses is like. Nor, for that matter, do most people. Drug use and young people go hand in hand and I've seen many, many people whose lives have been ruined by this involvement. I've also had friends die and become mentally and physically ill through drug use. However, it isn't the drugs themselves which cause the problem, by and large it's the legal system and lifestyle people have to adopt which causes the poverty, crime, illness, addiction and overdoses.

Making and keeping drugs illegal will never, and has never, stopped people taking them. To a certain degree the very illegal nature creates a glamour which attracts people to drugs. This is a very big can of worms to untangle and views vary widely on it. All I can say is I have reached my conclusions through many years of seeing the drug world at first hand, initially through my own experiences and those of friends, and later from working with drug users.

Unfortunately, when it comes to addictions, some people have addictive personalities and if they aren't addicted to one thing then it will be another. Believe it or not you have to try *very* hard to get addicted to heroin. Tobacco and alcohol are far more damaging drugs than heroin and kill hundreds of thousands of people a year. Yet the same people who rant and rave about heroin, cannabis etc are the same people who smoke 20 a day and are down the pub a few nights a week. I find that a disgusting hypocrisy, both on their part and on the part of the government who profits from these legal drugs. People should look into the history of drugs and when and why they became illegal. It's most instructive as it's invariably to do with personal beliefs of politicians, treaties with other countries or – worst of all - social engineering to stop youth movements. I now manage fifteen staff and a 40-bed hostel.

SM: On the assumption that Gaynor is a "believer", how do you juxtapose her views with yours? Or is it comparable to two people living in the same house, one who votes Labour and the other Conservative?

AR: A believer in what exactly? People should remember Gaynor was a child when she had her UFO experiences and a young teenager during the Green Stone (and other Psychic Questing) events. That Gaynor 'believes' the experiences she's recounted happened to her is, I think, all that needs to be said on this. She has no interest whatsoever in the subject now, having been closely involved with, and at the heart of, ufology and occultism for so many years. She has met far too many nutters for her to hold anything but contempt for these subjects as they are practised. Knitting and painting by numbers are Gaynor's only vices these days and her devotion to Our Lady of the Sorrows can't be faulted. I thank the Lord I've found a good Christian woman at last.

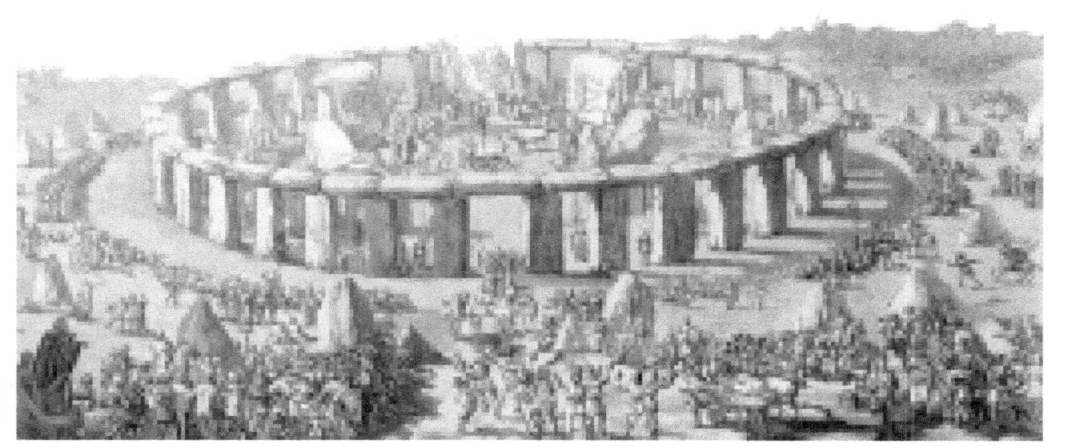

BY THE SAME AUTHOR

BOOKS

Catflaps: Anomalous Big Cats in the North. Brigantia Books, 1986/CFZ 2001
Phantoms of the Sky (with David Clarke), Robert Hale, 1990
Earthlights Revelation (contributing author), Paul Devereux, Blandford, 1991
Ghosts & Legends of Yorkshire, Jarrold, 1992
Twilight of the Celtic Gods (with David Clarke) Blandford, 1996/97
The UFOs That Never Were (with Jenny Randles & David Clarke - Feb. 2000)
Out of the Shadows (with David Clarke), Piatkus, 2002
Strange Secrets (with Nick Redfern), Paraview, 2005
The Flying Saucerers (with David Clarke), Heart of Albion, 2007
Albion Dreaming: A Social History of LSD in the UK (Marshall Cavendish, 2008)

In addition I have contributed chapters to the following anthologies:

UFOs 1947-87, Fortean Tomes, 1987
Phenomenon, Macdonald & Co., 1988
Fortean Studies 3, John Brown Publishing, 1996
Fortean Studies 5, John Brown Publishing 1999
Be Glad For The Song Has No Ending, Adrian Whittaker, Helter Skelter, 2008

TV

The Isle Is Full Of Noises, Everyman, BBC1, November 1992
Down To Earth, Discovery channel, also shown on C4, 1995
Origin Unknown, Granada, Jan/Feb 1999
The Haunted Valley Granada, November 2000
Timewatch, BBC1, January 9, 2004
Danny Wallace's Hoax Files, Sky 1, December 2005
Britains Closest Encounters, C4, August 2008

THE CENTRE FOR FORTEAN ZOOLOGY

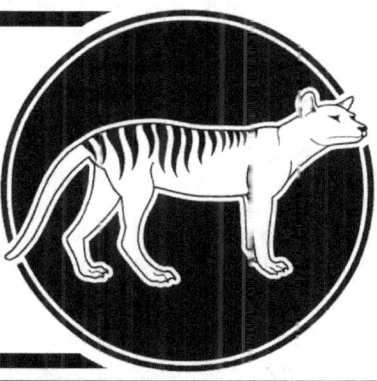

So, what is the Centre for Fortean Zoology?

We are a non profit-making organisation founded in 1992 with the aim of being a clearing house for information, and coordinating research into mystery animals around the world. We also study out of place animals, rare and aberrant animal behaviour, and Zooform Phenomena; little-understood "things" that appear to be animals, but which are in fact nothing of the sort, and not even alive (at least in the way we understand the term).

Why should I join the Centre for Fortean Zoology?

Not only are we the biggest organisation of our type in the world, but - or so we like to think - we are the best. We are certainly the only truly global Cryptozoological research organisation, and we carry out our investigations using a strictly scientific set of guidelines. We are expanding all the time and looking to recruit new members to help us in our research into mysterious animals and strange creatures across the globe. Why should you join us? Because, if you are genuinely interested in trying to solve the last great mysteries of Mother Nature, there is nobody better than us with whom to do it.

What do I get if I join the Centre for Fortean Zoology?

For £16 a year, you get a four-issue subscription to our journal *Animals & Men*. Each issue contains 60 pages packed with news, articles, letters, research papers, field reports, and even a gossip column! The magazine is A5 in format with a full colour cover. You also have access to one of the world's largest collections of resource material dealing with cryptozoology and allied disciplines, and people from the CFZ membership regularly take part in fieldwork and expeditions around the world.

How is the Centre for Fortean Zoology organised?

The CFZ is managed by a three-man board of trustees, with a non-profit making trust registered with HM Government Stamp Office. The board of trustees is supported by a Permanent Directorate of full and part-time staff, and advised by a Consultancy Board of specialists - many of whom who are world-renowned experts in their particular field. We have regional representatives across the UK, the USA, and many other parts of the world, and are affiliated with other organisations whose aims and protocols mirror our own.

I am new to the subject, and although I am interested I have little practical knowledge. I don't want to feel out of my depth. What should I do?

Don't worry. We were *all* beginners once. You'll find that the people at the CFZ are friendly and approachable. We have a thriving forum on the website which is the hub of an ever-growing electronic community. You will soon find your feet. Many members of the CFZ Permanent Directorate started off as ordinary members, and now work full-time chasing monsters around the world.

I have an idea for a project which isn't on your website. What do I do?

Write to us, e-mail us, or telephone us. The list of future projects on the website is not exhaustive. If you have a good idea for an investigation, please tell us. We may well be able to help.

How do I go on an expedition?

We are always looking for volunteers to join us. If you see a project that interests you, do not hesitate to get in touch with us. Under certain circumstances we can help provide funding for your trip. If you look on the future projects section of the website, you can see some of the projects that we have pencilled in for the next few years.

In 2003 and 2004 we sent three-man expeditions to Sumatra looking for Orang-Pendek - a semi-legendary bipedal ape. The same three went to Mongolia in 2005. All three members started off merely subscribers to the CFZ magazine.

Next time it could be you!

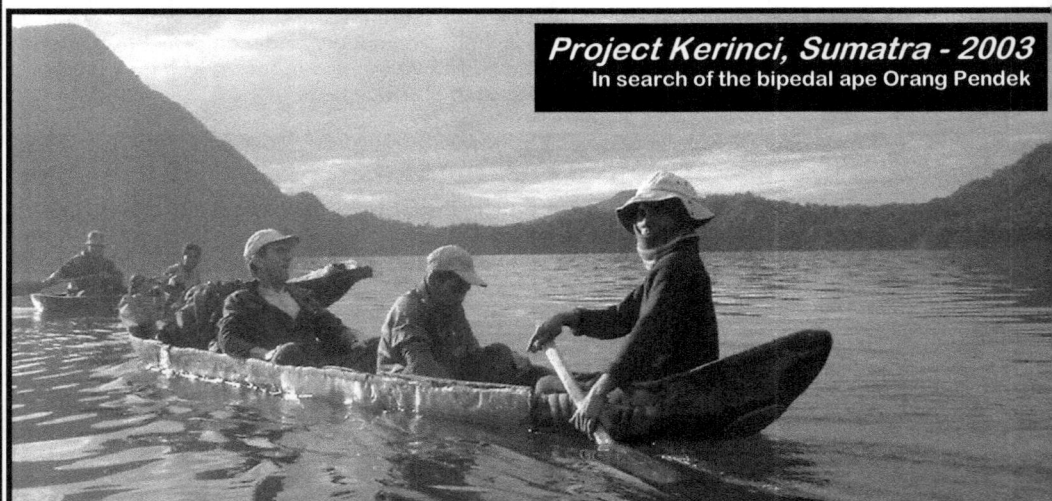

Project Kerinci, Sumatra - 2003
In search of the bipedal ape Orang Pendek

How is the Centre for Fortean Zoology funded?

We have no magic sources of income. All our funds come from donations, membership fees, works that we do for TV, radio or magazines, and sales of our publications and merchandise. We are always looking for corporate sponsorship, and other sources of revenue. If you have any ideas for fund-raising please let us know. However, unlike other cryptozoological organisations in the past, we do not live in an intellectual ivory tower. We are not afraid to get our hands dirty, and furthermore we are not one of those organisations where the membership have to raise money so that a privileged few can go on expensive foreign trips. Our research teams both in the UK and abroad, consist of a mixture of experienced and inexperienced personnel. We are truly a community, and work on the premise that the benefits of CFZ membership are open to all.

What do you do with the data you gather from your investigations and expeditions?

Reports of our investigations are published on our website as soon as they are available. Preliminary reports are posted within days of the project finishing.

Each year we publish a 200 page yearbook containing research papers and expedition reports too long to be printed in the journal. We freely circulate our information to anybody who asks for it.

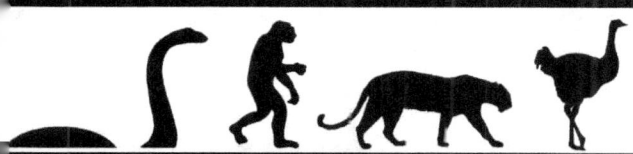

No. Each year since 2000 we have held our annual convention - the *Weird Weekend* - in Exeter. It is three days of lectures, workshops, and excursions. But most importantly it is a chance for members of the CFZ to meet each other, and to talk with the members of the permanent directorate in a relaxed and informal setting and preferably with a pint of beer in one hand. Since 2006 - the *Weird Weekend* has been bigger and better and held in the idyllic rural location of Woolsery in North Devon. The 2008 event will be held over the weekend 15-17 August.

Since relocating to North Devon in 2005 we have become ever more closely involved with other community organisations, and we hope that this trend will continue. We also work closely with Police Forces across the UK as consultants for animal mutilation cases, and we intend to forge closer links with the coastguard and other community services. We want to work closely with those who regularly travel into the Bristol Channel, so that if the recent trend of exotic animal visitors to our coastal waters continues, we can be out there as soon as possible.

We are building a Visitor's Centre in rural North Devon. This will not be open to the general public, but will provide a museum, a library and an educational resource for our members (currently over 400) across the globe. We are also planning a youth organisation which will involve children and young people in our activities.

Apart from having been the only Fortean Zoological organisation in the world to have consistently published material on all aspects of the subject for over a decade, we have achieved the following concrete results:

- Disproved the myth relating to the headless so-called sea-serpent carcass of Durgan beach in Cornwall 1975
- Disproved the story of the 1988 puma skull of Lustleigh Cleave
- Carried out the only in-depth research ever into the mythos of the Cornish Owlman
- Made the first records of a tropical species of lamprey
- Made the first records of a luminous cave gnat larva in Thailand.
- Discovered a possible new species of British mammal - the beech marten.
- In 1994-6 carried out the first archival Fortean zoological survey of Hong Kong.
- In the year 2000, CFZ theories where confirmed when an entirely new species of lizard was found resident in Britain.
- Identified the monster of Martin Mere in Lancashire as a giant wels catfish
- Expanded the known range of Armitage's skink in the Gambia by 80%
- Obtained photographic evidence of the remains of Europe's largest known pike
- Carried out the first ever in-depth study of the *ninki-nanka*
- Carried out the first attempt to breed Puerto Rican cave snails in captivity
- Were the first European explorers to visit the `lost valley` in Sumatra
- Published the first ever evidence for a new tribe of pygmies in Guyana
- Published the first evidence for a new species of caiman in Guyana

EXPEDITIONS & INVESTIGATIONS TO DATE INCLUDE:

- 1998 Puerto Rico, Florida, Mexico *(Chupacabras)*
- 1999 Nevada *(Bigfoot)*
- 2000 Thailand *(Giant snakes called nagas)*
- 2002 Martin Mere *(Giant catfish)*
- 2002 Cleveland *(Wallaby mutilation)*
- 2003 Bolam Lake *(BHM Reports)*
- 2003 Sumatra *(Orang Pendek)*
- 2003 Texas *(Bigfoot; giant snapping turtles)*
- 2004 Sumatra *(Orang Pendek; cigau, a sa-bre-toothed cat)*
- 2004 Illinois *(Black panthers; cicada swarm)*
- 2004 Texas *(Mystery blue dog)*
- Loch Morar *(Monster)*
- 2004 Puerto Rico *(Chupacabras; carnivorous cave snails)*
- 2005 Belize *(Affiliate expedition for hairy dwarfs)*
- 2005 Loch Ness *(Monster)*
- 2005 Mongolia *(Allghoi Khorkhoi aka Mongolian death worm)*
- 2006 Gambia *(Gambo - Gambian sea monster , Ninki Nanka and Armitage's skink*
- 2006 Llangorse Lake *(Giant pike, giant eels)*
- 2006 Windermere *(Giant eels)*
- 2007 Coniston Water *(Giant eels)*
- 2007 Guyana *(Giant anaconda, didi, water tiger)*
- 2008 Russia *(Almasty)*
- 2009 Sumatra *(Orang pendek)*
- 2009 Republic of Ireland *(Lake Monster)*
- 2010 Texas *(Blue dogs)*

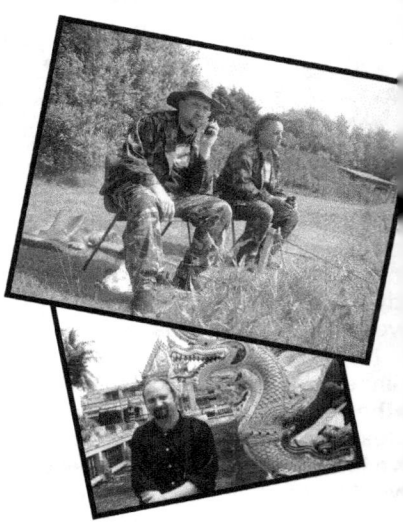

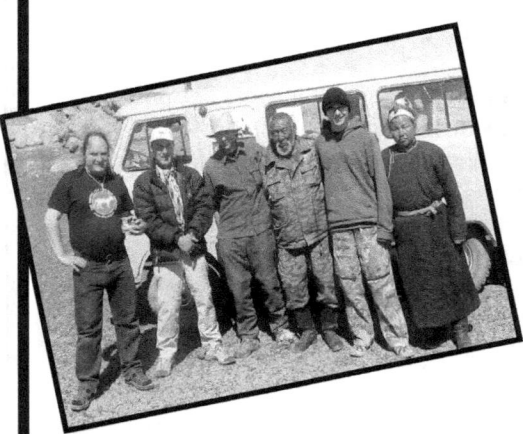

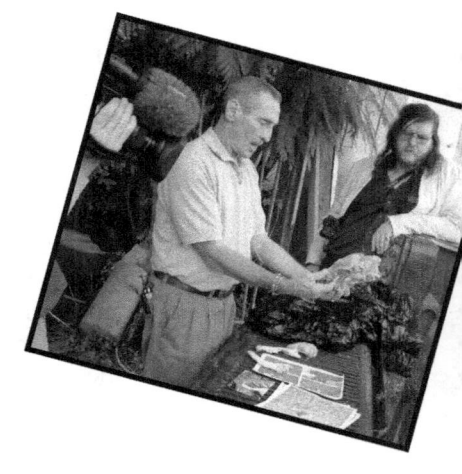

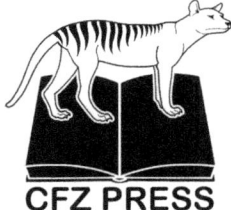
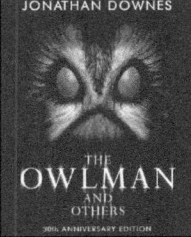
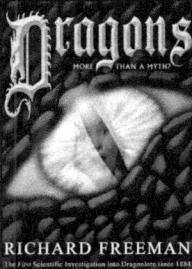
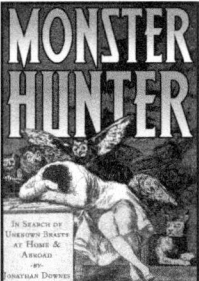
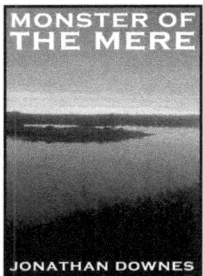

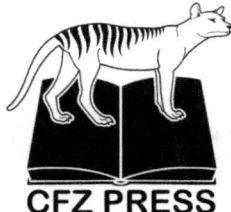
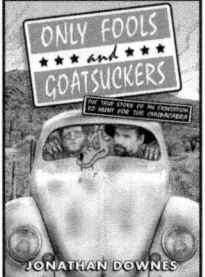
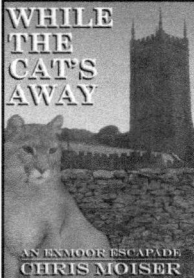
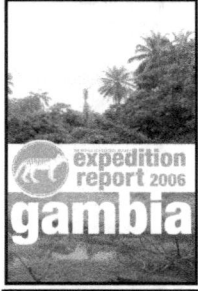
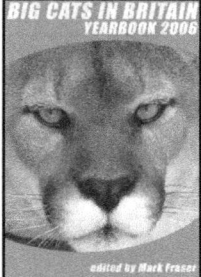

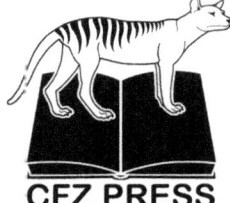
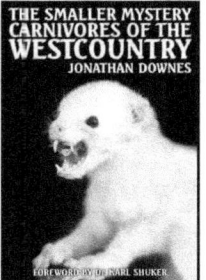
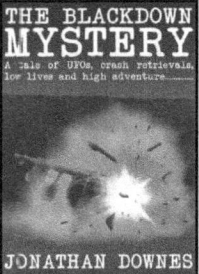
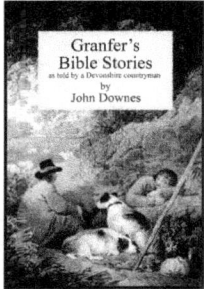
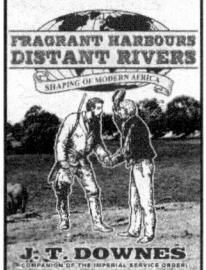

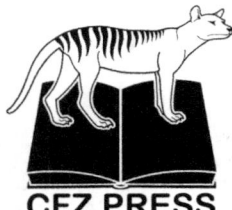
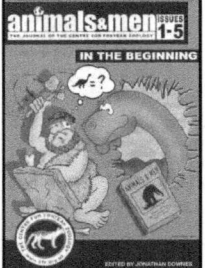
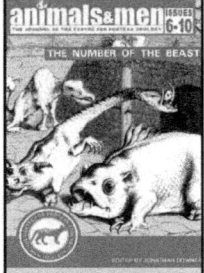
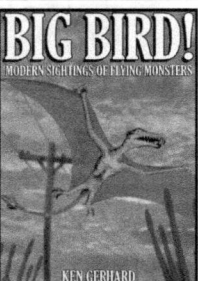
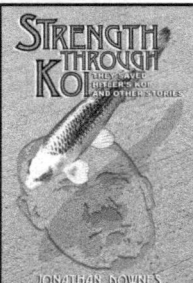

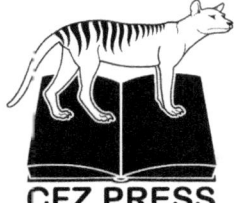

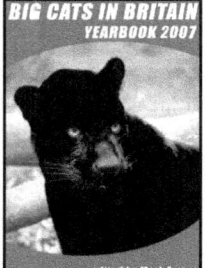
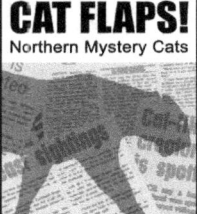
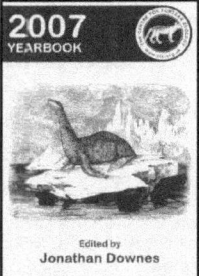
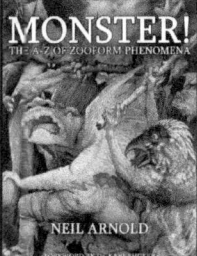

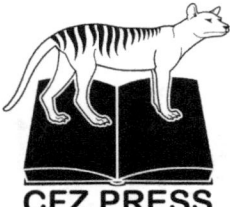
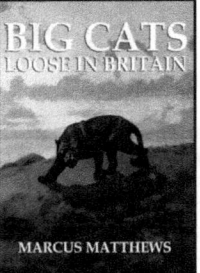
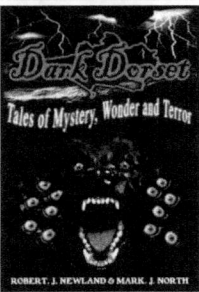
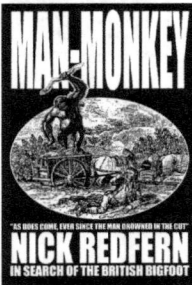
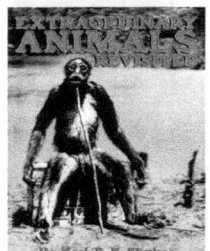

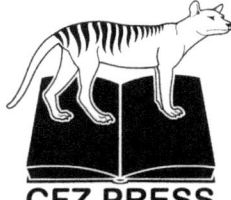
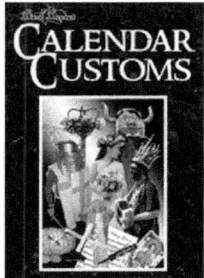
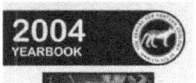
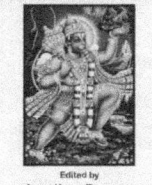
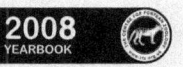
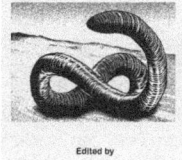
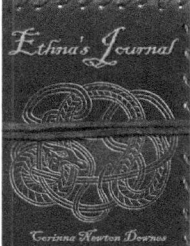

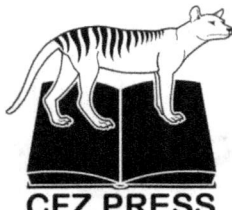

Other books available from
CFZ PRESS

CFZ PRESS

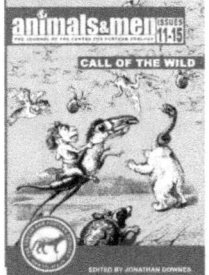

ANIMALS & MEN - Issues 11 - 15 - The Call of the Wild
Jonathan Downes (Ed) - ISBN 978-1-905723-07-2

£12.50

Since 1994 we have been publishing the world's only dedicated cryptozoology magazine, *Animals & Men*. This volume contains fascimile reprints of issues 11 to 15 and includes articles covering out of place walruses, feathered dinosaurs, possible North American ground sloth survival, the theory of initial bipedalism, mystery whales, mitten crabs in Britain, Barbary lions, out of place animals in Germany, mystery pangolins, the barking beast of Bath, Yorkshire ABCs, Molly the singing oyster, singing mice, the dragons of Yorkshire, singing mice, the bigfoot murders, waspman, British beavers, the migo, Nessie, the weird warbling whatsit of the westcountry, the quagga project and much more...

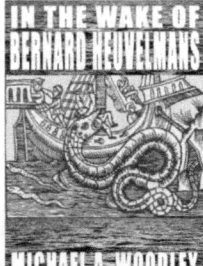

IN THE WAKE OF BERNARD HEUVELMANS
Michael A Woodley - ISBN 978-1-905723-20-1

£9.99

Everyone is familiar with the nautical maps from the middle ages that were liberally festooned with images of exotic and monstrous animals, but the truth of the matter is that the *idea* of the sea monster is probably as old as humankind itself.

For two hundred years, scientists have been producing speculative classifications of sea serpents, attempting to place them within a zoological framework. This book looks at these successive classification models, and using a new formula produces a sea serpent classification for the 21st Century.

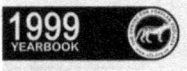
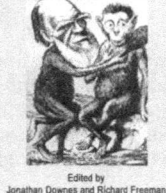

CENTRE FOR FORTEAN ZOOLOGY 1999 YEARBOOK
Edited by Jonathan Downes
ISBN 978 -1-905723-24-9

£12.50

The Centre For Fortean Zoology Yearbook is a collection of papers and essays too long and detailed for publication in the CFZ Journal *Animals & Men*. With contributions from both well-known researchers, and relative newcomers to the field, the Yearbook provides a forum where new theories can be expounded, and work on little-known cryptids discussed.

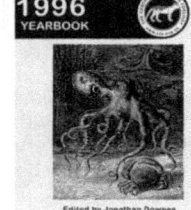

CENTRE FOR FORTEAN ZOOLOGY 1996 YEARBOOK
Edited by Jonathan Downes
ISBN 978 -1-905723-22-5

£12.50

The Centre For Fortean Zoology Yearbook is a collection of papers and essays too long and detailed for publication in the CFZ Journal *Animals & Men*. With contributions from both well-known researchers, and relative newcomers to the field, the Yearbook provides a forum where new theories can be expounded, and work on little-known cryptids discussed.

**CFZ PRESS, MYRTLE COTTAGE,
WOOLFARDISWORTHY BIDEFORD,
NORTH DEVON, EX39 5QR
www.cfz.org.uk**

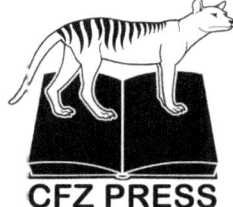
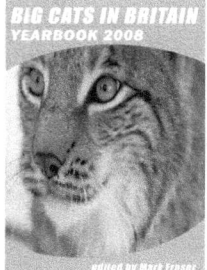
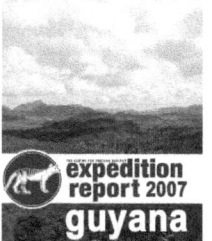
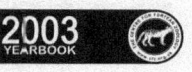
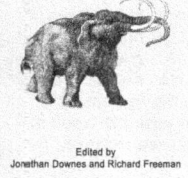
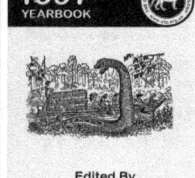

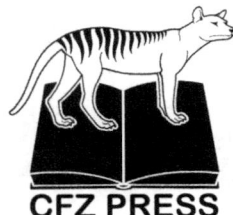
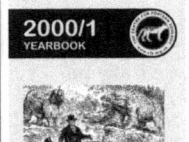
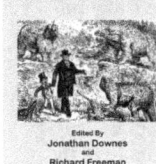
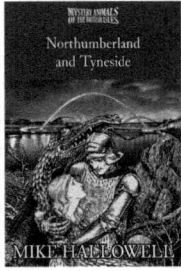
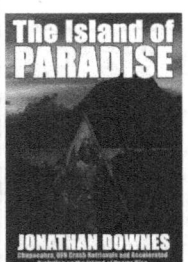
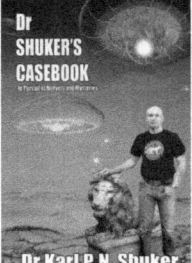

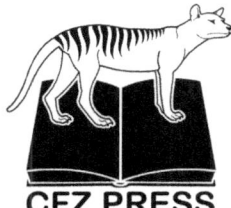
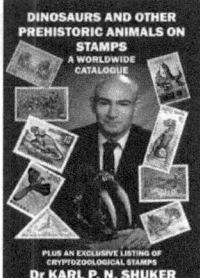
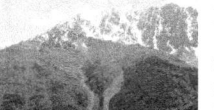
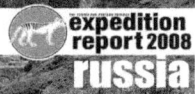
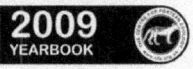
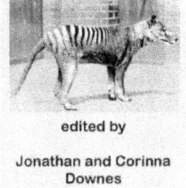
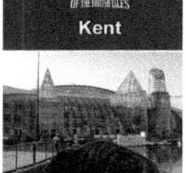

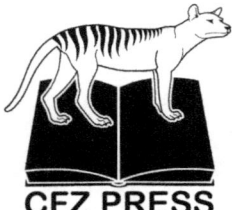

Other books available from
CFZ PRESS

CFZ PRESS

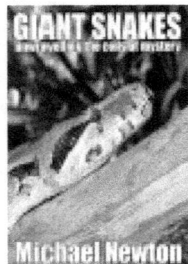
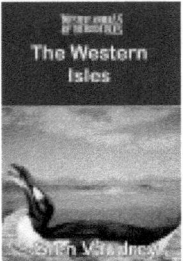
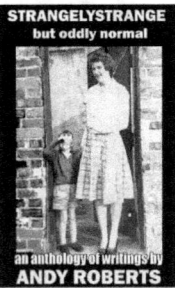
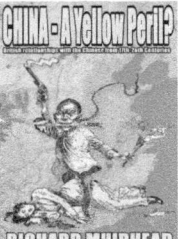